The 'cursus laborum' of
Roman Women

Also available from Bloomsbury

A Cultural History of Childhood and Family in Antiquity
edited by Mary Harlow and Ray Laurence
A Cultural History of Women in Antiquity edited by Janet H. Tulloch
Women in Ancient Rome by Bonnie MacLachlan
Women's Life in Greece and Rome by Mary R. Lefkowitz and Maureen B. Fant

The 'cursus laborum' of Roman Women

Social and Medical Aspects of the Transition from Puberty to Motherhood

Anna Tatarkiewicz

Translated into English by Magdalena Jarczyk

BLOOMSBURY ACADEMIC
LONDON • NEW YORK • OXFORD • NEW DELHI • SYDNEY

BLOOMSBURY ACADEMIC
Bloomsbury Publishing Plc
50 Bedford Square, London, WC1B 3DP, UK
1385 Broadway, New York, NY 10018, USA
29 Earlsfort Terrace, Dublin 2, Ireland

BLOOMSBURY, BLOOMSBURY ACADEMIC and the Diana logo are trademarks of
Bloomsbury Publishing Plc

First published in Great Britain 2023
Paperback edition published 2025

Copyright © Anna Tatarkiewicz, 2023

Anna Tatarkiewicz has asserted her right under the Copyright, Designs and Patents Act, 1988, to be identified as Author of this work.

For legal purposes the Acknowledgements on p. xii constitute an extension of this copyright page.

Cover image: Ancient Roman relief carving of a midwife attending a woman giving birth. Wellcome Collection. Attribution 4.0 International (CC BY 4.0)

All rights reserved. No part of this publication may be reproduced or transmitted in any form or by any means, electronic or mechanical, including photocopying, recording, or any information storage or retrieval system, without prior permission in writing from the publishers.

Bloomsbury Publishing Plc does not have any control over, or responsibility for, any third-party websites referred to or in this book. All internet addresses given in this book were correct at the time of going to press. The author and publisher regret any inconvenience caused if addresses have changed or sites have ceased to exist, but can accept no responsibility for any such changes.

A catalogue record for this book is available from the British Library.

Library of Congress Cataloging-in-Publication Data
Names: Tatarkiewicz, Anna, author. | Jarczyk, Magdalena, translator.
Title: The 'cursus laborum' of Roman women : social and medical aspects of the transition from puberty to motherhood / Anna Tatarkiewicz ;
translated into English by Magdalena Jarcyzk.
Description: London ; New York : Bloomsbury Academic, 2023. |
Includes bibliographical references.
Identifiers: LCCN 2022046405 | ISBN 9781350337398 (hardback) |
ISBN 9781350337435 (paperback) | ISBN 9781350337411 (epub) |
ISBN 9781350337404 (ebook)
Subjects: LCSH: Childbirth–Rome–History. | Pregnancy–Rome–History. |
Reproductive health–Rome–History. | Women–Rome–Social conditions. |
Motherhood–Rome–History. | Mothers–Rome–Social conditions.
Classification: LCC RG513 .T38 2023 | DDC 362.1984009456/32—dc23/eng/20221018
LC record available at https://lccn.loc.gov/2022046405

ISBN:	HB:	978-1-3503-3739-8
	PB:	978-1-3503-3743-5
	ePDF:	978-1-3503-3740-4
	eBook:	978-1-3503-3741-1

Typeset by RefineCatch Limited, Bungay, Suffolk

To find out more about our authors and books visit www.bloomsbury.com and sign up for our newsletters.

Contents

List of Illustrations	vi
List of Abbreviations and Editions	vii
Acknowledgements	xii
Introduction	1
1 Marriage: The Institution that Makes One a Mother	14
2 Women Preparing to Be Mothers	35
3 Specialized Care for the Would-be Mother	68
4 Pregnancy and Its Course	81
5 Parturition	106
6 *Dies lustricus*: The Birth of ... a Mother?	137
Conclusion	153
Notes	159
Bibliography	221
Index	237

Illustrations

1	Roman doll	48
2	Terracotta uterus models	65
3	A swaddled child. A votive offering	66
4	A tombstone from Ostia. Scribonia Attice, a midwife, at work	73
5	Pregnant woman (a votive offering?)	104
6	Pregnant woman. A votive offering found in Suffolk	105
7	Birth scene	110
8	Terracotta image of a placenta with the umbilical cord	112
9	Roman surgical instruments – different hooks	127
10	*The Birth of Caesar.* A woodcut from Suetonius' *Lives of the Twelve Caesars*, published in 1506	129
11	Plaque in tomb relief showing mother and child	139
12	A mother feeding a swaddled infant	148

Abbreviations and Editions

Amm. Marc. – Ammianus Marcellinus, *History*, ed. and transl. J. C. Rolfe, Cambridge 1950 (Loeb Classical Library).
Apul. Apol. – Apuleius, *Apologia. Florida. De Deo Socratis*, ed. and transl. Ch. P. Jones, Cambridge 2017 (Loeb Classical Library).
Apul. Met. – Apuleius, *Metamorphoses (The Golden Ass)*, ed. and transl. J. A. Hanson, Cambridge 1996 (Loeb Classical Library).
Artem. – *Artemidori Daldiani Onirocriticon libri V*, ed. R. Ambrose, Leipzig 2011 (Bibliotheca scriptorum Graecorum et Romanorum Teubneriana).
Cael. Aurel. – *Gynaecia: Fragments of a Latin Version of Soranus' Gynaecia from a Thirteenth Century Manuscript, Caelius Aurelianus*, ed. M. F. Drabkin, I. E. Drabkin, Baltimore 1951.
Cass. Dio – Dio Cassius, *Roman History, Volume V*, transl. E. Cary, H. B. Foster, Cambridge 1917 (Loeb Classical Library).
Dio Cassius, *Roman History, Volume VII–VIII*, transl. E. Cary, H. B. Foster, Cambridge 1924 (Loeb Classical Library).
Catullus Carm. – *Catullus*, ed., transl. and comm. G. P. Goold, London 1983.
Celsus, De medicina – Celsus, *On Medicine*, transl. W. G. Spencer Cambridge 1935 (Loeb Classical Library).
Cens. – *Livre de Censorinus sur le jour natal*, transl. J. Mangeart, Paris 1843.
Cic. De leg. – Cicero, *On the Republic. On the Laws*, transl. C. W. Keyes, Cambridge 1928 (Loeb Classical Library).
Cic. Att. – Cicero, *Letters to Atticus*, ed. and transl. D. R. Shackleton Bailey, Cambridge 1999 (Loeb Classical Library).
Cic. De div. – Cicero, *On Old Age. On Friendship. On Divination*, transl. W. A. Falconer, Cambridge 1923 (Loeb Classical Library).
Cic. Fin. – Cicero, *On Ends*, transl. H. Rackham, Cambridge 1914 (Loeb Classical Library).
Cic. pro Cluentio – Cicero, *Pro lege Manilia. Pro Caecina. Pro Cluentio. Pro Rabirio Perduellionis Reo*, transl. H. Grose Hodge, Cambridge 1927 (Loeb Classical Library).
M. Tullius Cicero. *The Orations of Marcus Tullius Cicero*, lit. transl. C. D. Yonge, B. A. London. Henry G. Bohn, York Street, Covent Garden. 1856.

Cic., Tusc. – Cicero, *Tusculan Disputations*, transl. J. E. King, Cambridge 1927 (Loeb Classical Library).
Cyranides – *Die Kyraniden*, ed. D. Kaimakis, Hain, Meisenheim am Glan 1976.
Dig. – *Corpus Iuris Civilis, t. 1, Institutiones. Digesta*, ed. P. Krueger, Berlin 1922. S. P. Scott, *The Civil Law*, III–IV, Cincinnati 1932.
Dion. Hal. Ant. Rom. – Dionysius of Halicarnassus, *Roman Antiquities*, transl. E. Cary, Cambridge 1937 (Loeb Classical Library).
Diosc. – *Estudios y traduccion Dioscorides. Sobre los remedios medicinales. Manuscrito de Salamanca*, transl. A. López Eire, F. Cortés Gabaudan, Salamanca 2006.
Galen, Hyg. – Galen, *Hygiene*, ed. and transl. I. Johnston, Cambridge 2018 (Loeb Classical Library).
Garg. – *Plinii Secundi, quae fertur una cum Gargilii Martialis, Medicina*, ed. V. Rose, Lipsiae 1875.
Gell. – *A. Gellii Noctium Atticarum libri XX*, ed. M. Herz, C. Hosius, Lipsiae 1903 (Bibliotheca scriptorum Graecorum et Romanorum Teubneriana). Gellius, *Attic Nights*, transl. J. C. Rolfe, Cambridge 1927 (Loeb Classical Library).
H. A. – *Scriptores Historiae Augustae*, ed. E. Hohl, Leipzig 1965 (Bibliotheca scriptorum Graecorum et Romanorum Teubneriana).
Hor. Od. – Q. Horatius Flaccus (Horace), *Odes*, ed. J. Conington. Horace, *Odes and epodes*, ed. N. Rudd, Cambridge 2004 (Loeb Classical Library).
Hyginus, Fabulae – Hygin, *Fables*, transl. J.-Y. Boriaud, Paris 2012 (Les Belles Lettres). Hyginus, Fabulae from *The Myths of Hyginus*, ed. and transl. M. Grant. University of Kansas Publications in Humanistic Studies, no. 34.
Iuv. Sat. – Juvénal, *Satires*, transl. P. De Labriolle, F. Villeneuve, Paris 2004 (Les Belles Lettres).
Lucr. – *T. Lucreti Cari De rerum natura libri sex*, ed. J. Martin, Leipzig 1953 (Bibliotheca scriptorum Graecorum et Romanorum Teubneriana). Lucretius, *De Rerum Natura*, ed. W. E. Leonard, E. P. Dutton. 1916.
Macrob. Sat. – Macrobe, *Les Saturnales*, transl. Ch. Guittard, Paris 1997 (Les Belles Lettres). *Ambrosii Theodosii Macrobii Saturnalia*, ed. J. Willis, Leipzig 1994 (Bibliotheca scriptorum Graecorum et Romanorum Teubneriana).
Mart. – Martial, *Epigrams, Volume II–III*, ed. and transl. D. R. Shackleton Bailey, Cambridge 1993 (Loeb Classical Library).

Musc. – *La Gynaecia di Muscione: manuale per le ostetriche et le mamme del VI sec. d.C.*, ed. R. Radicchi, Pisa 1970.

A. Prenner, *Mustione 'traduttore' di Sorano di Efeso. L'ostetrica, la donna, la gestazione*, Napoli 2012.

Ovid. Ars am. – Ovid, *L'Art d'aimer*, ed. and transl. H. Bornecque, Paris 2011 (Les Belles Lettres).

Ovid. Fasti – Ovid, *Fasti*, transl. J. G. Frazer, Cambridge 1931 (Loeb Classical Library).

Ovid. Amores – Ovid, *Heroides. Amores*, transl. G. Showerman, Cambridge 1914 (Loeb Classical Library).

Diosc. – Pedanii Dioscuridis Anazarbei, *De materia medica*, ed. M. Wellmann, Berlin 1907

Pedanius Dioscorides of Anazarbus, *De materia medica*, transl. L. Y. Beck, Hildesheim 2005.

Pers. Sat. – Pers, *Satires*, ed. and transl. A. Caretault, Paris 2002 (Les Belles Lettres).

Plaut. Aul. – Plautus, *Amphitryon. The Comedy of Asses. The Pot of Gold. The Two Bacchises. The Captives*, ed. and transl. W. de Melo, Cambridge 2011 (Loeb Classical Library).

Plaut. Capt. – Plautus, *Amphitryon. The Comedy of Asses. The Pot of Gold. The Two Bacchises. The Captives*, ed. and transl. W. de Melo, Cambridge 2011 (Loeb Classical Library).

Plin. Ep. – *Plinius Caecilius Secundus Gaius: Epistularum libri novem. Epistularum ad Traianum liber. Panegyricus*, ed. M. Schuster, R. Hanslik, Lipsiae 1958 (Bibliotheca scriptorum Graecorum et Romanorum Teubneriana).

Pliny the Younger. *Letters, Volume II: Books 8–10. Panegyricus*, transl. B. Radice, Cambridge 1969 (Loeb Classical Library).

Plin. HN – Pliny, *Natural History, Volume III: Books 8–11*, transl. H. Rackham, Cambridge 1940 (Loeb Classical Library).

Pliny, *Natural History, Volume VI: Books 20–23*, transl. W. H. S. Jones, Cambridge 1951 (Loeb Classical Library).

Pliny, *Natural History, Volume VII: Books 24–27*, transl. W. H. S. Jones, A. C. Andrews, Cambridge 1956 (Loeb Classical Library).

Pliny, *Natural History, Volume VIII: Books 28–32*, transl. W. H. S. Jones, Cambridge 1963 (Loeb Classical Library).

Plut. *De amore prolis*

Plut., *De liberis educandis* – Plutarch. *Moralia*, transl. Frank Cole Babbitt.

Cambridge, MA. Harvard University Press. London. William Heinemann Ltd. 1927.

Plutarch, *Moralia, Volume VI: On Affection for Offspring*, transl. W. C. Helmbold. Cambridge 1939 (Loeb Classical Library).

Plut. Rom. – Plutarch, *Lives, Volume I: Theseus and Romulus. Lycurgus and Numa. Solon and Publicola*, transl. B. Perrin, Cambridge 1914 (Loeb Classical Library).

Propert. – *Sexti Properti Elegiarum libri IV*, ed. P. Fedeli, Leipzig 2006 (Bibliotheca scriptorum Graecorum et Romanorum Teubneriana).

Quint. Decl. min. – Quintilian, *The Lesser Declamations*, ed. and transl. D. R. Shackleton Bailey, Cambridge 2006 (Loeb Classical Library).

Sen. Controv. – Seneca the Elder, *Controversiae*, transl. M. Winterbottom, Cambridge 1974 (Loeb Classical Library).

Sen. Helv. – Seneca, *Moral Essays, Volume II: De Consolatione ad Helviam*, transl. J. W. Basore, Cambridge 1932 (Loeb Classical Library).

Sen. Marc. – Seneca, *Moral Essays, Volume II: De Consolatione ad Marciam*, transl. J. W. Basore, Cambridge 1932 (Loeb Classical Library).

Sen. QN – Seneca, *Natural Questions, Volume I–III*, transl. T. H. Corcoran, Cambridge 1971 (Loeb Classical Library).

Solinus – *Solinus: Wunder der Welt. Collectanea rerum mirabilium. Lateinisch und Deutsch*, ed. Kai Brodersen, Darmstadt 2014.
Gaius Iulius Solinus, the Polyhistor, transl. Arwen Apps https://topostext.org/work/747 (accessed on 20 December 2020).

Soranus – *Sorani Gynaeciorum libri IV*, ed. Johannes Ilberg, Leipzig/Berlin 1927.
Soranus of Ephesus, Soranus' Gynecology, ed. and transl. O. Temkin, Baltimore 1991.

Stat. Silvae – Statius, *Silvae*, ed. and transl. D. R. Shackleton Bailey, Cambridge 2015 (Loeb Classical Library).

Suet. – Suétone, *Vie des douze Césars*, transl. H. Ailloud, Paris 1931–2 (Les Belles Lettres).
Suetonius, *Lives of the Caesars, Volume I: Julius. Augustus. Tiberius. Gaius. Caligula*, transl. J. C. Rolfe, Cambridge 1914 (Loeb Classical Library).

Tac. Ann. – Cornelius Tacitus (I): *Annales*, ed. E. Koestermann, Leipzig 1960 (Bibliotheca scriptorum Graecorum et Romanorum Teubneriana).
Tacitus. *Histories: Books 4–5. Annals: Books 1–3*, transl. C. H. Moore, J. Jackson, Cambridge 1931 (Loeb Classical Library).

Terent. Adelph. – Terence, *Phormio. The Mother-in-Law. The Brothers*, ed. and transl. J. Barsby, Cambridge, 2001 (Loeb Classical Library).
Terent. Andr. – Terence, *The Woman of Andros. The Self-Tormentor. The Eunuch*, ed. and transl. J. Barsby, Cambridge 2001 (Loeb Classical Library).
Tert. *De anima* – Tertullianus, *De anima*, ed. J. H. Waszink, Amsterdam, 1947.
Th. Prisc. – *Theodori Prisciani Euporiston libri III cum Physicorum fragmento et additamentis pseudo-Theodoreis*, ed. V. Rose, Leipzig 1894.
Varro, *De agri.* – Varro, *On Agriculture*, transl. W. D. Hooper Cambridge 1934 (Loeb Classical Library).
AE – *L'Année épigraphique*
CIL – *Corpus Inscriptionum Latinarum*
CIPRBU – *Corpus de inscripciones romanas de la provincia de Burgos. Fuentes epigráficas para la historia social de Hispania romana*
Dig. – *Digesta Iustiniani*
PIR – *Prosopographia Imperii Romani*

Acknowledgements

If I were to list by name all the people who supported me, encouraged me, and cheered me on while I was writing this book, I would have to cover several pages more. Still, I hope none of them will feel insulted if I express my gratitude collectively: for the conversations and the encouragement – thank you all.

However, there are a few institutions and persons I must mention. I would like to thank the Dean of the Faculty of History, Adam Mickiewicz University Poznań, Professor Józef Dobosz, for the funds which made an English translation of this book possible, and Magdalena Jarczyk for the translation itself, which I believe excellent.

I will always have fond memories of my visits to the library in Kiel; I would like to thank the Board of Christian-Albrecht University of Kiel for the invitations and financial aid. During my visits in Kiel I could always count on the help of the International Center, and particularly Isolda Ritter and Andreas Ritter. But I feel especially grateful to Professor Andreas Luther (and his family members, who were extremely kind) for his incredible commitment to providing me with excellent working conditions at the library. Thank you so much! It was great to feel in Kiel as if one were . . . in Poznań.

The manuscript has benefited immensely from the helpful suggestions of the anonymous reviewers. My gratitude extends also to Alice Wright and Lily Mac Mahon. Thanks are also owed to Merv Honeywood, Moira Eagling and everyone working on the publication of this book.

I would never have finished the book without the support of my family. Jaś, if it were not for your presence in my life, the subject of this book would be altogether different! I am grateful to you and Witas for your angelic patience, magnanimity and trust that I would finish one day. This book would not exist without your help.

Introduction

Cursus laborum feminae Romanae[1]

In 1994, Danielle Gourevitch published an unusual paper in the *Acta Belgica Historiae Medicinae*. Indicating she had used narrative, epigraphic and medical sources available, she created the fictional character of Vipsania, not so much a woman as a girl. Vipsania's narrative, put into the form of a diary, is written in the first person. The reader may well identify with the girl, who lives in Rome in the second century CE. She recounts her childhood, puberty, and conversations with her mother and nurse regarding her changing body and first menstruation; she also gives an account of her emotions in relation to marriage, and shares her apprehension and fear of pregnancy and childbirth with her physician, Soranus.[2]

Every historian working on ancient Rome, social history, or the history of family and of women dreams of discovering such a direct account. However, none exists (or at least, none has been found). We do not have an extant diary, memoir or life account of a Roman woman penned by herself, and the great majority of the preserved accounts, even if they are about women, were written by men and present a male point of view.[3] Thus the Vipsania created by Gourevitch does not speak to us in the voice of a Roman girl or woman either; hers is a man's voice and reflects how men saw women's world. It is a kind of mental trap from which we cannot free ourselves due to the lack of sources. Still, Gourevitch's idea seems incredibly interesting: while it presents us with the male perspective of Roman womanhood once again, it also alerts us to the fact that at least some aspects of a woman's (biological) life were not taboo to men – physicians, politicians, or ordinary fathers and husbands – as well as the fact that women – not only their character, behaviour, looks and so on, but also their biological affairs – were of importance to men. Not that it should be surprising; taking care of a woman began the moment a female infant was born. Men – fathers, brothers and husbands – had considerable influence on the lives of girls and women.

The *cursus laborum* of women comprised a few more or less distinct stages: being 'accepted' into the family, childhood, betrothal, marriage, childbirth, motherhood and life after the husband's death or divorce, or marrying again. Marriage and the birth of children were breakthrough moments, which determined and defined the woman's position in the family and society. From the men's perspective marriage was necessary for the birth of legitimate children but, for the women, it was something more: a rite of passage. By marrying, a woman became a matron and later, inevitably, a mother.

Aulus Gellius writes that the word *matrona* refers to a woman who has married a man, so long as she remains married to him, even if no children have been born of the union yet:

> 'matronam' dictam esse proprie quae in matrimonium cum viro convenisset, quoad in eo matrimonio maneret, etiamsi liberi nondum nati forent, dictamque ita esse a matris nomine, non adepto iam, sed cum spe et omine mox adipiscendi, unde ipsum quoque 'matrimonium' dicitur ...

> 'matron' was properly applied to one who had contracted a marriage with a man, so long as she remained in that state, even though children were not yet born to them ...[4]

The author goes on to state the word *matrimonium* (marriage) has the same origin, which could be said to answer the question of why Romans married. It may seem a platitude but, although the power lay with men, they did depend on women, since only women could provide them with descendants. First of all, however, every politician, military commander or father of a family – every man – had a mother.

Being born a girl made it extremely likely they would one day be a mother. In her book on the history of women in the Victorian era, A. Gromkowska-Melosik ventured the claim that

> in all cultures, locations, and times, being born a woman predetermines the biography and life options available to an individual ... with marriage being among the most important social roles a woman can play.[5]

In other words, becoming a mother was no trifle:[6] it defined the Roman woman. Her biological role was also her most important social role, and motherhood elevated her standing, particularly for mothers of male children.[7]

In other words, in the Roman view of women's *cursus laborum*, marriage and motherhood were closely related, and as girls grew up, they faced the prospect of marrying and giving birth to a child as a fundamental life mission. Women from all social groups were in that situation but, since it was mostly daughters of Roman elite families who were seen as future mothers, they were also the ones particularly responsible for procreation. Or at least that is the impression we are left with as, regrettably, mothers from lower social strata are near-invisible in the sources.[8] In general, however, we do not get to see things from the woman's and mother's perspective, regardless of her social standing, and details regarding her daily perceptions of the realities of motherhood are unknown as well. Unlike the historians who study the mothers and motherhood of other periods, we have at our disposal no letters, diaries, memoirs, or books written by mothers. All we know is how mothers were seen by politicians, philosophers and physicians – but also husbands and sons – both what they believed mothers were actually like, and what they thought they ought to be like.[9]

While writing this book, I taught a class at my university.[10] We were discussing the *cursus honorum* of Roman officials when a student asked why it was only men we were talking about. I replied that while many Roman women did have a *cursus*, it was one of *laborum* (toil). In my opinion, the word demonstrates women's strength. Plutarch stresses the power of maternal love, able to overcome pain and suffering. When he wants to highlight the role of Empona, Sabinus' wife, who hid with him under the city, he recounts her ability to cope with the pain of a twin birth and compares her to a lioness, a symbol of strength.[11]

Women

The history of women, which includes the history of motherhood, has for decades been part of social history (and gender studies).[12] It is also researched by historians of antiquity, although, as Martha Nussbaum notes,

> the techniques most often used by ancient historians, which focused on textual and inscriptional evidence, were insufficient to write the lives of women. The reading of documentary papyri is a highly specialized skill possessed by only a handful of experts, none of whom had been interested enough in women to use it extensively to that end.[13]

However, an overview of the intensive research into women in antiquity leaves one with the irresistible impression that Nussbaum's diagnosis is by now (fortunately) obsolete. The roles women played in Roman society have been a popular research topic. Over the last thirty years, hundreds of books and thousands of papers have been written throughout the world, demonstrating unflagging interest in that aspect of antiquity. The research focuses on women who were active participants in Rome's public life: priestesses, administrators of estates, entrepreneurs and funders of public buildings, involved in the well-being of their local and supra-local communities.[14] Many studies have also appeared on women's bodies, sexuality and parenthood.[15]

Mothers

Research into motherhood in ancient Rome was pioneered by Susan Dixon. Her two books, *The Roman Mother*[16] and *The Roman Family*,[17] provide some fundamental observations on the role of mothers and their relationship with their children in Roman society. In these two studies, Dixon looks into the major questions surrounding the place of motherhood in the Roman family – its legal implications, the relations between the Roman mother and her older children – both sons and daughters – as well as the mother–child relationship formed in infancy and early childhood. The year 2009 saw the publication in Spain of *Madres y maternidades: Construcciones culturales en la civilización clásica*, a collection of essays born of a conference on motherhood, depicting motherhood as a construct created by men to confirm and legitimize their power over women. Then there is a 2012 collection, likewise resulting from a conference, which mostly focuses on the social, cultural and symbolic aspects of being a mother in classical antiquity,[18] and A. Augoustakis's monograph on the image of mothers and their political influence in the Flavian period as reflected in the literary sources from that era.[19]

In the conservative and patriarchal society of ancient Rome, where the rights of the father (*patria potestas*) were supposed to be absolute, motherhood took on complicated aesthetic, moral and political meanings in literary discourse. These diverse meanings and aspects of motherhood in the poetry of the early Empire are discussed by Mairéad McAuley in *Reproducing Rome: Motherhood in Virgil, Ovid, Seneca, and Statius*, while Anna L. Morelli tries to demonstrate motherhood was a useful element of propaganda, one which defined the role of a woman as that of a mother – a vital element, since it guaranteed dynastic continuity.[20] Another work to focus on various aspects of, and perspectives on, motherhood is the article collection *Maternal Conceptions in Classical Literature and Philosophy*, which addresses motherhood in classical literature, philosophical texts, inscriptions and poetry.[21]

There have been plenty of new books and articles on various aspects of motherhood in recent years, and the subject matter I have decided to pursue is an integral part of a broad spectrum of research into women's history, but the overwhelming majority of that research has been into women whose status as mothers is already beyond any doubt. The process of *becoming* a mother, meanwhile – the whole range of phenomena which determine that – is usually treated as marginal or a mere introduction to research into the history of children and childhood. It is only very rarely that it is considered as a separate research topic.

In statu nascendi

I do not propose here to examine the construct of a mother who has and brings up children, mourns dead children or raises the children of another, or the mother's position in the family, or her role in local or pan-Roman politics. Instead, I am interested in the mother *in statu nascendi*,[22] a woman at the moment she becomes a mother. Several such moments can be singled out and, in my opinion, they form a logical series. The first is the birth of a girl, seen as a (future) mother; next, marriage (becoming a matron, with the hope of becoming a mother); then pregnancy (where losing the pregnancy, be it due to miscarriage or abortion, is depriving the father of a descendant, so the woman is by then treated as a mother); labour and actual, physical childbirth;[23] and finally, the *dies lustricus*, which can be considered the legally sanctioned *social* birth, of both the child and the mother.

It is therefore natural that the broadly conceptualized reproductive health of women is the leitmotif of this study. It was, after all, very significant socially (but also politically and in terms of propaganda) and so, alongside those multiple moments of becoming a mother, another issue of interest to me here is how women were taken care of and what kind of interest there was in their (reproductive) health – that is, what was known at the time about puberty, sexual maturation, pregnancy hygiene and the safety of labour and puerperium, as well as the treatment of the dangers of miscarriage and issues related to contraception and abortion.

The problems of pregnancy, labour, postpartum period and, more broadly, of women's health were of interest to Danielle Gourevitch, the author of a comprehensive study into the health of Roman women, *Le mal d'être femme. La femme et la médecine dans la Rome antique*,[24] whereas Veronique Dasen's research combines her interest in the history of women with that of early childhood. In her search for the relationships and connections between mothers and children, Dasen uses the results of anthropological and ethnographic studies as well as traditional sources.[25] The problems of women's health were of interest to Rebecca Flemming, the author of a most comprehensive study into the reproductive health of Roman women: *Medicine and the Making of Roman Women: Gender, Nature, and Authority from Celsus to Galen*.[26] Two decades ago an interesting study appeared whose author, Angelika Dierichs, depicted parturition in a twofold manner, setting the mythical births of gods against knowledge of obstetrics and the experiences of women in antiquity.[27]

The great interest in the issue of reproductive health of women in the ancient world is best evidenced by the bibliography collected by Y. Panidis. There one can find information about many monographs as well as articles devoted to this topic.[28]

The transition from puberty to motherhood: Women's reproductive health

Reproductive health was defined fairly recently at the 1994 Cairo International Conference on Population and Development. The term featured in its final Programme of Action, in the sense of the state of complete physical, mental and social well-being in all matters to do with the reproductive system and its functions and processes, which phrasing was approved the following year in Beijing.[29] Thus, according to the Programme of Action, reproductive health means, among other things, that human beings are capable of reproducing and are free to decide whether to have children, when and how many. The definition includes a wide range of aspects: from family planning methods, through health services, care of the pregnant woman, prenatal care, safe childbirth, care following childbirth, care of the infant, breastfeeding, prevention and treatment of infertility, preventing unwanted pregnancy, safe abortion options, to treatment of genital infections and, generally speaking, access to healthcare at every stage of life.[30] In other words, the term covers all the issues surrounding the human reproductive system throughout a person's life. The scope of reproductive healthcare clearly shows that the term is semantically rich, including social and cultural as well as medical aspects; however, this spurs debates in some circles due to differences in world view.[31] The difficulty may arise from the term's broad range of meaning in English, which then leads to translation problems, and so semantic problems in national languages.

Of course, the term *reproductive health* did not exist in the ancient world, but it does not follow that no issues covered by it existed. Because of its broad range of meaning, because not all of the problems recognized today were known in antiquity, and because of the specific sociocultural conditions of the era, I shall include in it, as far as ancient Rome is concerned, issues related to be widely understood as fertility and infertility, care for the woman during pregnancy and labour, and care for the newborn infant – but also contraception and pregnancy termination.[32]

The premise

Looking into the reproductive health of people who lived two thousand years ago is no easy task. It is not my goal to create a universal model of women's reproductive health in the Roman world, as that would simply not be possible due to the scope and nature of the sources (scattered in both time and space). Or rather, it would be possible to create an artificial model, but it would be unlikely to accurately reflect the realities of the time. Having no (or very few) direct accounts by women, we have to look at how men viewed the health of the women who would bear their children, and how those women were cared for.

Interpreting the words of Aulus Gellius quoted above, S. Treggiari wrote, 'Matrimonium is an institution involving a mother',[33] and it is that notion that Chapter 1, 'Marriage: The Institution that Makes One a Mother', discusses. The ceremony of marriage was among the moments a Roman mother was born, and the Romans themselves, as they swore their oath before the censors, declared they were marrying *liberorum procreandorum causa*, as only children born of marriage were legitimate in the eyes of Roman law. Plutarch leaves his reader with no illusions: social considerations were important in a man's choice of wife. A good mother should come from a respectable family and have an immaculate moral reputation. So, his advice is:

τοῖς τοίνυν ἐπιθυμοῦσιν ἐνδόξων τέκνων γενέσθαι πατράσιν ὑποθείμην ἂν ἔγωγε μὴ ταῖς τυχούσαις γυναιξὶ συνοικεῖν, λέγω δ' οἷον ἑταίραις ἢ παλλακαῖς· τοῖς γὰρ μητρόθεν ἢ πατρόθεν οὐκ εὖ γεγονόσιν ἀνεξάλειπτα παρακολουθεῖ τὰ τῆς δυσγενείας ὀνείδη παρὰ πάντα τὸν βίον καὶ πρόχειρα τοῖς ἐλέγχειν καὶ λοιδορεῖσθαι βουλομένοις.

and I should advise those desirous of becoming fathers of notable offspring to abstain from random cohabitation with women; I mean with such women as courtesans and concubines. For those who are not well-born, whether on the father's or the mother's side, have an indelible disgrace in their low birth, which accompanies them throughout their lives.[34]

A child may have been a value in itself, and the desire to have one could have stemmed from a biological need to feel parental love, but actually the hope for offspring had a much broader social and cultural context. Children promised the continuity not merely of the nation, but also of the family name, as well as ensuring they would take over the family's business. Of course periods occurred when the state tried to interfere in citizens' private lives by introducing a system of rewards and punishments meant to encourage reproductive success on the scale of the state. For example, quoting the number of citizens in his *Res gestae divi Augusti*, Octavian emphasized the success of his 'reproductive policies'. But having children was not necessarily everybody's wish, for a variety of reasons. For the society elite, too many children could have led to fragmentation of property and family strife with its concomitant weakening of the family's economic and political influence, resulting in them limiting (or trying to limit) the number of prospective heirs. Among the less wealthy, interest in contraception and abortion may have been due to economic reasons (that is, inability to feed another child) or social ones (such as not wanting to give birth to an illegitimate child). Still, the Romans did know that not every woman had the prospect of motherhood open to her; this is discussed in Chapter 2, 'Women Preparing to Be Mothers'.

The accounts left by Roman physicians leave no room for doubt. A suitable background, being part of the elite, education and family history did not guarantee fertility in the slightest. Advising his reader on the choice of a fertile wife, Soranus lists those elements of a woman's appearance, behaviour or even lifestyle which could be indicative of health, increasing the chances of conception. Somewhat paradoxically, he believes retaining virginity is better for a woman's health, claiming that pregnancy and labour risk her health and damage the body.[35] He clearly emphasizes that, while both menstruation and pregnancy were natural phenomena and necessary for the creation of new life, they were dangerous and harmful to the woman.[36] With that in mind, the Romans tried various methods of treating infertility, their last resort being petitioning the gods to intercede in the hope that they would grant them the child they wanted. While awareness existed that it was possible for men to be infertile, in the common opinion it was chiefly the woman who was responsible for lack of offspring. A woman believed infertile faced social exclusion; she was unlikely to be able to marry again (say, after a divorce ruled because of that very affliction).

Chapter 3, 'Specialized Care for the Would-be Mother', is concerned with the people who helped and advised women on reproductive health, primarily midwives. Some midwives were so highly educated they were called *medicae*. In medical texts authored by men, references to women regarded as authorities in the field are frequent.[37] One such figure was believed to be Metrodora; although today she is usually considered to have only lived and practised in the twelfth century, she does have to be mentioned, at least in this introduction, if only because of the many years of scholarly debate surrounding her life. She was reputedly the first female author of a medical treatise,[38] a gynaecological work that discussed diseases of the uterus. The drugs it listed were mostly contraceptives, but also those which increased fertility. It described the course of a pregnancy and other issues, including diseases of the breast. Some researchers suppose Metrodora could have lived and written at the same time as Soranus of Ephesus wrote his *Gynaikeia*, treated as a 'handbook for midwives'.[39]

We also know that in extreme cases, such as when complications arose during labour, a male doctor was called in to see to the woman. The husband was excluded from the women-only birth circle (as were other men).[40] However, like the physician, he probably had the right to interfere in some cases, following a well-defined procedure. Sources that broach the subject are imprecise and even fewer than those on a male physician's presence. The husband of the woman giving birth is mentioned, for instance, in Pliny's *Natural History* in the context of traditions and magical practices to do with inducing labour:

> Partus accelerat et mas, ex quo quaeque conceperit, si cinctu suo soluto feminam cinxerit, dein soluerit adiecta precatione, et cinxisse eundem et soluturum, atque abierit.
>
> If the man by whom a woman has conceived unties his girdle and puts it round her waist, and then unties it with the ritual formula: 'I bound, and I too will unloose,' then taking his departure, childbirth is made more rapid.[41]

In Chapter 4, 'Pregnancy and Its Course', I discuss symptoms of pregnancy, its duration, the course of a normal pregnancy and advice for pregnant women, but also anomalous and multiple pregnancies as well as ones which ended in miscarriage or even the woman's death.

Chapter 5, 'Parturition',[42] deals with the biological process of becoming a mother – that is, the birth itself. It is concerned with such issues as caring for the woman, preparations for childbirth, monitoring its course, methods of inducing labour and of alleviating pain. It is also in Chapter 5 that I write of unusual and difficult births.

A woman did not become a mother in the social sense of the word as soon as her child was born. The time immediately following childbirth is discussed in

Chapter 6, '*Dies lustricus*: The Birth of . . . a Mother?' The time between the baby's birth and the eighth or ninth day after was filled with closely caring for both the woman and the child, as, formally speaking, the social birth of the mother took place on the *dies lustricus*, a very important celebration for the Roman family, but most of all for the woman. A pregnant woman had already lost her previous standing, but had not yet become a mother. Pregnancy was a liminal phase: a time of preparation for her new role. If we assume that until the *dies lustricus* the infant was not a truly separate entity, remaining instead part of the woman, then she too was still in a transitional state and it was only from the *dies lustricus* that she could claim to be a mother.[43]

Sources

The most detailed medical discussion that we have on the subject of Roman women's reproductive health is the work of the physician Soranus,[44] who came from Ephesus, studied in Alexandria and practised medicine in Rome during the reigns of Trajan and Hadrian. His most famous text is the *Gynaecology* (*Τὰ Γυναικεῖα*), only known from Caelius Aurelianus' Latin translation, until in 1830 F. Dietz discovered a Greek version dated to the late fifteenth century (Paris Ms. Gr. 2153). I have used Soranus' treatise in J. Ilberg's edition.[45] An English translation by O. Temkin exists.[46]

The excerpts I draw on in the text come from that translation, so I will be using the numbering of books, sections and paragraphs it employs.

Soranus offered advice (and criticisms) on presumably all matters related to reproductive health: from choosing the optimal time to have intercourse (if the goal is for the woman to conceive), through diagnosing pregnancy, pregnant women's diet and the delivery itself, all the way to taking care of the newborn child. The treatise also discusses anatomy, women's diseases, the hygiene and care of babies, as well as a midwife's duties. The question remains, however, who the intended (and the possible) audience was. The author clearly stated his textbook need not be limited in its use to midwives, it was also addressed to people wanting to know how to pick the best midwife. That *may* have meant women, although M. Green thinks more likely it was men, masters of the house, who employed midwives to take care of their pregnant wives. Thus the treatise could have been known to educated and well-to-do citizens. Most of the poor inhabitants of cities, however, could not afford the time needed for all the procedures, and especially the money necessary to carry out Soranus' recommendations on diet, bathing and massage the pregnant woman should follow. Either way, gynaecological and obstetric care was entrusted directly to women.[47]

Like Soranus' work before it, Caelius Aurelianus' later text was directed at women studying and practising midwifery.[48] Other late ancient authors of Latin adaptations of the Greek physician's treatise, Theodorus Priscianus[49] and Muscio,[50] likewise addressed their work to midwives. Priscianus did not try to explain the more complicated problems of obstetric practice in his text, arguing they should be learned from experience rather than reading, whereas Muscio lamented midwives' ignorance of Greek and unambiguously admitted to abridging Soranus' ample text to make a more easily digestible compendium so the midwives found it easier to understand. In any case, Muscio's work is a very interesting example of how earlier medical treatises written in Greek were 'recovered' and 'revived' in Latin through a conversion aimed at retaining all the basic content while simplifying the language. His remake of Soranus then became a textbook addressed to Latin-speaking midwives in North Africa.[51]

Narrative sources that mention broadly conceptualized aspects of reproductive health are scattered and varied. I have made use of the remarks on motherhood, usually fortuitous and of minor importance, encountered in Dionysius of Halicarnassus,[52] Tacitus,[53] Suetonius,[54] Plutarch,[55] Cassius Dio[56] and the *Historia Augusta*[57] alike, as well as Cicero's letters and speeches,[58] Pliny the Younger,[59] Apuleius,[60] *Natural History* by Pliny the Elder,[61] Solinus,[62] and the *Attic Nights* by Aulus Gellius[63] – texts which, while at times anecdotal, supply a wealth of useful information.

I further draw on remarks made by Quintilian,[64] Seneca the Elder[65] and Seneca the Younger,[66] as well as Ammianus Marcellinus.[67] I have also found worthwhile the works of Artemidorus,[68] Censorinus,[69] Pedanius Dioscorides[70] and Gargilius.[71]

Lucretius' poetry was meant to 'free' his readers from unjustified belief in gods and divine control over the universe and the fate of individuals, including future parents.[72] One other author who ought not to be omitted in a book on women is Ovid,[73] and topics to do with having offspring were taken up by Horace[74] and Propertius.[75]

Martial's[76] and Juvenal's[77] social commentary is scathing at times and certainly exaggerates and distorts the realities of their time, also as regards mothers, but if the vicious derision was to be understood by their contemporaries, their texts must have been based on the real life of the elite in Rome. Justinian's surviving

Digest[78] is another invaluable source, which makes it possible to understand numerous legal regulations.

Inscriptions and anatomical votive offerings are a source as valuable as narrative material, or indeed more so, as they often provide data on social classes other than the upper. Most of my sources can be dated to between the first century BCE and the third century CE, but occasionally I have made use of earlier or slightly later material, although it represents a fraction of the whole. I have also decided not to use any Christian sources, deliberately.[79]

Limitations and expectations: A summary

On the first page of the preface of her book, S. Dixon makes the fairly depressing remark that after researching the history of women for twenty years she was more sceptical about extracting satisfactory data from the surviving sources than she had been at the beginning of her research career.[80] As I have stressed more than once, those sources reflect men's ideas of women's reproductive health. Our knowledge regarding the reproductive health of Roman woman cannot but, for the most part, remain shaped by the men of the Roman elite. As A. Richlin notes, the works of the male authors are always shot through with fear of men's helplessness regarding controlling women's fertility. Fertility, of course, was an important bargaining chip of Roman women: birthing healthy children who would live to adulthood remained the simplest way a woman could raise her standing, both in the close circle of family and friends and in the wider social context. That male fear is clearly visible in the excerpt from Ovid's *Fasti* where the abducted Sabine women bore no children, and later, during the women's 'reproductive' strike. Richlin believes men emphasizing their power by belittling, mocking, intimidating and continuously judging women to be a 'defensive response'.[81] Thus the emphasis on women's reproductive role: a man will not bear a child; he will never be a mother (unless he is Zeus, who gave birth to Athena and was 'pregnant' with Dionysus).[82]

Becoming a mother may be interesting in that pregnancy does not discriminate between social groups. It is a universal experience of all the women who go through it (even though, naturally, no two pregnancies are alike and neither are any two births). Does that absolve us of the need to carry out research? Hardly. But there seems to be no hope of creating a single universal canon or model of becoming a mother. The question remains of *when* a woman became a mother. With the role being culturally determined, did it happen as soon as a female child was born, or at the moment the woman married? When pregnancy was diagnosed, or biologically, at the moment of giving birth, or perhaps only after the newborn had survived their own birth to be given a name and so, legally speaking, became a person? The problem is more complex than that. Any of those moments in a woman's life can be regarded as crucial and decisive for considering her a potential/future/biological/legal mother.

***

I tried to write my book so it would be a voice in the discussion on the subject and of interest to an expert, but also of use to students of classics and researchers into the history of medicine, as well as laypeople passionate about women's history and ancient history in general, and that is why I quote texts in Latin and Greek in the footnotes. Where passages are important for the flow of my reasoning, the originals are featured in the main text, however, accompanied by English translations. The source quotation style was a conscious choice. To students and laypeople, it is the story that matters: the account in the body of the text, which provides them with the relevant excerpts in English translation. However, not all quotations are important to the account; some merely serve to verify specific information or the credibility of a source. Those were placed in footnotes and left in their original languages for more advanced readers, who ought to be able to check them against the sources themselves. I make use of some less-known and less-available sources, as well as works of ancient authors who do not at first glance belong in women's studies. The quotation method I adopted makes it possible to look up the context quickly and verify the information according to the *read-and-check* principle.

All abbreviations of the titles of works I have used can be found in the section 'Sources (Abbreviations and Editions)', which also contains information on editions and translations.

1

Marriage: The Institution that Makes One a Mother

'Matrimonium is an institution involving a mother, mater'[1]

Liberorum procreandorum causa

In the Roman elite, marriages were made so that children could be born of them. Dionysius of Halicarnassus reports that Romulus' legislation already contained regulations obliging citizens to marry and have offspring,[2] as the censors conducting the census asked each citizen whether he had married for the purpose of having children.[3] There are also mentions of such a solution in Aulus Gellius' *Attic Nights*,[4] and a marriage contract from Roman Egypt contains characteristic phrasing, which expresses the same thing:

> [C(aius) Antistius Nomissianus filiam suam] Zenarion uirginem e lege Iuliạ
> [quae de maritandis ordinibus(?)]
> [lata est liberorum procrea(?)]ṇdorum causa in matrimonio [eam collocauit, uxorem eam(?)]
> [duxit M(arcus(?)) Petronius Seruilliu]ṣ

> Nomissianus [in accordance with the Julian law], which has [been] enacted concerning marriage arrangements, has given his maiden daughter [Zenarion] in marriage for the sake [of begetting children] and M. Petronius Servillius [has taken her as his wife].[5]

Macrobius actually claimed it was holy to marry for the sake of having children,[6] and similar sentiments had been voiced by Suetonius[7] and Tacitus,[8] while mentions of children as the main reason for marriage can even be found in Plautus' comedies.[9] Soranus is of the same opinion, considering as he does the primary reason for marrying to be τέκνων ἕνεκα καὶ διαδοχῆς, that is: children and succession (of one's family). Although the physician repeatedly says in his treatise that pregnancy endangers the woman's life and health, and may cause her to age early, he ultimately gives in to social pressure and agrees with the opinion held among the Roman elite, emphasizing that children are chiefly important for the sake of διαδοχή, or the continuity of the family for the purpose of succession in terms of the name, property and citizenship.

The connection between marriage and procreation was also seen as integral and in accordance with natural law. As Ulpian wrote, it was the reason why the union of a man and a woman known as *marriage* even took place – because it resulted in procreation and bringing up children.[10] The poet and philosopher Lucretius went even further in his reflection, saying:

> mulier coniuncta viro concessit in unum (…)
> cognita sunt, prolemque ex se videre creatam,
> tum genus humanum primum mollescere coepit
>
> woman mated with man moved into one …
> and they saw offspring born of them,
> then first the human race began to grow soft[11]

Thus he sees the origin of civilization in connection with the union between a man and a woman and the birth of their children. A similar association was exploited by Cicero, who claimed a wise man ought to desire to live according to nature, that is, to marry and sire offspring with his wife.[12] He also understood having children as a sign one cared for one's family's future,[13] but it was a fairly widespread belief that for a Roman citizen, having heirs was actually 'patriotic duty'. Livy cited a speech given in 131 BCE by the censor Quintus Metellus, which urged the audience to marry and have children.[14] Metellus himself, naturally, was a model father and grandfather,[15] and the speech would reputedly be quoted by Augustus to point out he was not the first to care about the birthrate in the state:

> Etiam libros totos et senatui recitavit et populo notos per edictum saepe fecit, ut orationes Q. Metelli 'de prole augenda' et Rutili 'de modo aedificiorum', quo magis persuaderet utramque rem non a se primo animadversam, sed antiquis iam tunc curae fuisse.
>
> He even read entire volumes to the senate and called the attention of the people to them by proclamations; for example, the speeches of Quintus Metellus 'On Increasing the Family' … to convince them that he was not the first to give attention to such matters, but that they had aroused the interest even of their forefathers.[16]

Augustus and his reproductive policy

Octavian attempted to deliberately and comprehensively regulate Romans' rights and obligations in matters of marriage by having a series of laws concerned with those issues approved.[17] After he began to proclaim moral restoration, stressing the power and significance of the family, marriage and having children, a need arose for justification and social understanding of those ideas. As W. Suder writes, poets came to the rescue. Among them, Horace depicted the moral decline of the Roman society in order to justify why it was necessary to change things. In his own words,

> Fecunda culpae saecula nuptias
> primum inquinavere et genus et domos:
> hoc fonte derivata clades / in patriam populumque fluxit
>
> Generations prolific in sin first defiled marriage, the family, and the home. From this source is derived the disaster which has engulfed our fatherland and its folk.[18]

Such 'propaganda' was necessary as an explanation for the new laws, since in 28 BCE, when Augustus first proposed the marriage law introducing compulsory marriage and the obligation to have children, he subsequently decided to withdraw it, having met with strong social resistance. The draft only returned ten years later, in 18 BCE, and to avoid another failure, it was introduced by virtue of Augustus *tribunicia potestas* rather than as a law.[19] Officially, the *lex Iulia de adulteriis coërcendis* was aimed at putting an end to the increasing decline in morals. The emperor wanted to restore the by then forgotten *mos maiorum*, bringing back the old moral order. Then the *lex Iulia de maritandis ordinibus* introduced regulations regarding marriage in the various social groups, as well as the obligation to remain married, which applied to women aged twenty to fifty and men aged twenty to sixty. Should a marriage end, men were supposed to enter another immediately, while women had the right to wait – one year if their spouse had died, and half a year in the case of divorce. Contrary to Augustus' hopes, the laws were once again greeted coldly, and many protests occurred demanding they be relaxed. That did not happen; on the contrary, another law, the *lex Papia Poppaea* of 9 CE, further obliged citizens to have children. Punishments for breaking the regulation included receiving only half of any inheritance specified in a will, with the remaining property transferred to other inheritors listed by the will who did have children, or to the state.

Most scholars believe Augustus' main goal was to restore the morality and population of the Roman state,[20] with the marriage law meant to apply to all the social strata, not just the senatorial order, but as W. Suder emphasizes, 'the alleged moral decline, widespread bachelorhood, and unwillingness to have children brought up by some poets, not least of them Horace, cannot really be confirmed in non-Augustan literary sources or in demographic analysis. In fact, neither demographic analysis nor archaeological sources confirm any depopulation of Italy under the late Republic or early Empire.'[21] Suder further points out that in that period, women of the senatorial order generally bore around three children, and in the legislators' opinion, three births were enough for satisfactory demographic development. Still, present-day researchers maintain it would have taken five to six children born per marriage, with presumably only half of them living to adulthood, for the population to increase by 0.5 per cent yearly, considering the high mortality rate.[22] W. Suder does not suggest there are reasons to think in terms of a fertility crisis in Rome in the first century CE, and believes the introduction of marriage laws to have been a purely propaganda-oriented move, intended mostly to legitimize Augustus' power, in part through the moral renewal of the Roman society he proclaimed, for which the laws were merely to serve as additional legal superstructure.[23]

The *ius trium liberorum*

In 9 CE, proclaiming the *lex Papia Poppaea*, which made marriage and children compulsory, Augustus sanctioned it not merely with many penalties, but also privileges for those who could meet the reproductive expectations,[24] especially if they boasted many children (three in Rome itself, four in Italy, or five in the provinces). Those included preferential treatment for candidates for various offices,[25] provincial governorship nominations, and even the right to assume an office before reaching the requisite age.[26] In criminal trials, having many children was considered an extenuating circumstance and might result in a lighter sentence.[27] Interestingly, the emperor could specially grant the privileges defined by that law to people who did not qualify, having fewer children than three or, in some cases, no children at all. One of those was Martial, who not only had no children, but also, as is suspected, no wife.[28] Pliny the Younger, whose attempts at having offspring remained futile, received the licence from the emperor Trajan:

> Exprimere, domine, verbis non possum, quantum mihi gaudium attuleris, quod me dignum putasti iure trium liberorum.

I have no words to tell you, Sir, how much pleasure you have given me by thinking me fit for the privileges granted to parents of three children.[29]

The three children required by Augustus' legislation also granted special privileges and freedoms to women, removing them from under the legally mandated oversight of a man and allowing them to inherit from their children. Nor were they required to remarry.[30]

We have a surviving application for the privilege of 'the right of three children' submitted by an Aurelia Thaisus. It is an interesting example for how women made use of the opportunity. The text comes from Roman Egypt and is dated to 263 CE:

[..] .α[...] .. [.] ... [...,] δ[ιαση]/μότατε ἡγεμών, οἵτινες/ ἐξουσίαν διδόασιν ταῖς γυναι/ξὶν ταῖς τῶν τριῶν τέκνων/δικαίῳ κεκοσμημένα[ι]ς ἑαυ/τῶν κυριεύειν καὶ χωρ[ὶς] κυ/ρίου χρηματίζειν ἐν αἷς ποι/οῦν[τ]αι οἰκονομίαις, πο[λλ]ῷ/ δὲ πλέον ταῖς γρά[μ]ματα/ ἐπισταμέναις. καὶ αὐτὴ τοί/νυν τῷ μὲν κόσμῳ τῆς εὐ/ παιδείας εὐτυχήσασα,/ἐγγράμματος δὲ κα[ὶ ἐ]ς τὰ/ μάλιστα γράφειν εὐκόπως/ δυναμένη, ὑπὸ περισσῆς/ ἀσφαλείας διὰ τούτων μου/ τῷ[ν] βιβλειδίων προσφῶ/ τῷ σῷ μεγέθι πρὸς τὸ δύνα/σθαι ἀνεμποδίστως ἃς ἐν/τεῦθεν ποιοῦμαι οἰκ[ον] ομία[ς]/ διαπράσσεσθαι. ἀξιῶ ἔχε[ιν]/ αὐτὰ ἀπροκρίτως .τρ[ῖς δι]/καίοις μ[ο]υ ἐν τῇ σῇ τοῦ [δια]/σημοτάτου τ[ά]ξι, ἵν' ᾧ β[εβο]/ηθ[η]μένη κ[α]ὶ εἰ[σ]αεί σ[οι]/ χάριτας ὁμολογήσω. διευτ[ύ]χ[ει.]/ Αὐρηλία Θαϊσ[ο]ῦς ἡ καὶ Λολλ[ι]/ ανὴ διεπεμψάμην πρὸς ἐ/πίδοσιν. ἔτους ι Ἐπεὶφ β[ ]/ἔσται σο[ῦ] τὰ βιβλία ἐν τῇ [τάξει.]

[Laws long ago have been made], most eminent prefect, which empower women who are adorned with the right of three children [5] to be mistresses of themselves and act without a guardian in whatever business they transact, especially those who know how to write. [10] Accordingly, as I too enjoy the happy honour of being blessed with children and as I am a literate woman able to write with a high degree of ease, [15] it is with abundant security that I appeal to your highness by this my application with the object of being enabled to accomplish without hindrance whatever business I [20] henceforth transact, and I beg you to keep it without prejudice to my rights in your eminence's office, in order that I may [25] obtain your support and acknowledge my unfailing gratitude. Farewell. I, Aurelia Thaisous also called Lolliane, have sent this for presentation. Year 10, Epeiph 21. 30 (Annotation) Your application shall be kept in the [office].[31]

As a well-educated woman (or at least, one who stressed her literacy), Aurelia was certainly aware that freeing her from a man's obligatory guardianship went beyond the prefect's remit. After 212 CE, every woman with three children acquired the *ius liberorum ex necessitate legis*. M. Jońca and P. Szarek believe Aurelia may have requested an authenticated copy of her application to use it each time there was doubt as to her legal capacity, so she would not have to present her children. In their opinion, the papyrus demonstrates that even the women the *ius trium liberorum* applied to needed something to verify it if they wanted to avoid unnecessary complications as they carried out legal transactions or official formalities.[32] Thus in this specific case, the official petition for the *ius trium liberorum* could have been the excuse the applicant used to obtain a certificate which would make her life considerably easier as she went about her business in various public offices.

Does everyone want to have children?

Although the many literary sources mentioned above do demonstrate that the desire to have children can be natural and harboured by both genders, other authors express the opinion that children, wives and even marriage itself are an exhausting burden to a man, wanted only by the hopelessly naive, completely unaware of what they actually mean.[33] Children can be ungrateful and the reward for the hard work of raising them uncertain. Juvenal, for instance, says men, motivated by emotions and urges, want marriage and a wife who could give them children, but the investment is very unreliable:

> carior est illis homo quam sibi. nos animorum/ inpulsu caeco vanaque cupidine ducti coniugium petimus partumque uxoris, at illis/ notum qui pueri qualisque futura sit uxor.

> While we are led by our blind emotional impulses and by empty desire to seek marriage and children from a wife, it is the gods who know who our boys will be and what kind of wife she'll be.[34]

Seneca the Elder, meanwhile, mentions a man for whom his wife's fertility became more of a curse than a blessing: he describes the man's children as three monsters.[35] Indeed, the cost of raising one's children and either setting the sons on a political career path or setting aside the daughters' dowries was high, as Marcus Hortalus discovered, so that he begged Tiberius for financial aid:

> nepos erat oratoris Hortensii, inlectus a divo Augusto liberalitate decies sestertii ducere uxorem, suscipere liberos, ne clarissima familia extingueretur. igitur

quattuor filiis ante limen curiae adstantibus ... ad hunc modum coepit: 'patres conscripti, hos, quorum numerum et pueritiam videtis, non sponte sustuli sed quia princeps monebat; simul maiores mei meruerant ut posteros haberent ... iussus ab imperatore uxorem duxi. en stirps et progenies tot consulum, tot dictatorum ... Q. Hortensii pronepotes, divi Augusti alumnos ab inopia defende.'

Augustus, by the grant of a million sesterces, had induced him to marry and raise a family, in order to save his famous house from extinction. With his four sons, then, standing before the threshold of the Curia, he awaited his turn to speak; then, directing his gaze now to the portrait of Hortensius among the orators (the senate was meeting in the Palace), now to that of Augustus, he opened in the following manner:— 'Conscript Fathers, these children whose number and tender age you see for yourselves, became mine not from any wish of my own, but because the emperor so advised, and because, at the same time, my ancestors had earned the right to a posterity. For to me, who in this changed world had been able to inherit nothing and acquire nothing, — not money, nor popularity, nor eloquence, that general birthright of our house, — to me it seemed enough if my slender means were neither a disgrace to myself nor a burden to my neighbour. At the command of the sovereign, I took a wife; and here you behold the stock of so many consuls, the offspring of so many dictators! I say it, not to awaken odium, but to woo compassion. Some day, Caesar, under your happy sway, they will wear whatever honours you have chosen to bestow: in the meantime, rescue from beggary the great-grandsons of Quintus Hortensius, the fosterlings of the deified Augustus!'[36]

That story of the fall of house Hortensia, found in Tacitus, illustrates the financial difficulties arising from raising children. Hortalus was so poor he needed (and received) extra money to marry and have children. As he himself said, the marriage was very successful in reproductive terms, as the couple had four children of both genders;[37] however, Hortalus also thought he and his wife had proven too fertile. In his request for financial help, addressed to Tiberius and the senate, he stresses the children were not his idea at all.

Contraception and abortion

'In the human race the males have devised every out-of-the-way form of sexual indulgence, crimes against nature, but the females have invented abortion.'[38]

Dionysius of Halicarnassus noted it was Romulus who decreed Romans must acknowledge all their male offspring and at least their first daughter. It was also forbidden to kill a child under the age of three unless they were deformed.[39] Since Augustus openly compared himself to the legislator and wished to be seen as the new Romulus, one can suppose (as K. Milnor did) that the decree attributed to Romulus was in fact a pure figment of propaganda created for Augustus' purposes,[40] and Dionysius' account was only meant to legitimize his reform,[41] as in the light of the emperor's legislation, the point of marriage was to serve the interests of the state, meaning its basic purpose was to provide that state with enough citizens. Therefore women of the Roman elite who were of reproductive age, but refused to bear children, were accused of not wanting to damage their figure and so either avoiding becoming pregnant or trying to terminate their pregnancy. The criticism of childless women concentrates mostly on their vanity: their unwillingness to ruin their bodies, fear of feeling unwell and fear of childbirth pain.[42] The philosopher Favorinus even claimed Roman women had abortions for aesthetic reasons, not wanting their abdomens to wrinkle and sag.[43] Still, such motivation was often ascribed primarily to wealthy women from great houses, since, as the satirist Juvenal notes, 'hardly any woman lies in labour on a gilded bed'.[44] Even so, is it surprising that women were afraid of their appearance changing, and is the Roman men's shock not hypocritical? Men's descriptions of women considered unattractive or old prove that worship of a young, firm, smooth body was quite alive in Rome as well.[45] It was the same men who wrote that pregnancy cut a woman's youth short, wrinkled her belly and made her breasts lose their firmness. In one of his works, Statius implored the goddesses of childbirth to protect the beauty of the body and face of a friend's pregnant wife.

A wish to limit the number of children, however, could also have stemmed from the need to control the total number of offspring or to erase evidence of illegal unions, that is, pregnancies resulting from adultery. One of the most interesting and rarest reasons for an abortion is mentioned in Quintilian. In one of his declamations, he recounts the story of a woman who married a man with three sons of his own. After she had an abortion, her husband sent her away.

> Quod primum pertinet ad pudorem huius feminae, non adulterium obicitur, non aliqua adversus maritum licentia. Necesse est plurimum eius moribus tribuat ex qua liberos quaerit ... 'Sterilitatis medicamentum bibit.' Si tu liberos non haberes, poteram tamen illa dicere: periculum timuit, documentis quarundam infeliciter parientium mota est, fortasse male sensit de temporibus ipsis, vidit eam luxuriam, ea vitia, ut paene educare liberos amentis esset. Tu porro in uxore nihil aliud spectas quam fecunditatem? 'Non parit.' Sed obsequium, sed fidem praestat. Sed iam tempus est propriis eam rationibus

defendi. Bibit illud cum tres liberos haberes. Nec statim hoc amore et adfectu defendo; interim tamquam ambitiosam tuebor. Voluit effugere fabulas novercarum, voluit se adversus casus etiam praeparare, voluit nihil in domo habere propter quod privignis invideret. Quid si fecit hoc non modo novercae sed etiam uxoris optimae animo? Plenam invenerat domum, plenum testamentum. 'Quid mihi' inquit 'cum partu erat? Dederat mihi Fortuna iuvenes; neque maritus eius aetatis est ut concupiscere novos liberos possit. Ne fraternitatis quidem eadem iura futura erant [inter tam dissonantes tamque discordes].' At nunc expellitur et, quoniam bona fuit noverca, nec liberos habitura est nec virum.

What is first relevant to the honor of this woman, she is not taxed with adultery or any license against her husband. He must needs think highly of the character of a woman from whom he wants children. The whole reason for divorce lies in one charge. What sort of charge, we shall see later; meanwhile, it is the only one. What mortal is so fortunate? And I am not speaking of a woman, whose is the weaker sex, but even in those who are accustomed to boast of their prudence and wisdom repentance has a place. But [this] one charge, let it be grave, let it be criminal (and upon my word that will be believable in a woman who had three stepsons): I expect one of those step motherly acts. Did she prepare poison, did she plot against your children, or, what is the least of them, did she try to turn your mind against them? None of these. The charge is novel, never before heard of: a stepmother is said to love her stepsons too much. 'She drank a drug causing sterility.' If you didn't have children, I could still say that she feared the danger, was upset by certain examples of women unfortunate in childbirth, perhaps had a bad opinion of the times we live in—she saw such loose living, such vices, that it was well-nigh madness to bring up children. Moreover, do you think of nothing in a wife except fecundity? 'She does not produce a child.' But she gives obedience, gives loyalty. But now it's time she be defended by arguments special to her case. She drank that drug when you had three children. I am not defending this straight away by love and affection: for the present I shall say on her behalf that she was eager to shine. She wanted to escape the stories about stepmothers, wanted to prepare herself too against ill chances, wanted to have nothing in her home to make her jealous of her stepsons. What if she did it not only in the spirit of an excellent stepmother but of an excellent wife? She had found a full home, a full will. 'What had I to do with childbearing?' she says. 'Fortune had given me sons; and my husband is not of an age that he can form a desire for new children. Nor would the laws of brotherhood have remained the same [among persons so dissonant, so discordant].' But now she is expelled, and because she was a good stepmother, she will have neither children nor husband.[46]

Her defence focuses on the reasons why she decided to abort. Among them are listed her love for her stepsons and fear a child of her own would make her into a stereotypical stepmother. The author also remarks her husband is of an age when one no longer wants to take on raising another child, depicting her as someone who entered an excellent family as a spouse and stepmother and really wanted to become part of it, with the abortion being due to her fear of destroying that good set-up. Even so, the woman was sent away. Quintilian then asks her husband, 'Moreover, do you think of nothing in a wife except fecundity?' Although there is no comment directly to that effect, one may observe the woman's only offence was that she took the decision herself. That, in fact, may well have been what alarmed Roman men the most: independent decisions regarding reproductive health over which they had no control.

One can similarly interpret Ovid's mention of Corinna's abortion: one gets the impression the heaviest charge against her is that she 'dared' decide without consulting her lover.[47]

Men's fear of having no influence over women's actions is even clearer in Book One of the *Fasti*, where Ovid recounts a 'strike' held by women:

> nam prius Ausonias matres carpenta vehebant
> (haec quoque ab Euandri dicta parente reor);
> mox honor eripitur, matronaque destinat omnis
> ingratos nulla prole novare viros.
> neve daret partus, ictu temeraria caeco
> visceribus crescens excutiebat onus.
> corripuisse patres ausas immitia nuptas,
> ius tamen exemptum restituisse ferunt,
> binaque nunc pariter Tegeaeae sacra parenti
> pro pueris fieri virginibusque iubent.

> For of old Ausonian matrons drove in carriages ... Afterwards the honour was taken from them, and every matron vowed not to propagate the line of her ungrateful spouse by giving birth to offspring; and lest she should bear children, she rashly by a secret thrust discharged the growing burden from her womb. They say the senate reprimanded the wives for their daring cruelty, but restored the right of which they had been mulcted; and they ordained that now two festivals be held alike in honour of the Teagean mother to promote the birth of boys and girls.[48]

Although the Roman society was by all accounts patriarchal, with men controlling women's lives to a considerable degree, when it came to propagating the species they were vulnerable: they needed heirs, but were unable to birth them themselves. Perhaps it is this vulnerability, this fear of women's reproductive power, that lies behind those descriptions of the selfishness of women, who want flat stomachs and involve their husbands in bringing up children they had not sired.

The 'strike' of women perfectly illustrates men's anxiety regarding women's actions which might potentially threaten their families, themselves and even Roman society itself,[49] a perspective clearly discernible in the defence of Aulus Cluentius Habitus. In it, Cicero adduces the story of a woman from Miletus who brought about artificial miscarriage pharmacologically. The orator stresses she was then sentenced to death, a verdict he deems just, because

> quandam mulierem ... quod ab heredibus [secundis] accepta pecunia partum sibi ipsa medicamentis abegisset, rei capitalis esse damnatam; nec iniuria, quae spem parentis, memoriam nominis, subsidium generis, heredem familiae, designatum rei publicae civem sustulisset.

> a certain woman of Miletus, who had accepted a bribe from the alternative heirs and procured her own abortion by drugs, was condemned to death: and rightly, for she had cheated the father of his hopes, his name of continuity, his family of its support, his house of an heir, and the Republic of a citizen-to-be.[50]

Thus Cicero regarded the abortion as a murder of a future Roman citizen.[51]

It is actually quite frequently that abortion was depicted in ancient sources not so much as a personal matter, but rather as neglecting the interests of the state. Ovid's tone is similar when he writes that if every woman had the right to take decisions about her body herself, the earth could even depopulate:

> si mos antiquis placuisset matribus idem,
> gens hominum vitio deperitura fuit,
> quique iterum iaceret, generis primordia nostri
> in vacuo lapides orbe, parandus erat
> quis Priami fregisset opes, si numen aquarum
> iusta recusasset pondera ferre Thetis?
> Ilia si tumido geminos in ventre necasset,
> casurus dominae conditor Urbis erat.
> si Venus Aenean gravida temerasset in alvo,
> Caesaribus tellus orba futura fuit.

> If vicious ways like this had found favour with mothers of olden time, the race of mortal men would have perished from the earth, and someone must have been

found to cast abroad a second time in the vacant world the stones that were the first beginnings of our kind. Who would have crushed the might of Priam if divine Thetis of the waves had refused to bear the burden hers by due? Had Ilia slain the twins in her swelling bosom, 'twould have been doom to the founder of the City that rules the earth; had Venus laid rash hand to Aeneas in her heavy womb, the world to come would have been orphaned of its Caesars.[52]

However, it was only Septimius Severus and Caracalla who banned abortion by married women. The relevant imperial decrees declared a woman inducing miscarriage as grounds for divorce or banishment,[53] and those who supplied the drugs necessary for inducing the miscarriage were to be punished as well, with either compulsory mining labour or exile; should the woman die due to the miscarriage, they were tried as if for murder.[54]

Contraception methods

While it is often assumed people in antiquity did not distinguish between contraception and abortion, it should be noted the issue and the difference were, in fact, considered in medical circles.[55] Soranus clearly indicated there was a distinction between contraceptive and abortifacient drugs,[56] as well as pointing out it had long been discussed whether pregnancy termination was acceptable from the perspective of medical ethics. He himself believed prevention safer than abortion.[57]

If a woman wished not to conceive, she ought to avoid intercourse during the time doctors believed the best for conception, that is, directly before and after her menses, while during the coupling itself, she should hold her breath and pull away a little as the man is about to ejaculate, so the sperm cannot reach the uterus, then immediately rise and 'sneeze while kneeling up, carefully wash out her vagina or drink some cold water'.[58]

Conception could also be made more difficult by rubbing into the exit of the uterus stale olive oil, honey, cedar resin, or Arabian balsam tree balm with either white lead or wax ointment mixed in. Other contraceptives included a wad of soft wool inserted deep into the vagina and special suppositories intended to block off the entrance to the uterus.[59] By causing a contraction, closing off and cooling down, those measures were supposed to block the entrance and stop the semen from getting into the uterus. Soranus believed them irritants that could cause muscle spasms, which not only hindered 'semen staying in the uterus, but also extracted liquid from it'.[60] In that group, he included pine bark and Sicilian sumac bark, to be ground in wine and applied with a tampon two or three hours before intercourse. He also recommended mixing Cimolian earth[61] and fennel root with water or grinding a pomegranate, possibly adding some dissolved alum, and dipping a scrap of wool in that to be inserted in the vagina before sex. One other method involved grinding unripe galls, pomegranate and ginger (two drachms of each) with wine, forming the mass into pellets the size of a pea, drying them and 'using as suppositories before intercourse'. Dried figs ground with natron were used in similar ways, and so was pomegranate peel mixed in equal parts with resin and rose oil.[62]

Soranus also quoted what advice he knew from other experts, although he noted he did not always believe in the efficacy of the medication they recommended. This included:

ἐνίοις δὲ ἔτι δοκεῖ καὶ ἅπαξ τοῦ μηνὸς ὀπὸν Κυρηναϊκὸν πίνειν ὅσον ἐρεβίνθου πλῆθος ἐν δυσὶ κυάθοις ὕδατος ὡς καταμήνιον ἐπισπώμενον. ἢ ὀποπάνακος καὶ ὀποῦ Κυρηναϊκοῦ καὶ πηγάνου σπέρματος ἀνὰ ὀβολοὺς δύο [λειώσαντα] καὶ περιπλάσαντα κηρῷ διδόναι καταπίνειν, εἶτα κραμάτιον ἐπιρροφεῖν ἢ ἐν κραματίῳ πίνειν. [ἢ] λευκοΐου σπέρματος καὶ μυρσίνης ἀνὰ τριώβολον, σμύρνης δραχμήν, πεπέρεως λευκοῦ κόκκους δύο μετ᾽ οἴνου ἐφ᾽ ἡμέρας τρεῖς διδόναι πίνειν. ἢ εὐζώμου σπέρματος ὀβολὸν ἕνα, σπονδυλίου ἡμιώβολον πιεῖν μετὰ ὀξυμέλιτος. ταῦτα δὲ οὐ μόνον κωλυτικὰ συλλήψεως ὑπάρχει, ἀλλὰ καὶ φθαρτικὰ τῆς ἤδη συνεστώσης.

Once during the month to drink Cyrenaic balm to the amount of a chick-pea in two cyaths of water for the purpose of inducing menstruation. Or: Of panax balm and Cyrenaic balm and rue seed, of each two obols, [grind] and coat with wax and give to swallow; then follow with a drink of diluted wine or let it be drunk in diluted wine. [Or:] Of wallflower seed and myrtle, of each three obols, of myrrh a drachm, of white pepper two seeds; give to drink with wine for three days. Or: Of rocket seed one obol, of cow parsnip one-half obol; drink with oxymel. However, these things not only prevent conception, but also destroy any already existing.[63]

Soranus considered the above-mentioned drugs dangerous, because they ruined the stomach, induced vomiting, made the head heavy, and caused general weakness. Among safe measures, he counted amulets (containing a female mule's uterus or earwax),[64] but many more pieces of folk advice of that kind survive,[65] so it is possible many Roman women not only knew of such methods, but also used them. Female mule's earwax does come up in later texts, including the *Cyranides*:

τῆς οὖν μούλας ὁ ῥύπος ὁ ἐν τῷ ὠτίῳ ἀσύλληπτον ἄκρως ἐστίν, ἐν δέρματι αὐτῆς περιαφθείς. ἐὰν δὲ τὸν ῥύπον δῷς λάθρα ἐν ποτῷ γυναικί, οὐ συλλήψεταί ποτε. οὕτω δὲ καὶ ἐὰν ἐκ τῆς μήτρας αὐτῆς συνεψήσας μεθ' ἑτέρων κρεῶν δῴης λάθρα γυναικὶ φαγεῖν, οὐδέποτε συλλήψεται. ὁμοίως καὶ οἱ ὄνυχες αὐτοῦ κεκαυμένοι τὸ αὐτὸ ποιοῦσιν.

Female mule's earwax is a very efficient contraceptive when carried in a pouch made of its hide worn around the neck. If you stealthily add some female mule's earwax to a woman's drink, she will never conceive. Likewise, if you cook a mule's uterus with other meat and give a woman to eat, she will never conceive either. The same effect is obtained from burnt hooves.[66] (retransl. from a Polish translation by E. Żybert)

The collection has more such 'dietary supplements': 'if a woman drinks the marrow of eagle, and then places a small amount of it in her vagina, she will become infertile'.[67] Also 'the seeds (of eruca) drunk in wine are a contraceptive',[68] while a mule's testicle tied in mule leather and worn next to the body as an amulet makes conception impossible. 'Cut off the weasel testicles when the moon wanes, and the weasel, release live. Give the testicle to a person to carry around in mule hide; it is the best contraceptive measure'.[69] 'If you take a piece of a dog's dried penis, you will have an amulet to prevent pregnancy'.[70]

Another method employed by women who wanted to avoid pregnancy was the right behaviour during intercourse. Lucretius, for instance, claimed prostitutes had their ways of not getting pregnant with their clients, as pregnancy would have deprived them of their livelihood for a while:

nam mulier prohibet se concipere atque repugnant,
clunibus ipsa viri Venerem si laeta retractat
atque exossato ciet omni pectore fluctus;
eicit enim sulcum recta regione viaque
vomeris atque locis avertit seminis ictum.
idque suacausa consuerunt scorta moveri,
ne complerentur crebro gravidaeque iacerent.

For a woman forbids herself to conceive and fights against it, if in her delight she thrusts against the man's penis with her buttocks,[a] making undulating movements with all her body limp; for she turns the share clean away from the furrow and makes the seed fail of its place. Whores indulge in such motions for their own purposes, that they may not often conceive and lie pregnant.[71]

Another alternative was for the women to have sexual congress with eunuchs. That is what Juvenal suggests:

sunt quas eunuchi inbelles ac mollia semper oscula delectent
et desperatio barbae et quod abortiuo non est opus.

> Some women are delighted by un-macho eunuchs with their ever gentle kisses and their unfulfilled beard—and there's no need to use abortion drugs.[72]

Due to the Roman understanding of fertility and pregnancy, those Roman women who wished to control the matter through a calendar-based method would have encountered considerable problems, as at the time it was universally believed that conception was most likely at the onset or end of menstruation. The belief had a twofold result: couples who looked forward to pregnancy and a baby may have missed the fertile window, while those trying to prevent pregnancy or simply not looking forward to it involuntarily increased their chances of conceiving by having intercourse at other times. Still, for most couples who had sex regularly, the woman would likely eventually become pregnant provided both parties were fertile.

Abortion methods

Soranus reports that if the drugs suggested as contraceptives failed and one wanted to miscarry, then in the first thirty days one should make sudden movements, be shaken about riding a cart on bumpy roads, jump, lift heavy objects, drink diuretic decoctions, empty one's stomach, anoint one's body, particularly the lower abdomen and hips, and bathe in warm water every day 'so that the seed separates'. One ought to spend a long time in the bath, drinking some light wine and eating spicy dishes beforehand.[73] Other measures advocated included 'hip-baths in a decoction of linseed, fenugreek, hollyhock, mallow and artemisia, and injecting into the birth canal stale olive oil, wormwood with honey or opopanax, or Syrian oil'.[74] If none of those worked, 'one ought to use lupin flour mixed with a bull's bile and wormwood, as well as other, similar poultices'.[75]

Should a woman want to induce miscarriage, she should bathe often, eat little, apply suppositories which softened the genitals, and have her blood let.[76] In encouraging those, Soranus drew on Hippocrates:

> τὸ γὰρ ὑπὸ Ἱπποκράτους εἰρημένον ἐν τοῖς Ἀφορισμοῖς εἰ καὶ μὴ ἐπὶ στεγνοπαθούσης, ἀλλὰ [καὶ] ἐπὶ ὑγιαινούσης ἀληθές· 'γυνὴ ἐν γαστρὶ ἔχουσα φλεβοτομηθεῖσα ἐκτιτρώσκει.' ὡς γὰρ ἱδρὼς κινεῖται καὶ οὖρον ἢ σκύβαλον ὑπερχαλωμένων τῶν περιεχόντων τὴν οὐσίαν αὐτῶν, οὕτως καὶ τὸ συλληφθὲν ἐκπίπτει προδιισταμένης τῆς μήτρας. μετὰ δὲ τὴν φλεβοτομίαν καὶ ζευκτῷ

κατασειστέον (ἐνεργέστερος γὰρ νῦν ὁ βρασμὸς ἐπὶ προητονηκόσιν τοῖς τόποις) καὶ πεσσοῖς δὲ μαλακτικοῖς χρηστέον. εἰ δὲ πρὸς τὴν φλεβοτομίαν ἀλλοτρίως ἔχοι τις καὶ ἄτονος εἴη, προανιέναι μὲν τοὺς τόπους ἐγκαθίσμασι καὶ λουτροῖς καὶ πεσσοῖς μαλακτικοῖς καὶ ὑδροποσίᾳ καὶ ὀλιγοσιτίᾳ καὶ κοιλιολυσίᾳ καὶ κλύσμα τι προστίθεσθαι μαλακτικόν, μετὰ ταῦτα πεσσὸν φθόριον.

For a woman who intends to have an abortion, it is necessary for two or even three days beforehand to take protracted baths, little food and to use softening vaginal suppositories; also to abstain from wine; then to be bled and a relatively great quantity taken away. For the dictum of Hippocrates in the 'Aphorisms', even if not true in a case of constriction, is yet true of a healthy woman: 'A pregnant woman if bled, miscarries.' For just as sweat, urine or faeces are excreted if the parts containing these substances slacken very much, so the fetus falls out after the uterus dilates. Following the venesection one must shake her by means of draught animals (for now the shaking is more effective on the parts which previously have been relaxed) and one must use softening vaginal suppositories.[77]

If, however, a woman was too weak for bloodletting. the focus should be on the right diet, baths, enemas and softening suppositories. The latter must not be too strong, or they might cause fever or a major inflammation. Soranus lists myrtle oil, *matthiola* seed, and a mixture of rue, myrtle and laurel leaves with wine. He thinks it is safe for the woman to apply a water-based suppository made of *matthiola*, bittercress, sulphur, wormwood and myrtle.[78]

Of course, parallel to the recommendations of specialists there was a whole array of 'magical' and folk remedies believed to spend the foetus. For example, it was thought that 'if one were to swallow a part of [a dog's dried penis], that would be an abortifacient for a foetus three months into the pregnancy'.[79] Olympias of Thebes, quoted in Gargilius, believed 'mallows with goose fat placed next to the genitals cause miscarriage',[80] while 'the effect of the seeds [of garden cress] is so strong the foetus actually dies'.[81] Another abortifacient was supposedly 'a decoction of the prickly poppy',[82] while 'myrrh ... ground and placed inside the vagina, spends the foetus and induces menstruation'.[83]

Probably the largest arsenal of plant and mineral drugs which can, on their own or combined with others, cause the death of the foetus or induce miscarriage, known and used in antiquity, is presented in Dioscorides (see Table 1),[84] but the question remains of how effective those drugs were and if they worked as expected at all. J. Riddle argued Romans were actually able to limit the size of their families. Based on his findings, he believed many of the remedies recommended by authors such as Soranus, Pliny, or Dioscorides did have contraceptive or abortifacient properties. He stressed they cannot have been inefficient altogether, or else knowledge of them would presumably not have been so widespread or repeated so often in various sources.[85] Still, if plant-based drugs, pessaries, tinctures, hip-baths and even bloodletting failed, there were still mechanical methods. Soranus notes one should avoid not merely strong abortifacients, but also 'spending the foetus with sharp instruments; then there is the danger of injuring the adjacent parts'.[86] Surgical termination of pregnancy must have been a last resort, because the risk was well known; the same Soranus explains abortion is more dangerous to the woman's health than an ordinary miscarriage.[87] Ovid recounts an abortion carried out by his mistress Corinna, who put her own health at risk and was in danger of dying from it. Moreover, she did it without him knowing, which angered him.[88] In one of his satires, Juvenal mentions the many induced miscarriages of the foetuses Julia conceived with the emperor Domitian,[89] whereas Suetonius' account indicates it was an abortion that caused her death:

> mox patre ac uiro orbatam ardentissime palamque dilexit, ut etiam causa mortis extiterit coactae conceptum a se abigere;

> became the cause of her death by compelling her to get rid of a child of his by abortion[90]

Similar testimony of that event can be found in a letter by Pliny the Younger:

> Nec minore scelere quam quod ulcisci videbatur, absentem inauditamque damnavit incesti, cum ipse fratris filiam incesto non polluisset solum verum etiam occidisset; nam vidua abortu periit.

> He had violated his own niece³ in an incestuous relationship and ended by causing her death, for she died as the result of an abortion during her widowhood.[91]

Tacitus, meanwhile, mentions how the emperor Nero, meaning to get rid of Octavia, who was his legitimate wife, accused her of an abortion (among other things), even though he had himself previously accused her of infertility.[92]

K. Kapparis thinks abortion was too perilous to have been widely practised as a family planning method, being however the main option open to prostitutes, slaves and other women who wanted to terminate an illegal pregnancy, if not to monogamous wives.[93] Contraception and abortion were most likely used in the context of extramarital fertility. However, S. Dixon notes that it is on the whole the modern interest in ancient reproduction that drives present-day scholarship on contraception and abortion, obscuring the efforts to ensure fertility, much stronger back then. To Roman families, Dixon argues, having too few children was much more of a problem than having too many unwanted pregnancies.[94]

Table 1. Plants and compounds used, according to Dioscorides, to prepare drugs (oils, ointments, incense powder, etc.) with abortifacient applications[95]

	Greek term	Latin term	English equivalent	Reference
1	ἶρις	*Iris pallida*	sweet iris	I, 1, 3
2	καρδάμωμον	*Elettaria cardamomum* (L.)	true cardamom	I, 6
3	κινάμωμον (κιννάμωμον)	*Cinnamomum cassia* (L.)	Chinese cinnamon	I, 14, 4
4	βάλσαμον	*Commiphora gileadensis* (L.)	Arabian balsam tree	I, 19, 4
5	ἀσπάλαθος	*Alhagi maurorum* (Medik.)	camelthorn bush	I, 20
6	ἰρίνου στῦψις	*Iris florentina* extract		I, 56, 3
7	σμύρνα	*Commiphora myrrha* (Ness.) Engl.	Myrrh	I, 64, 3
8	λίβανος	*Boswellia carterii* Birdw.	Frankincense	I, 68, 2
9	πίτυς	*Pinus pinea* (L.)	stone pine	I, 69, 1
10	βράθυ	*Juniperus sabina* (L.)	savin juniper	I, 76
11	κέδρος	*Juniperus oxycedrus* (L.)	prickly juniper	I, 77, 3
12	ὀξυάκανθα	*Cotoneaster pyracantha* (L.) Spach.	scarlet firethorn	I, 93
13	ὄρχις κάστορος	*Castor fiber*	Eurasian beaver (its testicle)	II, 24, 1
14	οἴσυπος	Oesypum	oesypum (refuse from wool)	II, 74, 4
15	ἐρέβινθος	*Cicer arietinum* (L.)	Chickpea	II, 104
16	θέρμος	*Lupinus albus* (L.)	white lupin	II, 109, 1
17	σίον	*Sium angustifolium* L.)	lesser water-parsnip	II, 127
18	κάρδαμον	*Lepidium sativum* (L.)	garden cress	II, 155, 1

19	θλάσπι	Capsella bursa-pastoris (L.) Medicus	shepherd's purse	II, 156, 2
20	στρούθιον	Saponaria officinalis (L.)	common soapwort	II, 163
21	δρακοντία μεγάλη	Dracunculus vulgaris (Schott)	dragon arum	II, 166, 2–3
22	κισσός	Hedera helix (L.)	common ivy	II, 179, 3
23	γεντιάνη	Gentiana purpurea (L.)	purple gentian	III, 3, 2
24	ἀριστολόχεια θήλεια	Aristolochia (L.)	Birthwort	III, 4, 4
25	κενταύριον (κενταύρειον) μέγα	Centaurea centaurium (L.)	Centaury	III, 6, 3
26	κενταύριον (κενταύρειον) μικρόν	Centaurium erythraea (Rafn.)	common centaury	III, 7, 2
27	γλήχων	Mentha pulegium (L.)	European pennyroyal	III, 31, 1
28	δίκταμον	Origanum dictamnus (L.)	dittany of Crete (hop marjoram)	III, 32, 2
29	καλαμίνθη	Calamintha officinalis Moench	lesser calamint	III, 35, 3
30	θύμος	Thymus capitatus (L.)	conehead thyme	III, 36, 2
31	βάκχαρις	Helichrysum sanguineum (Boiss.)	red cudweed	III, 44, 2
32	πάναξ	Opopanax hispidus (Friv.)	opopanax (all-heal)	III, 48, 4–5
33	σταφυλῖνος ἄγριος	Daucus carota (L.)	wild carrot (bird's nest)	III, 52, 2
34	σέσελι Μασσαλιωτικόν	Seseli tortuosum (L.)	seseli (moon carrot)	III, 53, 1
35	δαῦκος	Athamanta cretensis L.	Athamanta	III, 72, 2
36	σαγάπηνον	Ferula persica (Willd.)	fennel or giant fennel	III, 81, 2
37	χαλβάνη	Ferula galbaniflua (Mill.)	Galbanum	III, 83, 1–2

	Greek term	Latin term	English equivalent	Reference
38	Ἀμμωνιακή	Ferula marmarica (Asch. & Taub.)	–	III, 84, 2
39	κλινοπόδιον	Calamintha clinopodium (Spenner)	Clinopodium	III, 95
40	χαμαίδρυς	Teucrium chamaedrys (L.)	wall germander	III, 98, 2
41	βήχιον	Tussilago farfara (L.)	Coltsfoot	III, 112, 2
42	ἀρτεμισία πολύκλωνος	Artemisia campestris (L.)	field wormwood	III, 113, 2
43	κόνυζα μικρά	Inula graveolens (L.)	stinking fleabane	III, 121, 2
44	ὄνοσμα	Onosma echioides (L.)	Onosma	III, 131
45	ἀνθεμίς	Matricaria chamomilla (L.)	Chamomile	III, 137, 2
46	ἐρυθρόδανον	Rubia tinctorum (L.)	common madder	III, 143, 2
47	ἀνάγυρος	Anagyris foetida (L.)	Oro de Risco	III, 150, 2
48	ἄγχουσα	Alkanna tinctoria (L.)	dyers' bugloss	IV, 23, 2
49	μανδραγόρας	Mandragora sp.	Mandrake	IV, 75, 4
50	ἐλλέβορος λευκός	Veratrum album (L.)	European white hellebore	IV, 148, 2
51	ἐλατήριον	Ecballium elaterium (L.) A. Richard	squirting cucumber	IV, 150, 7
52	ἐλλέβορος μέλας	Helleborus niger L.	black hellebore	IV, 162, 3
53	σκαμμωνία	Convolvulus scammonia (L.)	Scammony	IV, 170, 4
54	θυμελαία	Daphne gnidium (L.)	flax-leaved daphne	IV, 172, 3
55	κολοκυνθίς	Citrullus colocynthis (L.) Schrader	Colocynth	IV, 176, 2
56	ἄμπελος λευκή	Bryonia cretica subsp. dioica (Jacq.) Tutin	white bryony	IV, 182, 3

57	ἄμπελος μέλαινα	*Tamus communis* (L.)	black bryony	IV, 183, 2
58	θηλυπτερίς	*Pteridium aquilinum* (L.) Kuhn	common bracken	IV, 185
59	φθόριος ἐμβρύων οἶνος	–	'abortifacient wine'	V, 67
60	ἐλλεβορίτης [οἶνος]	–	hellebore wine	V, 72, 3
61	στυπτηρία	–	astringents (alum)	V, 106, 6
62	θεῖον	–	Sulphur	V, 107, 2

2

Women Preparing to Be Mothers

'Now ripe for a husband, now of full age to be a bride'[1]

As mentioned in the previous chapter, marriage – a socially and legally sanctioned union aimed at reproduction – was a universal experience of Roman women.[2] Traditionally, we only see the process occur from men's points of view, which means we have no way of learning a young girl's feelings or her thoughts on marriage and becoming an adult. What information we have has been put together from the perspective of a grown man and how he saw his daughter, sister, mother, or wife.[3]

The transition from childhood, the state of full dependence on one's parents, to the adult life that came with marriage meant a change in identity. The girl became a wife, which involved moving house, possibly even to another town, entering a new network of social relationships, taking up new activities and assuming new social duties, not to mention embarking on her sexual life with its consequences. Most of all, however, marriage meant she was no longer a child. A *puella* (girl) quickly, unnoticeably, changed into a *virgo* (maiden) and then an *uxor* (wife).[4] Cicero's friend Atticus was already looking for an appropriate husband for his only daughter Attica when she was six.[5] Throughout her childhood, Attica knew her future would be that of a wife;[6] she was being prepared for the transformation from very early on. Pliny, in turn, describes a maiden of thirteen years as having an old woman's sense and a matron's seriousness, but accompanied by a girl's amiability and a virgin's modesty. In thus depicting Minicia, he also illustrates the meaning of the transformation a girl underwent into a Roman matron.[7]

According to M. Harlow, this suggests that socialization of girls and readying them for marriage sometimes started at a very young age.[8] Through marriages, the Roman elite made social and political ties. Finding a husband for a girl was legally speaking her father's duty, but the process of looking and choosing involved the whole family and their friends. Good family background and wealth were the most important criteria for creating marriage ties between socially similar families. In addition, the groom was expected to be of good moral character, looks and health, attributes 'exchanged' for the bride's virginity, modesty and diligence.[9] These were two of the reasons, Harlow thinks, that families wanted to marry their daughters off early: the fear of running out of suitable potential marital candidates and the fear their daughters might lose their virginity before they marry.[10]

Juridical texts define the minimum age of marriage as twelve years for girls and fourteen for boys, but they are normative and need not reflect everyday realities;[11] in general, Roman society preferred brides to be in their late teens or early twenties.[12] In girls from the elite, puberty often coincided with getting married.[13] Considering that natural birth control and effective contraception were either unavailable or unknown to many people, while awareness of expectations to provide the child so desired by the family was high, young women were likely to become pregnant quite quickly, which was particularly risky for teenagers. Many brides were not yet ready for marriage, pregnancy and childbirth, but since the main purpose of a Roman marriage was to produce legitimate children, Plutarch's final remark that the Greek way of marrying has more to do with the likelihood of siring children can be read as criticism of the Roman custom, which allowed for girls marrying at such a young age.[14]

Other authors wrote in a similar vein. In the context of Augustus' legislation of 17 BCE which forbade engagement longer than two years, Cassius Dio repeats that girls are considered of marriageable age when they are twelve,[15] while Tacitus notes Germans did not force their girls to marry quickly the way Romans did.[16] For the Roman *nobilitas*, the merits of an early marriage often outweighed the potential reproductive pitfalls, especially if the marriage was to be part of a contract or alliance between two great houses. In this case its theoretical objective of producing legitimate children came into conflict with another purpose: strengthening alliances between families of the elite. Early marriage and legitimate children followed from expectations that were not purely demographic in nature. As mentioned above, advantages such as fertility, chastity, modesty and the dowry to be brought in played an important part in arranging marriages.

Epigraphic documents confirm the young age of girls at the time of marriage, although the information is rarely listed directly; usually inscriptions note how old she was when she died and how many years she had been married.[17]

One intriguing example of an early betrothal is the case of the girl Insteia Polla, who was only seven when she was brought to C. Utianus Rufus' house. It is possible the inscription, which informs that the seven-year old girl was brought into the house of her would-be husband, merely referred to something along the lines of betrothal or promise, which did not equal an actual marriage or sexual initiation.[18] Perhaps Insteia lived and was educated there for some years before the marriage was properly finalized or consummated. Either way, the marriage resulting from the very early engagement proved excellent (*cum summo honore*) and, as the funder of the inscription claims, lasted fifty-five years.[19] Another epitaph from the same town attests to a marriage between a Figelius Atimetus and a Cisatia Polla, who was only ten. When she died at twenty-eight, she was commemorated by her husband and daughter.[20] Then there is the inscription from Ricini reporting the death, at only eighteen, of a Herennia Cervilla, but she had had three children already.[21]

As mentioned above, juridical texts set the lowest possible age of marriage at twelve for girls and fourteen for boys, but it would be an overgeneralization to claim it was widespread for very young girls to marry. The data supplied by inscriptions is often somewhat distorted by the so-called epigraphic habits: age at death and length of marriage were more likely to get mentioned if the person died particularly young or the marriage lasted unusually long – in other words, the information was listed because it was an exception rather than the rule.

Menstruation

'Woman is, however, the only animal that has monthly periods'[22]

τὸν μὲν ἄλλον χρόνον εἴθισται καὶ μεμελέτηκεν ἐμμήνοις ἡμερῶν περιόδοις ὀχετοὺς καὶ πόρους αὐτῷ τῆς φύσεως ἀναστομούσης ἀποχεόμενον τὸ μὲν ἄλλο σῶμα κουφίζειν καὶ καθαίρειν, τὴν δ'ὑστέραν οἷον ἀρότῳ καὶ σπόρῳ γῆν ἐν φυτοῖς ὀργῶσαν ἐν καιρῷ παρέχειν.

at other times it is Nature's custom and care to discharge the blood at monthly periods by opening canals and channels for it, to lighten and cleanse the rest of the body and in season to render the womb fertile ground for ploughing, as it were, and sowing.

These are Plutarch's words on menstruation.[23] Still, the monthly bleeding – on the one hand, believed to have 'life-giving powers' and on the other hand, considered a mystery[24] – was not a popular topic among Roman authors. Information on menstruation can mostly be found in medical texts and those which discuss the superstitions of 'folk medicine'.

Menstruation and its impact on women's health

'Menstruation, in most cases, first appears around the fourteenth year ... and so it finally comes to an end, usually not earlier than forty, nor later than fifty years.'[25] Naturally there is no menstruation during pregnancy; that would be in conflict with the belief that it was blood that the foetus fed on.[26] But if the woman is not pregnant, her period will return the next month (*mensis*), although occasionally it will be early or late. It was believed the onset could be predicted, as a few days in advance there would be a feeling of heaviness when moving around, heaviness in the hips, tiredness, yawning and flushed skin. There are also women for whom their period is preceded by lack of appetite and nausea.

Based on observation, it was known menstruation could stop or disappear because of illness or prolonged exertion, or it could be very copious. Ways were sought, some of them controversial, of 'treating' unusual periods. Gargilius believes:

> mirum est quod Xenocrates tradit, si unum seminis granum femina biberit, uno die ei menstrua contineri, biduo si duo, et totidem iam diebus quot grana sumpserit.

> Xenocrates recounts a remarkable thing: that if a woman swallows one grain, her menstruation is reduced to one day, two days if it is two grains, and as many days as the grains she eats.[27]

He also repeats a piece of advice attributed to Hippocrates, that women eat amaranth to stop excessive monthly bleeding,[28] while Pliny thought that *elaterium* (squirting cucumber) should be eaten if periods stop.[29]

There is nothing in the ancient sources to even hint that a menstruating woman was considered excluded from social life in Rome; on the contrary, Soranus writes that women who feel well during their menstruation and experience no anomalies should act as usual, merely slowing down a little, although they are advised against bathing during the first two days.[30] He is of the opinion that a normal menstruation is one during which the woman feels strong, breathes easily, keeps calm and retains her strength; if those criteria are not met, the menstruation is anomalous.[31] Even so, a menstruating woman can often be made to feel unwell by various seemingly trivial external factors. She might, for example, weaken from the smell of a beaver's hide:

> castoreoque gravi mulier sopita recumbit, et manibus nitidum teneris opus effluit ei, tempore eo si odoratast quo menstrua solvit.

The heavy scent of castor, makes a woman fall back asleep, dropping the dainty work from her tender hands, if she has smelt it at the time of her monthly courses.[32]

However, menstruation itself was regarded as harmful and likely to strongly impact one's general well-being, plaguing in particular women who were delicate and vulnerable to disease and sparing the strong and hardened ones. Soranus observed that among the women who did not menstruate (young girls, infertile women and elderly ones), there were many strong, healthy ones. In his own words:

πρὸς μόνον δὲ τὸ παιδοποιεῖν χωρὶς γὰρ τῆς καθάρσεως σύλληψις οὐ γίνεται;

virgins not yet menstruating would necessarily be less healthy; if, on the other hand, they enjoy perfect health, menstruation, consequently, does not contribute to their health, but is useful for childbearing only; for conception does not take place without menstruation.[33]

Thus he thinks menstruation has one purpose only: without it, there is no conception.

In his opinion, physicians exist who claim that absent or difficult periods contribute to diseases and excess weight, with sexual intercourse being the largest factr responsible for healthy periods,[34] as illustrated by cases of widows whose periods are scant and painful, but only until they remarry and resume a regular sex life. Even so, people recognized that menstruation was a very individual thing, its course and the woman's wellness dependent on many factors. For instance, the length of the bleeding and the volume of blood lost depended on the woman's age and figure; doctors of the time believed fat people bled less than slim ones. Lifestyle was another factor which could influence the menses: women who lived lazy, sedentary lives had a heavier flow than those who kept moving.[35] During the period, which lasts between one and seven days (Soranus thinks the average is three to four days), the woman loses around two *cotylae* (so, almost a pint, perhaps) of blood.

Unfortunately, no information survives in ancient authors on any objects or solutions employed by women during their periods to catch the flow. That is not surprising; if the subject of menstruation comes up at all, the author is a man, more likely to be interested in the medical or magical aspects of the phenomenon than the technicalities and actual measures women used. In the descriptions of gynaecological afflictions, one encounters mentions of various tampons soaked in medication; perhaps such woollen tampons were also used to stop menstrual bleeding, although pads cannot be ruled out either. In his *Life of Isidore*, Damascius recounts a story about Hypatia and a student who fell deeply in love with her. To discourage the obnoxious admirer, she reputedly resorted to the unusual act of showing him the cloth soaked in her menstrual blood (τῶν γυναικείων ῥακῶν, *women's rags*) and saying, 'indeed, this seems to be what you love, young man, not beauty!'[36] Perhaps the words were meant to express that the essence of womanhood includes all of the physicality of a woman's body, not necessarily attractive during menstruation, rather than simply her moral character and looks, but regardless of Hypatia's motives, it may well be the only mention in literature of a woman using anything like a pad.

Menstruation and magic

Even though it may seem menstruating women were not particularly stigmatized in Rome or excluded from daily life, menstrual blood must have caused some unease in the general population, as its properties were believed to be quite magical. The works of Pliny and of Solinus, who drew on him, are a treasure trove of knowledge about the superstitions surrounding menstruation.

Beneficial properties of menstrual blood

Menstrual blood could be used to treat gout, goitre, tumours near the ears, erysipelas, inflamed sores, and 'such a woman is to alleviate flow from the eyes by touching'. Pliny quotes the opinions of the midwives Lais and Salpe, who claimed that 'the bite of a mad dog, tertians and quartans were cured by the flux on wool from a black ram enclosed in a silver bracelet'.[37] In the opinion of Diotimus the Theban, wool from a black ram was not necessary, and any scrap of bloodstained cloth or even thread worn with the bracelet would do.[38] According to another midwife, Sotira, treating the same fevers required one to anoint the patient's feet with menstrual blood, and the results were best if the woman menstruating did it herself.[39] Then, if Pliny is to be believed, 'Icatidas the physician assures us that quartans are ended by sexual intercourse, provided that the woman is beginning to menstruate'.[40] Menstrual blood was also supposed to cure 'the fear of water and beverages from a dog's bite'.[41]

Apparently menstruation not only helped against some afflictions, but also had its uses in farming. Pliny writes it was believed that a menstruating woman walking naked in the fields helped purge the crop of any parasites: 'But at any other time of menstruation, if women go round the cornfield naked, caterpillars, worms, beetles and other vermin fall to the ground.'[42]

Harmful properties of menstrual blood

More often, however, it was ill influence that was attributed to menstrual blood. Solinus writes:

> mulier solum animal menstruale est, cuius profluuia non paruis spectata documentis inter monstrifica merito numerantur. Contactae his fruges non germinabunt, acescent musta, morientur herbae, amittent arbores fetus, ferrum robigo corripiet, nigrescent aera, si quid canes inde ederint in rabiem efferabuntur, nocituri morsibus quibus, lymphaticos faciunt. Bitumen in Iudaea quod Asphaltites gignit lacus adeo lentum mollitie glutinosa, ut a se nequeat separari, enimuero si abrumpere partem uelis, uniuersitas sequetur scindique non potest, quoniam in quantum ducatur extenditur. Sed ubi admota fuerint cruore illo polluta fila, sponte dispergitur, et adplicita tabe diducitur paulo ante corpus unum, fitque de tenacitate conexa contagione partitio repentina.

> Woman is the only 'monthly' animal. The monthly courses of women, as is observed by many, are justly to be accounted among the marvellous. The fruit of the earth, stained by menstrual blood, will not sprout; the new wine becomes sour, the turf dies, the trees lose their produce. Iron is attacked by rust, copper becomes black. If any dogs taste it, they become enraged into a frenzy; anyone injured by their bites becomes mad. But these are small things. Bitumen from Judaea, which is produced at Lake Asphaltites, is very sticky, and has a gluey pliability; it cannot be dissipated. It is impossible to divide it – if you wish to break it into parts, the whole will certainly stay together, as it extends as far as it is stretched out. But when the threads are brought near to the polluted blood, they are easily separated. When the noxious fluid is placed near any material, it is dissipated. The sudden division comes about through the tenacity being joined to the contagion.[43]

The list of disasters and crop failures attributed to menstruating women and their blood is expanded in Pliny,[44] who considers periods 'monstrous', because they 'portend things ugly and shameful'. He stresses that in order to write about them, he has to 'set his shame aside', and notes that because of them (sc. women on their menstrual periods)

> sementim enim arescere, item novella tactu in perpetuum laedi, rutam et hederam res medicatissimas ilico mori. multa diximus de hac violentia, sed praeter illa certum est apes tactis alvariis fugere, lina, cum coquantur, nigrescere, aciem in cultris tonsorum hebetari, aes contactu grave virus odoris accipere et aeruginem, magis si descrescente luna id accidat, equas, si sint gravidae, tactas abortum pati, quin et aspectu omnino, quamvis procul visas.

so that women walk, he says, through the middle of the fields with their clothes pulled up above the buttocks. In other places the custom is kept up for them to walk barefoot, with hair dishevelled and with girdle loose. Care must he taken that they do not do so at sunrise, for the crop dries up, they say, the young vines are irremediably harmed by the touch, and rue and ivy, plants of the highest medicinal power, die at once. I have said much about this virulent discharge, but besides it is certain that when their hives are touched by women in this state bees fly away, at their touch linen they are boiling turns black, the edge of razors is blunted, brass contracts copper rust and a foul smell, especially if the moon is waning at the time.[45]

Even worse, any woman dirtied with the menstrual blood of another must miscarry, claims Pliny, although it is enough for a pregnant woman to step over a bloodstain and that, too, will make her lose her pregnancy.[46] Abortifacient properties of menstrual blood were also mentioned by the midwives Lais and Elephantis, who thought 'the burning root of cabbage, myrtle, or tamarisk extinguished by the menstrual blood causes miscarriage',[47] while 'asses will not conceive for as many years as they have eaten grains of barley contaminated with it, or in their other portentous or contradictory pronouncements, one saying that fertility, the other that barrenness is caused by the same measures'. Pliny notes in such cases it is better to believe neither.[48]

Also mentioned in Pliny, Bithus of Dyrrachium says:

hebetata aspectu specula recipere nitorem [tradit] isdem aversa rursus contuentibus, omnemque vim talem resolvi, si mullum piscem secum habeant.

that a mirror which has been tarnished by the glance of a menstruous woman recovers its brightness if it is turned round for her to look at the back, and that all this sinister power is counteracted if she carries on her person the fish called red mullet.[49]

The effects of menstruation are most violent if the blood is from someone whose hymen has disappeared of itself or due to ageing.[50]

Pliny seems embarrassed, even in a sense disgusted when he discusses the properties of menstrual blood, since he concludes with these words:

Haec sunt quae retulisse fas sit, ac pleraque ex iis non nisi honore dicto, reliqua intestabilia, infanda, ut festinet oratio ab homine fugere.

This is all the information it would be right for me to repeat, most of which also needs an apology from me. As the rest of it is detestable and unspeakable, let me hasten to leave the subject of remedies from man.[51]

Ancient medicine attributed two distinctive features to women: the uterus and menstruation. The uterus is the most female of organs, and blood (menstrual blood) means women's nature. The two features converge in the process of reproduction, which was the basis of a woman's social standing in Rome, as clearly seen in the life stages of women put forward by S. Moraw: girl – woman – aged woman, where the researcher's primary criterion was reproductive ability. That in turn means the division should be read as follows: woman who cannot have children yet – woman who can have children – woman who cannot have children any more.[52] What does it mean, however: 'woman who can have children'? Is this moment biological (menarche), or is it more like a sort of rite of passage which ushers in and confirms maturity socially and culturally? Biologically speaking, the moments of transition in that model were menarche and the menopause, determining as they did the beginning and end of reproductive ability. Moraw emphasizes that in most patriarchal societies, the first rite of passage was marriage, a prerequisite for the main task of bearing legitimate children for one's husband and his family, but in the ancient world, that moment of social and cultural transformation coincided with the first period.[53] The same convergence is expressed by Soranus, who believes it is menstruation that guarantees fertility, and a woman who does not menstruate cannot get pregnant either.[54] He thought menstruation first appeared in girls around the age of fourteen and was related to other physical changes occurring at the time, such as breasts becoming larger, but also pain in the pubic symphysis and heaviness in the abdomen.[55] He confirms that moment is when one can consider a girl ready for marriage. That is why in his opinion it is so important for menarche to spontaneously appear before marriage.[56] Thus in order to advance the first period, he advocated that

> διὸ πρᾷος μὲν ὁ περίπατος ἔστω καὶ ὁμαλός, ἐπιμήκης δὲ ἡ αἰώρα καὶ ἀνειμένα τὰ γυμνάσια καὶ μετὰ πολλοῦ λίπους ἀναβεβλημένη ἡ τρίψις καὶ καθ' ἡμέραν τὸ λουτρὸν καὶ πᾶσα ψυχῆς διάχυσις.
>
> her walk should be easy and deliberate, passive exercise prolonged, gymnastics not forced, much fat applied in the massage, a bath taken daily and the mind diverted in every possible way.[57]

However, menarche and marriage did not mean the girl was ready to become a mother. It was believed such a young age was not suitable for bearing the first child, as the sex organs might not be ready yet for the girl to carry to term and give birth safely.[58]

Physicians did not advocate marrying early for biological reasons, particularly because the wife might not be ready to become pregnant.[59] For that reason Soranus believed girls ought to keep their virginity until they menstruated regularly,[60] which in his opinion demonstrated the uterus was ready to accept an embryo and keep the pregnancy. In other words, only after the cycle became fairly regular was the moment ripe for marriage. The physician is further of the opinion that in younger girls the uterus is not yet mature enough and should she conceive, she may have difficulties keeping the pregnancy or there may be complications during the pregnancy (such as deformation of the foetus) or during labour.[61] He also gives the same reasons for high mortality among younger mothers. Meanwhile, Pliny the Younger mentions two very young sisters of Helvidius dying in labour,[62] although we do not know the exact causes of their deaths. We may suspect perinatal complications, possibly due to their young age. Therefore Soranus advises women to marry at the age when 'space has already been formed for pregnancy' and they have some knowledge of their own bodies.[63]

Roman girls' sex education

In a letter to a grandfather of his very young wife, Pliny recounts the tragedy that miscarriage was to her:[64] 'In her naivety, she did not know she was pregnant.' What did that mean? Do we know who talked to adolescent girls, when and how about changes occurring in their appearance, menstruation, becoming sexually active, pregnancy and childbirth? We do not, and due to the lack of sources we cannot know if a teenage girl had any sexual experience whatsoever before marriage. She was most likely expected to have none. The sudden confrontation with sexuality on their wedding night probably constituted a drastic change in the lives of girls, who had only just commemorated their childhood the day before.[65] Still, could they have been prepared by conversations with their mothers, nurses, midwives, or other women who practised medicine?[66] Again, we have no sources that could answer the question directly. We keep searching for the answer: how was information passed on, how were girls taught about the changes going on in their bodies and their future life role?[67] Some researchers think girls may have been helped by dolls similar to that found in Creperia Tryphanea's tomb. In L. Caldwell's opinion, such dolls played a significant part in the socialization and sex education of young girls, allowing them to get used to the idea of taking on the role of a wife and mother.[68] They are interpreted today as a potential element in those girls' upbringing; through their lens, the girls learned about womanhood which was to inspire them or teach them by example. The dolls could also have been educational toys for acting out those future roles.[69] In a short mention in Persius, there is a reference to a *virgo*, an unmarried girl, who dedicated a doll to Venus before her marriage:

> at vos / dicite, pontifices, in sancto quid facit aurum?
> nempe hoc quod Veneri donatae a virgine pupae.
>
> But tell me, you priests, what good is gold in a sacred place?
> Exactly as much as the doll given to Venus by a little girl.[70]

Maybe the point of the doll was to serve as a sign of readiness for adult life.

Those who died young: 'wed to death'

Offspring born in a marriage were meant to guarantee the continuity of the family and *gens*; no wonder then that, as M. Kuryłowicz wrote, it was the duty of each *pater familias* to see to it that the family had an heir to take over the legacy and wealth accumulated by past generations.[71] Moreover, children were seen as carriers after a manner of memory; they could be brought up in the hope that they would venerate their great forefathers and would themselves grow up to be an example to future generations.[72] From a much more practical point of view, children, through their arranged marriages, gave the family the opportunity to ally itself to other aristocratic families. It is with that perspective in mind that one should see Pliny the Younger, who, in his many letters, paints himself as a matchmaker for his friends' children, regularly discussing the attributes of the relatives of both the fathers and mothers of potential candidates.[73]

Finally, it cannot be ruled out or dismissed that the Romans simply had parental instincts and loved their children, cherishing them for their own sake. Statius considers the birth of a son the greater for a father's glory, but thinks having a daughter is also a source of joy, because thanks to his daughter, who will marry younger than the sons, he will be a grandfather sooner:[74]

> macte, quod et proles tibi saepius aucta virili / robore! sed iuveni laetanda et virgo parenti / (aptior his virtus, citius dabit illa nepotes)
>
> Bravo too in that your stock has more often had increase in manly strength! But a maiden too brings happiness to a young parent (achievement belongs rather to them, but she will sooner give grandsons).[75]

Even so, some of the families preparing to marry their daughter off, and perhaps looking forward to the birth of the long-awaited grandchildren, would be disappointed. Examples are known for such plans being ruined by the would-be bride's sudden death. With her, the hope for grandchildren died as well.[76]

A friend of Pliny's, Fundanus, went from preparing a marriage ceremony to the unavoidable decision to hold the funeral of his daughter, Minicia Marcella, and in a letter to an acquaintance, Pliny wrote of the circumstances of her sudden death:[77]

> Fundani nostri filia minore defuncta. Qua puella nihil umquam festivius amabilius, nec modo longiore vita sed prope immortalitate dignius vidi. Nondum annos xiiii impleverat, et iam illi anilis prudentia, matronalis gravitas erat et tamen suavitas puellaris cum virginali verecundia ... Duravit hic illi usque ad extremum, nec aut spatio valetudinis aut metu mortis infractus est, quo plures gravioresque nobis causas relinqueret et desiderii et doloris. O triste plane acerbumque funus! o morte ipsa mortis tempus indignius! iam testinata erat egregio iuveni, iam electus nuptiarum dies, iam nos vocati. Quod gaudium quo maerore mutatum est! Non possum exprimere verbis quantum animo vulnus acceperim, cum audivi Fundanum ipsum, ut multa luctuosa dolor invenit, praecipientem, quod in vestes margarita gemmas fuerat erogaturus, hoc in tus et unguenta et odores impenderetur.

> The younger daughter of your friend Fundanus is dead ... She had hardly completed her fourteenth year, yet she possessed the prudence of old age and the sedateness of a matron, with the sweetness of a child and the modesty of a maiden ... What a sad, heart-rending funeral it was! The moment of her death seemed even more cruel than death itself, for she had just been betrothed to a youth of splendid character; the day of the wedding had been decided upon, and we had already been summoned to attend it. Think into what terrible grief our joy was changed! I really cannot tell you in words how acutely I felt it when I heard Fundanus himself, for one sorrow always leads on to other bitter sorrows - giving the order that the money he had intended to lay out upon wedding raiment, pearls and gems, should be spent upon incense, unguents and scents.[78]

A certain Trebia, daughter of Gaius, lived thirteen years. She was of marriageable age and ready for her wedding. When she died, she left behind her fiancé and would-be in-laws.[79] It was very painful for the family to lose their daughter before she had entered the next stage of her life. As in the case of Fundanus' daughter Minicia, joyous preparations and nuptial enthusiasm was replaced by grief over the death of a daughter and fiancée.[80] This is stressed by her epitaph, which mentions a wedding torch (a symbol of a girl's life changing) that was ultimately used as a funeral torch.[81]

A similar tragedy struck the family of a girl from Numidia, whose life-thread was cut short by the Fates. Julia Sidonia, a young priestess of Isis, died before she saw her wedding torches lit. A poetic sepulchral inscription commemorated her:

> Iulia Sidonia Felix, happy (*felix*) only in name. Alas, the Fates (Parcae) cut the thread of her life – oh, dreadful deed! – before the day her bridegroom touched the torches of Hymenaeus at the wedding. All lamented, the wood-nymphs mourned and Lucina wept the light of her torch tourned downwards, since the virgin was the only child of her parents. She has been a priestess of the goddess of Memphis with her rattle. Buried here, she is silent in the eternal gift of sleep. She lived nineteen years, four months and fourteen days. She lies here.[82]

Another bereft father, Gaius Gavius Daphnus, had a monument erected for his daughter. The inscription indicates Gavia Quadratilla had lived seventeen and a half years, and had been engaged for twenty days.[83]

Losing a daughter who was already preparing to get married may have felt to her family as a loss even greater than that of a child dying at any other point, especially if it happened suddenly and with no warning, as in the case of Opinia Neptilla, a daughter of Marcus Opinius Rufus and Gelia Neptilla, who died at fourteen, having fallen mortally ill right before her wedding.[84] Another girl we know of, Calliste, lived sixteen years, three months and six and a half hours. She was to marry on 15 October, but unfortunately died four days before the date. Her mother Puais had an inscription put up in which she emphasized her daughter's planned marriage.[85]

The graves of young girls often contained objects connected to the transition, violently interrupted by death, from childhood to being a wife (and a mother). Chief among them are golden hair nets, rings, other jewellery, small mirrors and elements of clothing which could have formed part of a bride's attire,[86] but also, as mentioned above, dolls.[87] As M. Harlow points out, the wealth of feminine elements in such tombs was not just a form of compensation for a life unlived, but also had a vital psychological part to play when it came to the bereft family, allowing the mourners to see the young girl as she would have been at the moment they had all awaited.[88] The tomb was often meant to reflect both her childhood and the maturity she had not reached, so becoming an expression of,

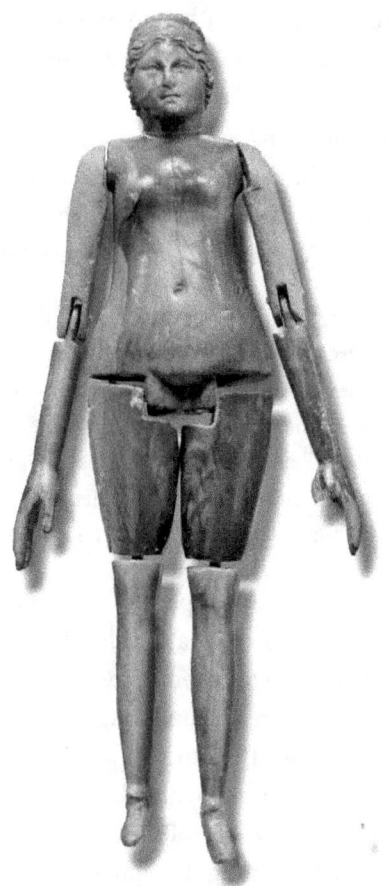

Figure 1 Roman doll © Public domain. From Wikimedia Commons, the free media repository.
Source: https://commons.wikimedia.org/wiki/File:Doll_Massimo_Inv168191_remade.jpg#filelinks

on the one hand, appreciation for what had been, and on the other, longing for what would never be. So prepared, the burial was in a sense intended as compensation.

According to Zahra Newby, dolls such as those mentioned above were to 'continue playing roles' after their owners' death as they had during their lives.[89] Being placed among the grave goods next to jewellery, cosmetics and other things used by grown women indicates, in Newby's opinion, that the dolls were not included in their capacity of favourite toys; rather, their presence was to do with the dead girls' status of eligible maidens. She does not think they were merely a symbol of virginity or a sign the dead girl had not lived long enough to offer the doll to the gods (as she would have when she married). Newby goes a step further in her interpretation, claiming the dolls were a kind of *alter ego* of their owners, or even the brides themselves in miniature. In her theory, she draws on the work of M. Bettini, who regards dolls as a peculiar type of items which can be dressed and moved, thus interacting with their owners in a special way.[90] He also highlights a play on words: in Latin, the word *pupa* means both *doll* and *girl*. Bettini believes for the future bride to offer her doll to the gods on the occasion of marriage also means to sacrifice to them the girl and the virginity she will then lose, since during her childhood the doll gave her a chance, and hope, to prepare for adulthood and married life. The doll represented its owner as she would be in the future: mature enough to marry, with an adult body ready to take on the tasks and duties of motherhood. By playing with dolls and animating them, girls gave them life; while they lived, the dolls were the girls in miniature, but more mature – their owners' projections of what they would one day become.

However, in Newby's opinion, that identification and relation changes. In life, the girl plays with a doll made of inanimate material (such as wood or ivory), but after the burial her body decays, while the material the doll is made of does not. Thus the doll does not represent the dead girl; instead, it stands for the girl as she was at the moment of death, the idea she then had of what she would look like in the future. That relationship offers hope that the girl will become the doll, taking on the role it stands for. In Newby's view, the doll and the girl swap places. After the child's death, the doll may have been something like a projection, an image of the life she and her family had aspired to.[91] The hopes for that future have been crushed by death, but the image suggests 'the bereft family hoped to see them'.[92]

A similar interpretation, which also refers to lost hopes, is put forward by M. Carroll,[93] who has analysed the images of women on sepulchral reliefs. Some of the women hold a newborn or older infant in their arms. Some inscriptions list the names of both the mother and the child, others only the woman's name. In Carroll's opinion, this may suggest the child died during birth or soon after, but before the *dies lustricus*, that is, before they were named. However, she also suggests another interpretation of the phenomenon: that the women holding a nameless child may never have given birth in the first place.[94] Rather, it was their own premature death which deprived those young women of their chance to have children, and their images as mothers are a symbolic fulfilment of the natural role expected of them in Roman society. In other words, just like the dolls placed in graves, the images of newborn babies could be symbolic compensation for goals not reached in life.

So go the theories. Only rarely is it possible to confront the tombstones discovered with the contents of the actual grave, but that is what happened in the case of the burial and monument of a woman called Bella, who died around 20 CE in Cologne.[95] On the slab of the gravestone, a young woman tightly hugs a child covered with its mother's cloak, as if for additional protection. The baby's name is not listed in the inscription,[96] which could indicate it died during the birth or right after, but before the naming. However, the excavations in the cemetery showed the grave held no remains of a child; there was only Bella's well-preserved skeleton. She was roughly twenty years old. Of course it cannot be ruled out that the image is one of a child born earlier, or that Bella did die in childbirth but the baby lived and the sepulchral image was only meant to commemorate the fact she had managed to become a mother. Carroll thinks in this case it may be guessed that although Bella is depicted as a mother, she never had a child, and the image of her holding one is only a compensation, a visual imagined by her family who paid for the stone of what their daughter's and wife's life would have looked like had she not died early.

Of course, theories are only that: theories. The extent to which we may go wrong in our search for an elaborate meaning of objects, gestures and events is illustrated by the story of a certain tomb and how it influenced interpretations which would then be current for a while. Towards the end of the 1920s, a doll was discovered by G. Mancini in an excavation in Tivoli of the tomb of the Vestal Virgin Cossina. For many years, the find had considerable impact on theories constructed to explain the dolls found among the grave goods in girls' graves. As the epitaph declares, Cossina was a Vestal for sixty-six years of her life. Girls were thought to offer dolls to the goddess before they married, so the doll in Cossina's grave was interpreted as indicative of her virginity.[97] It was only in 1983 that G. Bordenache Battaglia carried out another thorough analysis of the site and determined the doll was actually part of another, later burial, that of a young woman, near the spot Mancini had decided was part of Cossina's tomb.[98] In that way the discrepancy was also clarified between the Vestal's epitaph, dated to the first century CE, and the doll's hairstyle, which resembled that worn by Julia Domna in the second century CE. As Bordenache Battaglia sums up, Cossina was most likely cremated in the first century, whereas the doll found nearby came from a neighbouring grave, built one hundred years later.[99] A theory repeated for decades lay in ruins.

Fertility issues

'It is true that we did wish to have children, who had for a long time been denied to us by an envious fate'[100]

Fertility proven through the birth of a child determined and strengthened the marriage bond, granted satisfaction and respect, but also the tangible benefits offered to fertile spouses by the state. Meanwhile, when the married couple had no offspring, the political and legal difficulties could be bypassed, for example if the emperor himself granted them *ius trium liberorum*, although that was a privilege reserved for very few. Still, that imperial era grant only solved the legal issues, but could not meet the need for an heir or the emotional desire for having children.

In Rome, infertility was a gender-determined problem; blamed almost exclusively on women, it not so often applied to men – or at least not in the eyes of the public.[101] The belief was common, in fact, that should a man suspect his wife of infertility and be determined to sire children, he could divorce her, marry another, and try for children again with the new wife. The first wife had no such option, even if she suspected it was her husband's body, not hers, that was to blame for their childlessness. For a woman, especially a woman of the Roman elite, the label of infertility must have engendered feelings of failure, since marrying was practically her only job, and in that marriage she was supposed to conceive children regardless of whether or not she had the emotional need to do so. Seen from that angle, an infertile woman was simply socially useless.

According to the surviving accounts, divorce was defined unilaterally by one of Romulus' laws. Supposedly the king prohibited women from abandoning their husbands, but allowed men to send wives away if they committed adultery, had an abortion, or poisoned someone.[102] According to tradition, the first Roman man to send his wife off (that is, divorce her) was Spurius Carvilius Ruga,[103] who lived in the third century BCE, and it was because she was infertile:

> Spurius Carvilius, cui Ruga cognomentum fuit, vir nobilis, divortium cum uxore fecit, quia liberi ex ea corporis vitio non gignerentur, anno urbis conditae quingentesimo vicesimo tertio M. Atilio P. Valerio consulibus. Atque is Carvilius traditur uxorem, quam dimisit, egregie dilexisse carissimamque morum eius gratia habuisse, set iurisiurandi religionem animo atque amori praevertisse, quod iurare a censoribus coactus erat uxorem se liberum quaerundum gratia habiturum.

> Spurius Carvilius, who was surnamed Ruga, a man of rank, put away his wife because, owing to the some physical defect, no children were born from her; and that this happened in the five hundred and twenty-third year after the founding of the city, in the consulship of Marcus Atilius and Publius Valerius. And it is reported that this Carvilius dearly loved the wife whom he divorced, and held her in strong affection because of her character, but that above his devotion and his love he set his regard for the oath which the censors had compelled him to take, that he would marry a wife for the purpose of begetting children.[104]

Carvilius did all he could to avoid punishment, and while the reason he gave for sending his wife away was not listed in the king's law as 'just', it could not be questioned either, since it seemed in line with the best interest of the state as seen by the censors, which was focused on reproduction.[105] Carvilius explained he had sworn an oath to marry in order to make children, which was in fact part of the census declaration each citizen made when they were counted. As the officials in charge of morals, the censors also guarded the welfare and development of the state, that is, encouraging population growth by urging citizens to marry and have children. Carvilius made them face an exceedingly difficult choice, since they could either punish him as a divorcee, and so admit marriage need not serve reproduction at all, or allow the divorce, thus confirming that one might send one's wife away if she bore no offspring.

Infertility was also used by others as the excuse to divorce their wives: Dio recounts the divorce of emperor Caligula, who sent off Paulina. The pretext was that she was infertile; the real reason was that his mistress Milonia Caesonia had become pregnant and he wanted to formalize the union by marrying her.[106] In 62 CE, in turn, Nero desired to marry Poppaea Sabina, who had by then long kept him company at court as his mistress. The emperor's whim required a divorce again, this time from Octavia. Nero also gave infertility as the reason for the *repudium*; it was a tried and tested one (*exturbat Octaviam, sterilem dictitans*).[107] Under the principate, unilateral divorce was allowed, be it by the husband or the wife, and required no justification. If Nero did justify his decision, quoting infertility, it was probably because Octavia was extremely popular and divorcing her without giving any reason might have caused unrest.[108]

Still, Valerius Maximus' account indicates that earlier, in Carvilius' case, that kind of interpretation and decision regarding divorce met with public disapproval, as on the whole Romans believed a husband should not value his desire to have children over marital fidelity.[109] One such husband for whom it was more important to remain faithful was the funder of an inscription dedicated to his dead wife, known as the *Laudatio Turiae*. The married couple went together through a period of political storms, and Turia always stood by her husband's side, supporting him and even rescuing him from danger, but, as he mentions in the inscription:

> After peace was restored all over the earth and the republic was re-established, quiet and happy times came for us too. We did want children, but the envious fate had long denied us any. What would either of us have lacked for, had Fortune continued to favour us? But fate took a different course and put an end to our hopes.[110]

The man says that although his wife doubted her fertility and lamented his childlessness, she suggested they should get a divorce and he should entrust the household to another, fertile woman, lest staying in a childless marriage deprive him of the hope of children and so make him miserable. She also assured him she would consider his future offspring theirs and her own.[111] He repeatedly lists her virtues, underlining that she was devoted to him and wanted to be of use, and since she could not have children herself and 'felt bad with her infertility', she was going to give him children by divorcing him and choosing a new wife for him, a 'fertile woman':

> tibi vero quid memorabi[lius] quam inserviendo mihi c[onsilium cepisse] / ut quom ex te liberos ha[b]ere non possem per te tamen [haberem et diffi]/dentia partus tui alteriu[s c]oniugio parares fecunditat[em].

> But on your part, what could have been more worthy of commemoration and praise than your efforts in devotion to my interests : when I could not have children from yourself, you wanted me to have them through your good offices, and since you despaired of bearing children, to provide me with offspring by my marriage to another woman.[112]

How to choose a good wife – that is, a fertile wife

Soranus stresses that since most marriages are made for the sake of having children, less attention ought to be paid to the future wife's family background or wealth, and more to her build and age, which are the fundamental guarantees of fertility.[113] Following Diocles, he also observed those women found it easier to become pregnant whose

> loins and flanks are fleshy ... whereas those with contrary characteristics are sterile, namely: the undernourished, the thin or the very fat and those who are either too old or too young.[114]

Drawing on a metaphor, he emphasizes that

> καθάπερ ἐπὶ τῶν ἔξωθεν σπερμάτων οὐ πᾶς καιρὸς ἐπιτήδειος πρὸς τὸ κατὰ τῆς γῆς αὐτὰ βληθέντα καρποὺς ἐνεγκεῖν, οὕτως οὐδὲ ἐπὶ τῶν ἀνθρώπων [ὁ] πᾶς καιρὸς ἐπιτήδειος πρὸς σύλληψίν ἐστι τῶν ἐν ταῖς μίξεσιν μεθιεμένων σπερμάτων. ἵν' οὖν διὰ τῆς εὐκαιρίας τῆς χρήσεως τῶν ἀφροδισίων τὸ ζητούμενον ἔργον ἐπιτευχθῇ, χρήσιμον τὸν καιρὸν εἰπεῖν

> just as every season is not propitious for sowing extraneous seed upon the land for purpose of bringing forth fruit, so in humans too not every time is suitable for conception of the seed discharged during intercourse, it will be useful to state the proper time.[115]

It was believed the time right after menstruation was best for conception:

> κεκούφισται μὲν γὰρ ἡ μήτρα καὶ σύμμετρος παρέπεται θερμασία καὶ ὑγρασία. πάλιν γὰρ οὐκ ἐνδέχεται τὸ σπέρμα κολληθῆναι μὴ προτετραχυμμένης [καὶ οἷον] ἐξεσμένης κατὰ τὸν πυθμένα τῆς ὑστέρας.

> Uterus has been lightened and warmth and moisture are imparted in right measure. For again, it is not possible for the seed to adhere unless the uterus has first been roughened and 'scraped' as it were in its fundus.[116]

There should also be 'the urge and lust to couple'; Soranus believes that women cannot conceive without arousal, just as men cannot ejaculate without lust.[117] He also considers other factors important, such as comfort and a sense of well-being,[118] and finds appropriate the time of 'anointing the body which has consumed little food and is in the condition of full health'.[119] Women who want children should digest well and avoid diarrhoea, because in the physician's opinion, long-lasting indigestion hinders conception. It was, in fact, believed that trying for a child can be helped by changing the diet; people trying to make a baby ought to eat well, be healthy, and only drink alcohol in small quantities.[120]

Elsewhere, we read:

> ἔστω δὴ μήτε ἐνδεὲς τὸ σῶμα καὶ ἄτονον, τῷ γὰρ ὅλῳ καὶ τὰ μέρη συνατονεῖν εὔλογον. οὕτως δὲ καὶ τὴν ὑστέραν ἀτονωτέραν οὖσαν εἰκὸς καὶ περὶ τὴν ἐνέργειαν τοιαύτην ἔσεσθαι, τὸ δὲ συλλαβεῖν ὑστέρας ἔργον. μήτ' ἐνδεοῦς οὖν τοῦ σώματος ὄντος ἡ συνουσία παραλαμβανέσθω μήτε δὲ πάλιν βαρέος, [καὶ] ὁποῖον ἐν ἀπεψίαις ἐστὶ καὶ μέθαις. πρῶτον μέν, ὅτι κατὰ φύσιν διακείμενον τὸ σῶμα τῶν ἰδίων ἐνεργημάτων ἀποδοτικὸν γίνεται, κατὰ φύσιν δὲ οὐ διάκειται, καθ' ὃν καιρὸν ἐν μέθῃ καὶ ἀπεψίᾳ καθέστηκεν· ὡς οὖν οὐδὲ ἄλλο τι φυσικὸν ἔργον ἐν τοιούτῳ καταστήματι διοικεῖσθαι δύναται, οὕτως οὐδὲ ἡ σύλληψις. δεύτερον δέ, ὅτι κολληθὲν δεῖ τὸ σπέρμα διατρέφεσθαι, λαμβάνει δὲ τροφὴν

ἀπὸ τῆς ἐπιφερομένης ὕλης αἱματικῆς τε καὶ πνευματικῆς· ἐν δὲ ταῖς μέθαις καὶ ταῖς ἀπεψίαις πᾶς ἀτμὸς ἔφθαρται καὶ συντεθόλωται καὶ τὸ πνεῦμα· κίνδυνος οὖν ὑπὸ φαύλων τῶν ἐπιχορηγουμένων καὶ τὸ σπέρμα ἐπὶ τὸ φαυλότερον μεταβαλεῖν. εἶτα καὶ [ἡ] διὰ τὴν μέθην πολυυλία κωλυτικὴ [τῆς] πρὸς τὴν ὑστέραν γίνεται κολλήσεως τοῦ σπέρματος· ὡς γὰρ τὰ ἐπὶ τῶν μεθυόντων τραύματα δυσσύμφυτα ποιεῖ διὰ τὴν πολλὴν ἀναφορὰν ὁ οἶνος, οὕτως εὔλογον καὶ τὴν τοῦ σπέρματος κόλλησιν ὑπὸ τῆς αὐτῆς αἰτίας ἐπιταράττεσθαι.

the body must be neither in want nor weak, for it stands to reason that together with the whole the parts too are weak. Thus if the uterus is too weak it will be so, in all likehood, regarding its functions too, and conception is a function of a uterus. Thus intercourse shall be practised neither when the body is in want, nor, on the other hand, when it is heavy as it is in indigestion and drunkenness. First, because the body in a natural state performs its proper functions, but it is not in a natural state at the time of drunkenness and indigestion. And just as no other natural function can be effected in such a state, neither can conception. Second, because the seed when attached must be nourished, and take food from the substance containing blood and pneuma which is brought to it. But in drunkenness and indigestion all vapor is spoilt ant thus the pneuma too is rendered turbid. Therefore danger arises lest by reason of the bad material contributed the seed too change for the worse. Furthermore, [the] satiety due to heavy drinking hinders [the] attachment of the seed to the uterus.[121]

It is even possible to encounter the opinion that the man should not be under the influence of alcohol, as that may lead to character weaknesses in the children:

Ἐχόμενον δ' ἂν εἴη τούτων εἰπεῖν ὅπερ οὐδὲ τοῖς πρὸ ἡμῶν παρεωρᾶτο. τὸ ποῖον; ὅτι τοὺς ἕνεκα παιδοποιίας πλησιάζοντας ταῖς γυναιξὶν ἤτοι τὸ παράπαν ἀοίνους ἢ μετρίως γοῦν οἰνωμένους ποιεῖσθαι προσήκει τὸν συνουσιασμόν. φίλοινοι γὰρ καὶ μεθυστικοὶ γίγνεσθαι φιλοῦσιν ὧν ἂν τὴν ἀρχὴν τῆς σπορᾶς οἱ πατέρες ἐν μέθῃ ποιησάμενοι τύχωσιν. ᾗ καὶ Διογένης μειράκιον ἐκστατικὸν ἰδὼν καὶ παραφρονοῦν 'νεανίσκε' ἔφησεν, 'ὁ πατήρ σε μεθύων ἔσπειρε'.

It is that husbands who approach their wives for the sake of issue should do so only when they have either not taken any wine at all, or at any rate, a very moderate portion. For children whose fathers have chanced to beget them in drunkenness are wont to be fond of wine, and to be given to excessive drinking. Wherefore Diogenes, observing an emotional and crack-brained youth, said, 'Young man, your father must have been drunk when he begot you!'[122]

Physicians further stressed the importance of mental health and the right character traits, since, as Soranus wrote, 'Fertile women do not express with their countenance either joy or sadness'.

Female infertility

Romans had suspicions about many potential causes of infertility. Sometimes it may have been due to a decline in overall health, which in turn led to refraining from sex, but also due to not menstruating, the entrance to the uterus closing up, a distortion of the cervix, myomas, sores, ulcers, or blockage of the lumen of a fallopian tube:

> aut tamen sintexi vel habitudine quam cacexian vocant impediuntur, aut abstinentia menstruali, aut ore matricis clauso, aut collo inflexo vel carne aut membranulis obstruso aut duritia densato vel saxitate, quam Greci sclirosin vocant, aut ulcere aut horum similibus obstaculis, vel cecitate seminalium viarum, et propterea femina veluti eunucha permaneat aut, ut plerique memorant, luxuriosis moribus exercita nec regula vite servata ipsa sibi causa sit sterilitatis illate.

> or they are made difficult by atrophy or by the habit referred to as debauchery, or the absence of menses, or closee-off exit of the uterus, or the cervix being bent ot stopped up with muscular tissue or membranous fragments, or hardened or petrified, which the Greeks call *sclerosis*, or due to a wound and other such obstructions, or because the pathways for the seed [i.e. fallopian tubes] are stopped up, so that the woman emains like a eunuch, or, as many mention, obedient to licentious ways, or, observing no rules in her life, she herself will be the cause of her acquired infertility.[123] (retranslated from a Polish translation by W. J. Maciejewski)

Among the means of diagnosing any potential difficulty in conceiving were fumigation and suppositories. It was believed that the smell of the resin suppository, made of rue or garlic, appearing on the woman's breath could be indicative of her fertility.[124]

Unfortunately, no texts of Soranus survive in which he comes forward with direct advice for women trying and failing to have a child; in that matter one must rely on the aforementioned symptoms which could in his opinion result in either high fertility or trouble becoming pregnant.

Alongside general advice on health and lifestyle, one may find in ancient authors remarks regarding positions facilitating fertilization. In Lucretius' opinion, for example,

nam more ferarum
quadrupedumque magis ritu plerumque putantur
concipere uxores, quia sic loca sumere possunt,
pectoribus positis, sublatis semina lumbis.

> Another thing of very great importance is the position in which the soothing pleasure itself is taken; for wives are thought generally to conceive better after the manner of wild beasts and quadrupeds, because in that position, breast down and loins up, the seeds can occupy the proper places.[125]

Should there be difficulty conceiving, folk medicine was also another resort, most often recommending treatment with herbal extracts (for example, from pine twigs or white wine with cumin seeds) and cataplasms of stones,[126] with siderite being among the most popular solutions. Supposedly it gave hope for pregnancy and safe labour to women, who always carried a stone tied to their bodies.[127] Pliny claims infertile women ought to eat leeks (*allium porrum*) complete with the bulb, since already Hippocrates believed that 'leeks open up contracted uteri' and that 'food augments women's fertility'.[128] He also recommends a type of worm added to wine in fives or sevens to facilitate conception.[129]

Another specialist, Aëtius of Amida, reports a prescription for a vaginal suppository which should make conception easier (after first cleansing the uterus with other appropriate drugs). The medicine was to consist of hare's rennet and honey.[130] Another measure thought to facilitate conception was a pessary made of hare's bile, marrow and brain, mixed with *satyrios*, *althaea* (or *malva*) and olive oil.[131] Another recommended ingredient was bat's blood. 'If one soaks a kerchief in its blood, lays it beneath the head of a woman unaware of that, and then has intercourse with her, she will immediately conceive.'[132] Another pessary, made of fox faeces mixed with rose oil, had the same effect.[133]

Often the opinion was expressed that the most effective remedy against infertility may be to change sexual partners. 'Particular individuals may have a certain physical incongruity between them, and persons whose union is infertile may have children when they form other connexions—for instance Augustus and Livia.'[134] Augustus and Livia did in fact have children from previous marriages, but none from their joint one, even though it lasted many years. Suetonius writes that Augustus was quite disappointed that his union with Livia had proven childless, the only pregnancy in it ending, as he mentions, in premature labour ('one baby was conceived, but was prematurely born'),[135] although the event is not mentioned in any other text.

The advice to change partners was probably voiced fairly often. It does come up in Lucretius' poem:

> Nam multum harmoniae Veneris differre videntur.
> atque alias alii complent magis ex aliisque
> succipiunt aliae pondus magis inque gravescunt.
> et multae steriles Hymenaeis ante fuerunt
> pluribus et nactae post sunt tamen unde puellos
> suscipere et partu possent ditescere dulci.
> et quibus ante domi fecundae saepe nequissent
> uxoris parere, inventast illis quoque compar
> natura, ut possent gnatis munire senectam.
>
> For sexual harmony is seen to vary greatly. Some men more easily impregnate some women than others, some women more easily their burden from some than from others and become pregnant. Many women barren often enough in earlier wedlock, yet have found those from whom they could conceive children and be enriched with sweet offspring; and often men, in whose homes hitherto women though fruitful have been unable to bear a child, yet have found a natural mate, so that they could protect their old age with children.[136]

Pliny, and Solinus following him, stresses there is not a single infertility model typical of all women: some women are only infertile in their youth, while others only give birth once in their lifetime;[137] some are always infertile, and others regain fertility once they have a new husband; finally, some women bear only girls or only boys.[138]

In a passage dealing with infertility, Caelius Aurelius points out one other matter – namely, in some women the cause may lie in mental issues, which could have physical outcomes, leading to the body being ruined.

One crucial countermeasure when fighting stress, and so a factor conducive to conception, is relaxation. Soranus mentions that conception will be facilitated by bathing and anointing the body, because then

> ἀποπεφορτισμένων μὲν τῶν χθιζῶν ὡς ἄν εἴποι τις περιττωμάτων, διακεκαθαρμένου δὲ τοῦ σώματος καὶ πρὸς τὰς φυσικὰς οἰκονομίας εὐσταθῶς ἔχοντος.
>
> the food will give the inner turbulence an impetus towards coitus, the urge for intercourse not being diverted by appetite for food; while the rubdown will make it possible to lay hold of the injected seed more readily.[139]

This will be impossible without the right kind of effort. A woman trying for a baby should refrain from bathing and spend two days in her bed. During that time she must lie quietly, breathe and avoid all manner of jolts or else the semen might flow out. Solinus in turn points out that people who plan children should start by not sneezing after the intercourse, lest 'the sudden shock reject the semen before the paternal fluid can penetrate to the mother's inner parts'.[140]

Male infertility

Although blame for infertility was mostly placed on women, it is worth remembering Romans were aware that men can have fertility problems too.[141] Lucretius brings up reproduction towards the end of Book Four of *De rerum natura*. He begins with this suggestive description:

> Nec divina satum genitalem numina cuiquam
> absterrent, pater a gnatis ne dulcibus umquam
> appelletur et ut sterili Venere exigat aevom;
> quod plerumque putant, et multo sanguine maesti
> conspergunt aras adolentque altaria donis,
> ut gravidas reddant uxores semine largo.
> ne quiquam divom numen sortisque fatigant.

> It is not the divine powers that drive away the genital force from a man, so that he be never called father by sweet children and that he pass his days in barren wedlock, as men for the most part think, sorrowfully sprinkling their altars with much blood and making them burn with offerings, that they may make their wives pregnant with abundant seed. It is all vanity that they weary the gods' power and magic lots.[142]

The poet speaks of men who expend a lot of energy, and possibly money as well, on futile prayers to the gods so that they may be allowed to become fathers, but he is hardly understanding of their plight, and instead declares their approach incorrect outright, since it is not the gods who are responsible for their childlessness, but rather the men themselves or, more accurately, the quality of their sperm.[143] Namely:

> nam steriles nimium crasso sunt semine partim,
> et liquido praeter iustum tenuique vicissim.
> tenve locis quia non potis est adfigere adhaesum,
> liquitur extemplo et revocatum cedit abortu.
> crassius hinc porro quoniam concretius aequo
> mittitur, aut non tam prolixo provolat ictu
> aut penetrare locos aeque nequit aut penetratum

> aegre admiscetur muliebri semine semen.
> nam multum harmoniae Veneris differre videntur

> they are barren, some because too thick, others in turn because it is too watery and thin. The thin, because it cannot stick and adhere to the parts, at once flows away and departs withdrawn in untimely birth. That which is too thick, again, since it is emitted too closely clotted, either does not leap forward with so far-reaching a blow, or cannot equally well penetrate the part, or, although it penetrate, does not easily mix with the woman's seed.[144]

As the problem was considered serious, there were various attempts at clarifying and understanding it. Among other notions there was the fairly widespread belief that

> οὕτως καὶ τὰς σπερματικὰς δυνάμεις ἐν ἡμῖν τε καὶ τοῖς ἄλλοις ζῴοις αὔξεσθαι μὲν πληρουμένης τῆς σελήνης, ἐλαττοῦσθαι δὲ μειουμένης.

> as well as in other animals are said to increase with the waxing moon but to decrease with the waning moon.[145]

A man's fertility could also be weakened by debauchery and the concomitant venereal diseases, or, same as in women, general poor health, because

> [Semen may be] either weak and thin, or watery, or thick,[146] and either coldor hot, that is corrupt.

Permanent infertility could be caused by injury to or diseases of the sex organs, because

> aut si perseveraverint in corpore vitia, aut veretri caverna obliqua sit, aut non naturali loco constituta, aut ipsum veretrum adductione surreptum, aut in hiis quos Greci ypospadias vocant, non aliter generandi negant officium

> Or, should the defects persist in the body, or should the penis cavity be oblique, or positioned in an unnatural place, or should the penis itself retract as a result of tension, or should it [be as] in those the Greeks call *hypospadias* (almost eunuchs); it is in that exact way that they refuse the duty of conception.[147]

Impotence was another frequently mentioned cause of men's infertility.[148] As Justinian introduced a law which restricted divorce, he listed it among the possible reasons for dissolving a marriage. If a husband suffered from impotence continuously for the first two years of marriage, the wife's family had the right to demand their divorce (and keep the dowry).[149]

Of course impotence was a real problem, but also one of the subjects most frequently brought up by Martial's mocking poetry:

Omnes eunuchos habet Almo nec arrigit ipse:
et queritur, pariat quod sua Polla nihil.

Almo's household consists of eunuchs and he doesn't rise himself; and he grumbles because his Polla gives birth to nothing.[150]

Qua factus ratione sit requiris,
Qui numquam futuit, pater Philinus?
Gaditanus, Avite, dicat istud,
Qui scribit nihil et tamen poeta est.

You want to know how Philinus, who never fucks, became a father? Let Gaditanus answer that, Avitus, who writes nothing and yet is a poet.[151]

Juvenal, in a similar vein, writes:

Verum, ut dissimules, ut mittas cetera, quanto/metiris pretio quod, ni tibi deditus essem/devotusque cliens, uxor tua virgo maneret?/scis certe quibus ista modis, quam saepe rogaris/et quae pollicitus. fugientem nempe puellam/amplexu rapui; tabulas quoque ruperat et iam/signabat; tota vix hoc ego nocte redemi/te plorante foris. testis mihi lectulus et tu,/ad quem pervenit lecti sonus et dominae vox./instabile ac dirimi coeptum et iam paene solutum/coniugium in multis domibus servavit adulter./quo te circumagas? quae prima aut ultima ponas?/nullum ergo meritum est, ingrate ac perfide, nullum/quod tibi filiolus, quod filia nascitur ex me?/tollis enim et libris actorum spargere gaudes/argumenta viri. foribus suspende coronas:/iam pater est, dedimus quod famae opponere possis iura parentis habes, propter me scriberis heres,/legatum omne capis nec non et dulce caducum./commoda praeterea iungentur multa caducis,/si numerum, si tres implevero.

But though you ignore and disregard my other services, how do you value the fact that if I had not been your devoted and obedient client, your wife would still be a virgin? You know very well indeed how often you asked for that favour—the different ways you wheedled and the promises you made. Your bride was actually walking out on you when I grabbed her and embraced her. She'd even destroyed the contract and was already in the process of making a new arrangement. I spent the whole night on it and only just managed to retrieve the situation, with you sobbing outside the door. My witness is the couch—and you—you could surely hear the sound of the bed and its mistress' voice. There are many households where a lover has saved a marriage that's shaky and starting to fall apart and already more or less dissolved. Which way can you turn? What are your priorities? Is it no

> service, no service at all, you ungrateful cheat, that your little son or your daughter is my child? After all, you acknowledge them as your own and you're delighted to splash all over the newspapers the proofs of your virility. Hang the garlands over your doors: now you're a daddy—and it's me who's given you something to contradict the gossip. Because of me you possess the privileges of a parent, and you can be mentioned in people's wills, you can receive bequests intact, and some nice unexpected gifts too. What's more, many benefits will come along with those gifts if I make up the number to the full three.[152]

Romans tried to fight impotence with various drugs and other measures, mostly aphrodisiacs. Among the 'desire boosters' listed by Pliny there is the leek (which 'arouses amorous desires'),[153] the leaves and root of the terebinth,[154] asparagus (and wild asparagus, as well as the water from boiling it),[155] reed root[156] and *helichrysum* with vinegar.[157] Another popular aphrodisiac he mentions is garlic 'ground with fresh coriander, to be drunk with neat wine'.[158] A similar effect was promised from ingesting fennel seeds, also served with neat wine.[159] It was believed desire could be aroused by eating asparagus and carrots,[160] while turnips should be seasoned with rocket if they are to work.[161]

Another notion people had in antiquity is that chervil (*anthriscus*) 'fortifies the body weakened by sex and rouses men withered with old age to intercourse'.[162] Similar properties are attributed to wild kale, which 'has white flowers and is called *concilium*'.[163]

Not all the ingredients in the preparations to increase libido or prevent impotence were made of plants; they often included ground stones, and amulets were made of body parts from animals regarded as full of strength and vigour. One was, for example, advised to make an amulet from the testicles of a fox. Some such prescriptions are found in the *Cyranides*. For instance:

> the right testicle [of a fox], dried to powder and added to drink, is an aphrodisiac for women; the left, for men. The penis [of a fox] carried on one's person guarantees an enormous erection, as it does if dried to powder and mixed in with drink; the testicles, also dried and drunk in a beverage, do the same. Adding one spoon of the powder is enough, for the drug is most reliable, harmlessly inducing erection and intensifying true lust. But if you cut off a live animal's testicles, treat the animal, set it free, and hang them close on your body, you will immediately have an erection. If you wrap around the end of the penis a bladder or a piece of leather on which you write, with myrrh ink, the words *tin bib elithi*, and then hang it next to your body, you will be able to have intercourse safely... The kidneys of a fox, eaten or drunk, intensify desire.[164] (retransl. from the Polish transl. by E. Żybert)

We may guess an entire specialized market existed which offered stimulants and drugs to combat impotence. In that context, it is not surprising to learn that the physician Priscianus advised one other remedy against impotence, namely reading pornography: *suaviter fabulas amatorias describentibus*.[165]

Pliny the Younger, whose young wife Calpurnia miscarried, must have been very upset about it, but also reassured, in part at least, that she had conceived. He probably had some doubts as to his own virility and fertility or, worse, suspected others might have them. His previous marriage had lasted almost ten years and brought him no children. Therefore his vehement explanations to Calpurnia's grandfather Fabatus that the miscarriage proves she is in fact fertile and the promised great-grandchildren will be born soon, may point to a wish to justify himself and dispel the lingering doubts surrounding his own fertility. But, regardless of what he wrote in his letter to Fabatus, he must have also known that Calpurnia's ability to conceive was not definitive proof of her fertility. Pliny the Elder did mention in his work that there were women unable to carry to term, prone to frequent miscarriages and early births,[166] so Pliny the Younger likely did realize only the birth of a healthy child could prove Calpurnia's fertility. Still, by demonstrating his wife had been pregnant, he was able to absolve himself from any suspicions or blame for the childlessness of the marriage.

As Plutarch claims, 'no woman ever produced a child without the co-operation of a man'.[167] But while the ancient world did believe both men and women were necessary for reproduction and had a role to play in conception, infertility was usually blamed on the women.[168] In a society organized along patriarchal lines, where the purpose of marriage was to produce a legitimate child, a woman's infertility considerably lowered her standing and could even mean social death.[169] So, regardless of the era and social status, it was especially the women who had trouble conceiving who resorted to any means available, looking for divine aid as well as human, and even availing themselves of magic.[170]

Fertility and the gods

When no method approved by science, as it was then understood, worked, people asked the gods to bless them or intercede on their behalf.[171] In the Roman world, people worshipped and sacrificed to a variety of deities in charge of conception, the duration of pregnancy, the right course of labour and the development of the infant.[172] Paradoxically, we owe our modest knowledge about some of those deities – or, more specifically, their names and occasionally their sphere of influence – to writings of the Church Fathers, particularly Augustine of Hippo and Tertullian. And while those patristic authors mostly meant to fight superstition and abolish the traditional Roman religion, it is their works that provide us today with a lot of interesting information on the matter.[173] Augustine wrote that pagans assigned each stage of human life to the care of a different divine power.[174] Thus, he lists deities responsible for successful conception: Janus, who 'opens the door so the seed may be accepted'; Saturn, who gives of 'his fertility'; and Liber, who 'frees a man in the act of the man expending his seed'. Augustine also mentions a minor goddess, Mena, responsible for menstruation, while Tertullian emphasizes the significance of Fluvonia, who 'nourishes the infant in the womb'.[175]

However, for many Romans it was Juno Lucina who played the foremost role when it came to those delicate matters, *the* goddess of fertility and protectress of future mothers and women in labour. Under the empire she was greatly venerated by would-be parents, and information about her and the protection she extended to women is fairly common in numismatic, epigraphic and literary sources. Indeed, her role must have been significant, for a festival to her, the Matronalia, was held each year on 1 March.[176] During the festival, married women, mothers and pregnant women went to her temple in a procession.[177]

There is an account in Ovid of a dramatic situation in which Rome found itself shortly after it was founded. The threat of having no women around was avoided with the daring abduction ('rape') of Sabine maidens, but although time passed, most of the marriages then made remained childless.[178] In order to turn the course of fate in their favour, the married couples set off in a procession to a holy grove. Ovid's tale of the help the goddess granted the Sabines who wanted to give birth not only confirms that the worship of Juno Lucina in Rome was ancient, but also underlines her importance as a protectress of future mothers, who looked after women's fertility.[179]

Votive offerings and magic

In all the regions of the Roman world there are vestiges of shrines visited by people, mostly women, who came to ask for help and divine protection for the time between conception and birth and for health for themselves and the foetus (or infant). Among the votive offerings found in those places are objects resembling a woman's pubic triangle and women's breasts, but also the penis and testicles, made chiefly of stone and bronze.[180]

Many women believed in the beneficial effects of water from sacred springs. Already in the archaic period water stood for life, youth and eternity. It had the power to heal, rejuvenate and give life. Many votive items in the form of breasts were dedicated to Sequana, the goddess of the Seine.[181]

In the religious centre of Gravisca, the port town of Tarquinii, over two hundred clay figurines were found depicting uteri.[182] The goddess worshipped there was Uni (i.e. Juno). In total, over four hundred clay uteri from the vicinity of Gravisca and Vulci were x-rayed.[183] It turned out they all contained small clay balls (roughly 1 centimetre across), which were most likely meant to symbolize embryos.[184]

The most suggestive expression of the desire to conceive and have children, though, are votive images, usually made of stone or wood, of swaddled babies (that is, tightly wrapped all over with bandages).[185] It is possible some of those swaddled infant figurines were dedicated by parents praying for an ill child's health, but offerings in this form have mostly been discovered in shrines to water deities. The element of water granted (and represented) fecundity of the earth, so it seems likely votive offerings left for deities who had connections to water were brought there by men and women praying for 'the gift of life', that is, a child.[186]

Women who wanted children resorted to all manner of tricks to find out if they had a chance to bear a child. In his *De Divinatione*, Cicero uses the concept of fertility to criticize what he believes are the lies of dream interpreters.[187] He writes of a married woman who wanted to have a baby (*parere quaedam matrona cupiens*) but was not sure if she was pregnant. One night she dreamt her womb was sealed and asked to have the dream explained to her. The diviner told her she was infertile: if her womb was sealed, then conception was impossible. Since she was unhappy with the answer, she found another dream interpreter. This one

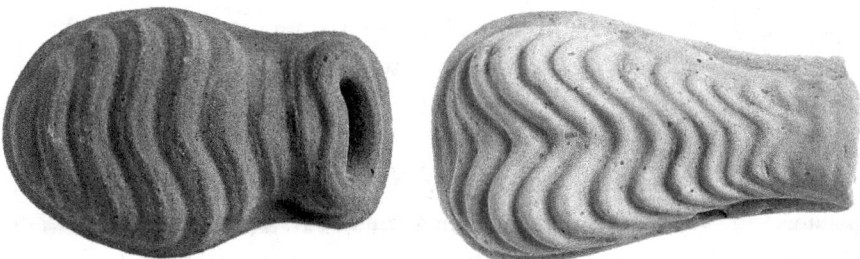

Figure 2 Terracotta uterus models © Wellcome Collection (CC BY 4.0). Source: https://wellcomecollection.org/works/xjfc6ara

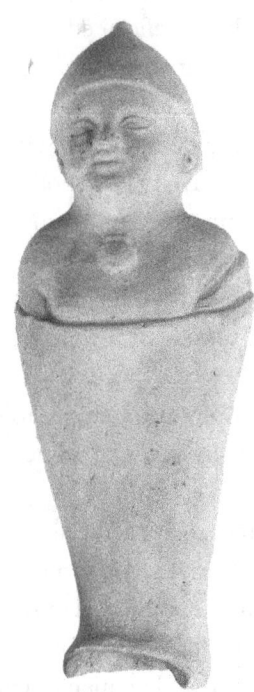

Figure 3 A swaddled child. A votive offering © Wellcome Collection (CC BY 4.0). Source: https://wellcomecollection.org/works/p992ghkb

told her she was, in fact, pregnant, as containers are not locked if empty. Cicero then asks his reader: what is a dream interpreter's skill if not clever deception? (*Quae est ars coniectoris eludentis ingenio?*) He tries to expose dream diviners as frauds by showing the same dream can have multiple meanings, naturally none of them true. It is interesting, however, that his example is a story of a woman who wanted to have a child, which may indicate it was a typical question to ask a dream interpreter. Magic and divination did not help, but they may have caused a placebo effect. We have a magic tablet from Novum near Parma, dated to the first century BCE, which reads, 'She who used to be infertile will give birth' (*[fe]ret quae ante sterilis fuit*), so outright attempts to command reality into shape were attempted as well.[188]

Thus diagnosis and advice regarding the best circumstances for conception included an evaluation of anatomy, menstrual issues, appearance, lifestyle, diet and even character traits of the future parents. It was that kind of holistic approach that was supposed to help people, especially women, looking forward to having offspring. Unfortunately sometimes the woman did not get pregnant, even though the circumstances were (theoretically) favourable, so it is no surprise that married couples desiring children asked the gods for the aid medicine was unable to give. Presumably their prayers were sometimes heard, and then

> μετὰ δέ τινα χρόνον κἀκ τοῦ τὴν ἐπίμηνον κάθαρσιν ἐπέχεσθαι ἢ ἐπ' ὀλίγον φαίνεσθαι, βαρυτέραν δὲ γίνεσθαι τὴν ὀσφὺν καὶ λεληθότως ἐπαίρεσθαι τοὺς μαστοὺς μετά τινος ἐπιπόνου συναισθήσεως, ὑπανατρέπεσθαι δὲ τὸν στόμαχον καὶ τὰ ἐπὶ τοῦ στήθους ἀγγεῖα κυρτὰ καὶ πελιὰ φαίνεσθαι καὶ τὰ κύλα τῶν ὀφθαλμῶν ὑπόχλωρα, ποτὲ δὲ καὶ σπίλους μελανίζοντας ἐπιπολῆς ταῖς ὄψεσιν ἐπιτρέχειν καὶ τὴν λεγομένην ἔφηλιν γενέσθαι· μετὰ δὲ ταῦτα τήν τε κίσσαν ἐπιφαίνεσθαι καὶ πρὸς λόγον τῆς τοῦ χρόνου προκοπῆς διογκοῦσθαι τὸ ἐπιγάστριον, εἶτα καὶ κινήσεως τοῦ κατὰ γαστρὸς ἀντιλαμβάνεσθαι τὴν κυοφοροῦσαν.

the monthly catharsis is held back or appears only slightly, that the loins feel rather heavy, that imperceptibly the breast swell, which is accompanied by a certain painful feeling, that the stomach is upset, that the vessels on the breast appear prominent and livid and the region below the eyes greenish, that sometimes darkish splotches spread over the region above the eyes and so called freckles develop.[189]

and

A conceptu decimo die dolores capitis, oculorum vertigines tenebraeque, fastidium in cibis, redundatio stomachi indices sunt hominis inchoati.

On the tenth day from conception pains in the pregnancy, head giddiness and dim sight, distaste for food and vomiting are symptoms of the formation of the embryo.[190]

3

Specialized Care for the Would-be Mother

'Canthara dear, quickly, run and fetch the midwife, so she doesn't keep us waiting when we need her'[1]

In ancient Rome, midwives and female physicians made a small group, which was, however, important to the society of the time. They were tasked with diagnosing illness, treatment and nursing care of their patients, most of whom were female.[2] Regrettably, our knowledge about the women who worked in medical professions then is not so much scant as very fragmentary. We do not have details regarding their education or career course. The sources are rather few, but they not only demonstrate the professions existed, but also indicate that men – physicians, teachers, husbands and fathers of the women referred to as *medicae* and *obstetrices*[3] – treated them with great respect and appreciated their professional skills. Their mere presence among their patients could have made Roman women trust medicine more, thus improving the standards of prevention and care of their reproductive health and life.[4]

Medicae

Unfortunately, it would be difficult, based on the extant sources, to fully demonstrate what *medicae* were in ancient Rome, and the problem is not limited to how the term *medica* ought to be understood. It is also unclear, in the case of some of the sources, if they qualify.[5] An example is provided by the inscription CIL VIII 806. The stone is damaged enough that the inscription was difficult to read when discovered, and it is not known where it is now. All we have is the record in CIL. It is usually read as put up in honour of a female physician, Geminia (*salus omnium medicine [?] Gemini*),[6] but sometimes it is reconstructed differently, to mean that no female doctor was intended; instead, it was the funder, a city magistrate and curator by name of Geminius Dativus (listed in the inscription), who was an educated physician.[7]

Luckily, most of the preserved inscriptions pose no such difficulties. We find in them the names of women of various social standings, both freeborn – such as Asyllia Polla,[8] Vibia Primilla,[9] Metilia Donata (who declares she had the inscription put up *de sua pecunia*),[10] Sextilia[11] and Scantia Redempta[12] – and not. In fact, Minucia Asste,[13] Venuleia Sosis,[14] Iulia Sophia,[15] Restituta[16] and Iulia Sabina[17] were almost certainly all freedwomen. In the cases of Sentia Elis,[18] Sarmanna,[19] Terentia Prima,[20] Iulia Saturnina,[21] Valeria Berecunda[22] and Valia Calliste,[23] it is believed more likely that they were freedwomen than born free,[24] whereas Iulia Pye[25] and Flavia Hedone[26] were probably imperial freedwomen. However, some of the women physicians known to us were slaves (examples include Melitine,[27] Secunda[28] and Ambata),[29] while the status of some others is impossible to determine due to the original quality of the inscription or its condition today.[30] In other cases we have visual material, but no way to learn the commemorated woman's name or social status.[31]

What do we know of the education those *medicae* had? Presumably the training of women doctors, same as that of their male counterparts, focused on practical aspects rather than on studying systematic theoretical foundations,[32] although regardless of gender, practitioners of medicine must have had some grounding in theory too.[33] One of the inscriptions refers to the woman listed in it as *medica philologa*;[34] another merely indicates the deceased woman was educated: *antistis disciplin[ae] / [in] medicina fuit*.[35]

We may suppose women doctors, like their male colleagues, mostly studied with and practised under the tutelage of other physicians, as did Restituta, a woman known from a Roman inscription. Restituta was a student of Claudius Alcimus, a physician of emperors.[36] Analysing the inscriptions leads one to suspect that in many cases the profession was inherited or in some way a family tradition. An interesting example of physicians within the same family being co-workers is provided by an inscription from Pergamon originating from the second century CE, dedicated to Panthea by her husband Glycon, also a doctor. The inscription enumerates the traits and merits Panthea had as a wife and mother, but Glycon also stresses that his wife could compete with him in medicine.[37] Another man to appreciate the professional skill of his wife was a certain Cassius Philippus, who mentions Iulia Saturnina was the better doctor.[38]

Obstetrices

The perfect midwife

Owing to the extant epigraphic and iconographic sources, but particularly owing to Soranus' *Gynaecology*, we can try to both describe that group in terms of professional qualifications required of women who cared after pregnant women, analyse the virtues expected of them, and define their background, social circumstances and occasionally even their family situation.[39]

Soranus emphasizes a person needs to be responsible, highly competent and educated in order to be a midwife. He points to literacy as an important skill and a good memory as an asset. A midwife should be healthy and strong, but also, he writes, honest and empathetic.[40] Still, interestingly, he remarks that in order to understand the woman giving birth and her needs, it is not at all necessary for the midwife have a child of her own. She should further take good care of her hands, so they are soft and cause the woman in labour no additional pain. Having listed those necessary requirements, he justifies in detail why they are so vital for the profession.[41] Among his reasons is the argument that the best midwives ought to be literate so they can broaden their education and read treatises on midwifery and paediatrics, which in turn might indicate such specialized texts meant for midwives existed. Soranus also notes that the professional background of midwives varies a great deal, since some of them have no theoretical education but do have a lot of practice, while others are well versed in the theory of gynaecology and obstetrics. Even so, the most highly valued midwives were practically equal to physicians and had comprehensive education covering pharmacology, nutrition and even surgery. Of particular interest is this passage on what makes 'the best' midwife:

> Τὰ συμπληροῦντα τὴν ἀρίστην μαῖαν εἰπεῖν ἀναγκαῖον, ἵνα αἱ μὲν ἄρισται γινώσκωσιν ἑαυτάς, αἱ δὲ ἀρτιμαθεῖς ὡς εἰς ἀρχετύπους ταύτας ἀποβλέπωσιν, ὁ βίος δὲ παρὰ τὰς χρείας εἰδῇ, τίνας δεῖ μετακαλεῖσθαι. κατὰ τὸ κοινὸν μὲν οὖν τελείαν φαμὲν τὴν μόνον τοῦ τέλους τῆς ἰατρικῆς ἐπιτυγχάνουσαν, ἀρίστην δὲ τὴν προσειληφυῖάν τι καὶ πρὸς ταῖς προστασίαις ἐν τοῖς θεωρήμασιν πολύπειρον. μερικώτερον δὲ λέγομεν ἀρίστην μαῖαν τὴν γεγυμνασμένην ἐν πᾶσι τοῖς μέρεσιν τῆς θεραπείας (τὰ μὲν γὰρ διαιτῆσαι δεῖ, τὰ δὲ χειρουργῆσαι, τὰ δὲ φαρμάκοις διορθώσασθαι) καὶ τὰ ὑγιεινὰ παραγγέλματα δοῦναι δυναμένην καὶ τὸ κοινὸν καὶ τὸ προσεχὲς ἰδεῖν καὶ τὸ συμφέρον ἐκ τούτου λαμβάνουσαν καὶ μήτ' ἀπὸ τῶν αἰτίων μήτ' ἀπὸ τῆς πλειστάκις τηρήσεως τῶν καθόλου συμ[βαινόν]των ἢ τινος τούτων· εἶτα κατὰ μέρος οὐ παρατυπουμένην ἐν ταῖς τῶν συμπτωμάτων μεταβολαῖς, παρηγοροῦσαν δὲ κατὰ τὴν πρὸς τὸ πάθος

ἀκολουθίαν, ἀτάραχον, ἀκατάπληκτον ἐν τοῖς κινδύνοις, δεξιῶς τὸν περὶ τῶν βοηθημάτων λόγον ἀποδιδόναι δυναμένην, παραμυθίαν ταῖς καμνούσαις πορίζουσαν, συμπάσχουσαν καὶ οὐ πάντως προτετοκυῖαν, ὡς ἔνιοι λέγουσιν, ἵνα συνειδήσει τῶν ἀλγημάτων ταῖς τικτούσαις συμπαθῇ, [οὐ] μᾶλλον γὰρ [τοῦτο] τετοκυίας· εὔτονον δὲ διὰ τὰς ὑπουργίας καὶ οὐ πάντως νέαν, ὥς φασίν τινες, καὶ γὰρ νέα τις ἄτονος καὶ οὐ νέα τοὐναντίον εὔτονος· σώφρονα δὲ καὶ νήφουσαν ἀεὶ διὰ τὸ ἄδηλον τῶν πρὸς τὰς κινδυνευούσας μετακλήσεων· ἥσυχον δὲ ἔχουσαν θυμὸν ὡς πολλῶν τῶν ἐν τῷ βίῳ μυστηρίων μετέχειν μέλλουσαν· ἀφιλάργυρον ὡς μὴ διὰ μισθὸν κακῶς δοῦναι φθόριον· ἀδεισιδαίμονα χάριν τοῦ μὴ δι᾿ ὄνειρον ἢ διὰ κληδόνας ἢ σύνηθές τι μυστήριον καὶ βιωτικὴν θρησκείαν ὑπεριδεῖν τὸ συμφέρον. ἐπιτηδευέτω δὲ καὶ τὴν τῶν χειρῶν τρυφερίαν, φυλαττομένη καὶ τὰς σκληρύνειν δυναμένας ἐριουργίας, διὰ χρισμάτων δὲ προσκατακτωμένη τὸ ἁπαλόν, εἰ μὴ πάρεστιν φυσικῶς, καὶ τοῦτο. τοιαύτην μὲν εἶναι δεῖ τὴν ἀρίστην μαῖαν.

It is necessary to tell what makes the best midwives, so that on the one hand the best may recognize themselves, and on the other hand beginners may look upon them as models, and the public in time of need may know whom to summon. Now generally speaking we call a midwife faultless if she merely carries out her medical task; whereas we call her the best midwife if she goes further and in addition to her management of cases is well versed in theory. And more particularly, we call a person the best midwife if she is trained in all branches of therapy (for some cases must be treated by diet, others by surgery, while still others must be cured by drugs); if she is moreover able to prescribe hygienic regulations for her patients, to observe the general and the individual features of the case, and from this to find out what is expedient, not from the causes or from the repeated observations of what usually occurs or something of the kind. Now to go into detail: she will not change her methods when the symptoms change, but will give her advice in accordance with the course of the disease; she will be unperturbed, unafraid in danger, able to state clearly the reasons for her measures, she will bring reassurance to her patients, and be sympathetic. And, it is not absolutely essential for her to have borne children, as some people contend, in order that she may sympathize with the mother, because of her experience with pain; for [to have sympathy] is [not] more characteristic of a person who has given birth to a child. She must be robust on account of her duties but not necessarily young as some people maintain, for sometimes young persons are weak whereas on the contrary older persons may be robust. She will be well disciplined and always sober, since it is uncertain when she may be summoned to those in danger. She will have a quiet disposition, for she will have to share many secrets of life. She must not be greedy for money, lest she give an abortive wickedly for payment; she will be free from superstition G so as not to overlook salutary measures on account of a dream or omen or some customary rite or vulgar superstition. She must also keep her hands soft, abstaining from such woolworking as may make them hard, and she must acquire softness by means of ointments if it is not present naturally. Such persons will be the best midwives.[42]

Even if a midwife was excellently prepared to do her job, she did not deliver children on her own. Rather, she was assisted by other women, who were to stand to the sides and behind the birthing chair. Soranus explains that their role included reassuring and calming the woman in labour. The person standing behind the chair needed to be strong enough to hold her up and control her movements, some of them violent or sudden. Meanwhile, the midwife herself sat in front of the woman giving birth and it was from there that she oversaw the course of the birth.[43]

When the child was born, one of the midwife's most important duties was to announce its gender. Before washing and swaddling the newborn, she would also determine whether the child was 'fit to be raised'. A test was used to that purpose, similar to present-day Apgar score.[44] First, the midwife would lay the child on the ground and evaluate its crying; loud cries indicated health, whereas sick babies cried weakly or not at all. Then she would check the orifices of the body and the ease with which the infant's limbs bent and straightened. By palpating the infant's skin, she would evaluate its sensitivity to tactile impulses.[45] It was most likely the midwife who, based on such an inspection and her own experience, decided how likely the baby was to live.

Soranus' depiction of midwives should probably be taken as idealized and divorced from the actual facts of the time. His requirements could hardly have been met by all the women who delivered babies in Rome. What, then, were they really like, those midwives who looked after the women giving birth? Did they meet the requirements outlined in Soranus' handbook? Unfortunately, the preserved body of sources is rather modest, just as in the case of *medicae*. We do not have a single extant biography of a female midwife, however brief. Our knowledge is mostly drawn from inscriptions and visual images.[46]

The iconography confirms Soranus' descriptions and recommendations fairly well.[47] For example, an ivory relief sculpture was found in Pompeii,[48] depicting four women: one giving birth in a chair, one assistant standing behind her, a midwife sitting on a low stool facing the woman giving birth, and a fourth woman standing behind the midwife.

A modest terracotta slab from a tomb in Ostia containing the remains of Scribonia Attice, wife of M. Ulpius Amerimnus, a surgeon, also depicts a birth

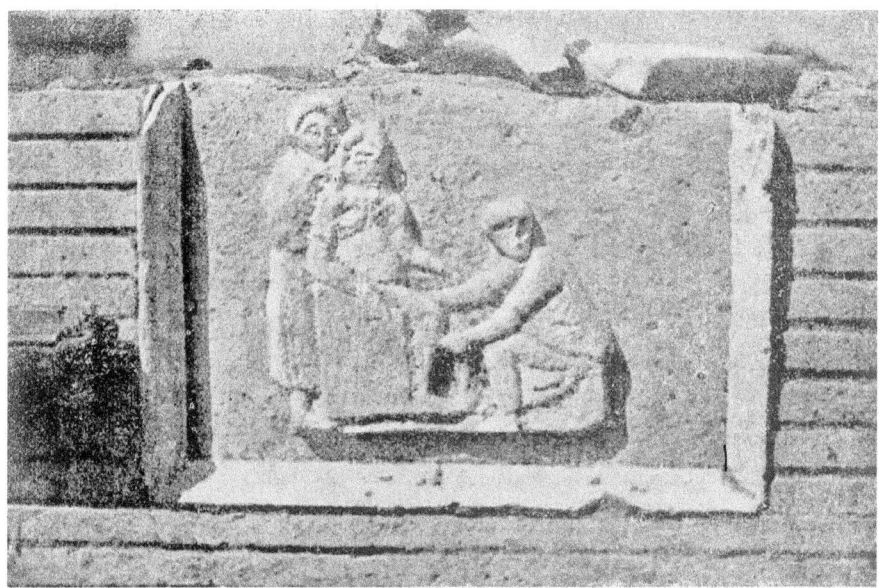

Figure 4 A tombstone from Ostia. Scribonia Attice, a midwife, at work. Picture from: *Aesculape: revue mensuelle illustrée des lettres et des arts dans leurs rapports avec les sciences et la médecine* © Wellcome Collection (CC BY 4.0).
Source: https://wellcomecollection.org/works/e52vpkpb/images?id=hstbkuz3

scene.[49] Scribonia worked as a midwife and the relief sculpture shows her at work (see photograph 4).

A joint medical practice of a male physician and a female midwife is mentioned by an inscription from Numidia,[50] which lists two slaves, the midwife Irene and the physician Faustus. Although the pair were not married, they may have been in some sort of informal relationship, and they plied their medical trade together.[51] Unfortunately when it comes to identifiable midwives (*obstetrices*), epigraphical sources are for the most part scant and even that amount of information is rare.[52]

Midwives' tombs were usually paid for by their fathers,[53] sons,[54] or husbands,[55] but there are cases where we do not know who the funder of the inscription was. Sometimes only the midwife's name survives; other times even that is lost.

We do know the names of a few midwives of presumably somewhat higher standing, who were in service with the imperial family. Two such women, Iulia [---]sia and Prima, worked for Livia Augusta, and Secunda of Sorrento may have been another.[56] Julia Augusta's midwife was Taxis Ionidis,[57] while Antonia Thallusae was a freedwoman and *obstetrix* of Antonia Augusta,[58] and Hygia a midwife of Claudia Marcella.[59]

It was not only women from the imperial family but also women from rich, influential Roman families who had their own midwives. Sempronia Peloris[60] was a freedwoman of Sempronia Atratina, a slave called Secunda was an obstetrix of Statilia Maior,[61] Hygia a slave of Flavia Sabina,[62] and Sallustia Athenais[63] and Sallustia Imerita[64] midwives among the slaves and freedwomen in the service of a Q. Sallustius.[65]

In a few cases, male doctors are listed alongside the midwives. Some researchers (such as A. Alonso Alonso) think they may have formed medical teams of sorts in the service of a family.[66] And so, in the columbarium of Sempronia Atratina (see above), there is a plaque for the physician L. Sempronius Sumphorus;[67] next to Statilia's slave Secunda, we have the name of a male physician, one Thyrsus;[68] and from the columbarium housing the remains of Q. Sallustius' freedmen, we know the epitaph for Diogenes, a physician of his.[69]

As can be deduced from these examples, midwifery was not, in Rome, a profession for free women. The *praenomina* of the women listed above clearly indicate they were all slaves, or at most freedwomen.[70] Some of them had typical Greek names, and the Latin names which did appear – Secunda, Imerita, Hilara, Veneria – were also characteristic of slaves. We should not be misled in this by the cases of Licinia Victoria from Utica or Caelia Victoria from Thagaste,[71] because, as A. Alonso Alonso notes, such *cognomina* were, in fact, typical of slaves and freedmen in the African provinces.[72]

The job of a midwife was handed down through generations and most likely became a family tradition of sorts, just as in the case of the *medicae* discussed above, the difference being that here, women were trained by their mothers rather than fathers. Perhaps some slaves learned by assisting their owners.

When it came to remuneration, Soranus admonishes midwives not to be to greedy,[73] while other texts imply the sums involved were not small, as midwives' pay was comparable to that of physicians (including men).[74] After all, the work carried with it a lot of responsibility. In Ulpian a midwife is mentioned who caused a female slave of someone else to die by administering wrong medication.[75] Meanwhile, a good, experienced midwife offered a makeshift sense of security which presumably not all Roman women could afford.

The question then remains of how poor women managed who could not afford the services of professional midwives. They probably asked female relatives for help, who did what they could to make it easier for them, but because of their lack of specialist training or experience, there was the danger of the birth ending in a tragedy. Unfortunately, we do not know if mortality rates of infants and mothers were any lower if they were in the care of skilled, educated midwives who followed the guidelines laid down in Soranus' textbook.[76]

Some of the women who worked as midwives must have enjoyed a high level of public trust. They would be summoned and consulted by the praetors, for example when it was necessary to determine if a woman was pregnant. They also oversaw birth and delivery in complicated family situations, making sure the baby would not be, say, taken away or replaced with another.[77]

'The other accounts given not only by midwives but actually by harlots'[78]

In contrast to the ideal picture of a midwife painted in Soranus and to the neutral messages of the inscriptions that mention midwives, the image to be found in Pliny the Elder seems alarmingly different. In his work, *obstetrices* have virtually no professional connection to childbirth or postpartum care, and only feature in the context of administering abortifacient drugs and libido enhancers. A certain Salpe, whom Pliny mentions as many as five times, suggested 'therapies' against eye diseases making use of human urine,[79] offered prescriptions for depilatories,[80] and allegedly even knew a formula to silence a barking dog.[81] According to Pliny, her works contained superstition-filled advice on using human saliva to dispel indisposition[82] and on increasing potency.[83]

The same Salpe and another midwife known by her presumably given name, Lais, both believed wool from a black ram soaked in menstrual blood would protect one from rabid dogs.[84] The midwife Sotira recommended rubbing the blood of a menstruating woman into the feet of a patient suffering from intestinal problems.[85] Alongside Lais, Pliny mentions Elephantis,[86] whose erotica were said to be known and liked by emperor Tiberius himself.[87] In other words, in the stories quoted by Pliny, midwives and their practices may well seem superstitions, and their actions resemble those of prostitutes.[88] He also points out that

> Lais et Elephantis inter se contraria prodidere de abortivo carbone e radice brassicae vel myrti vel tamaricis in eo sanguine extincto, itemque asinas tot annis non concipere, quot grana hordei contacta ederint, quaeque alia nuncupavere monstrifica aut inter ipsas pugnantia, cum haec fecunditatem fieri isdem modis, quibus sterilitatem illa, praenuntiaret, melius est non credere.

> Lais and Elephantis do not agree in their statements about abortives, the burning root of cabbage, myrtle, or tamarisk extinguished by the menstrual blood, about

asses' not conceiving for as many years as they have eaten grains of barley contaminated with it, or in their other portentous or contradictory pronouncements, one saying that fertility, the other that barrenness is caused by the same measures. It is better not to believe them.[89]

The content and context of that advice may suggest midwives sometimes took advantage of superstitions present in other professional groups and earned extra money by selling prescription ingredients, for example cauls to advocates (as they were said to bring good luck).[90] Thus the image painted by Soranus, who recommended that midwives be free of superstition, diverges from that in Pliny.

If the drugs administered by a midwife proved poisonous or harmed the patient in some other way, she could be tried. In their profession, criminal responsibility for medical errors applied too. Ulpian quotes the following principle:

> Ulpianus libro octavo decimo ad edictum: Item si obstetrix medicamentum dederit et inde mulier perierit, Labeo distinguit, ut, si quidem suis manibus supposuit, videatur occidisse: sin vero dedit, ut sibi mulier offerret, in factum actionem dandam, quae sententia vera est: magis enim causam mortis praestitit quam occidit.

> where a midwife administers a drug to a woman and she dies in consequence, Labeo makes a distinction, namely: that if she administered it with her own hands she is held to have killed the woman, but if she gave it to the latter in order that she might take it, an action *in factum* should be granted, and this opinion is correct; for she rather provided the cause of death, than actually killed the woman.[91]

Even though it was usually considered desirable to have a midwife present during childbirth, clearly not all the women in the profession enjoyed a good reputation. They are sometimes described as excessive drinkers or not reliable enough to be entrusted with a woman's first childbirth.[92] Another midwife turned out to be venal. As Ammianus Marcellinus recounts,

> nam et pridem in Galliis, cum marem genuisset infantem, hoc perdidit dolo, quod obstetrix corrupta mercede, mox natum praesecto plus quam convenerat umbilico, necavit.

> For once before, in Gaul, when she had borne a baby boy, she lost it through this machination: a midwife had been bribed with a sum of money, and as soon as the child was born cut the umbilical cord more than was right, and so killed it.[93]

Still, it would be hard to determine if the child's death was in fact paid for, or a result of an unintentional mistake due to poor education.

Obstetrix et medica – or, *obstetrix id est medica*?

In the case of the word *obstetrix* (or *opstetrix*) there is usually no doubt that it was used to refer to midwives whose task it was to take care of women while pregnant, in labour, and for a while after, but the interpretation of the term *medica*, also encountered in sources, does raise doubts. Although literally, the word *medica* tends to be rendered as *female physician*, it is often supposed the Roman *medicae* were simply relatively well-educated midwives, who had decent grounding in theory as well as a lot of professional practice.[94] Even so, this passage in *Pauli sententiae* indicates the two professions were frequently seen as identical:

> Quoties de mulieris praegnatione dubitatur, quinque obstetrices, id est [medicae], ventrem iubentur inspicere; et quod plures ex ipsis se agnovisse dixerint, hoc certissimum iudicatur.

> Whenever a woman's pregnancy is in doubt, five midwives, that is, female doctors, are told to inspect her belly, and whatever a majority among them say they have discerned, that is considered the most likely.[95]

However, another line remains unclear, this one stating: *Sed et obstetricem audiant, quae utique medicinam exhibere videtur.*[96] One possible translation is: 'But let them also listen to a midwife who at least seems to exhibit medical skill.'[97]

Scholars assuming *medicae* constituted a separate profession usually emphasize that while they mostly worked in gynaecology and obstetrics, it cannot be ruled out they also had the medical expertise to diagnose and treat other conditions. What is more, they treated and operated on men as well as women,[98] as indicated, for instance, by this passage in Apuleius' *Metamorphoses*: 'Instead of playing the dutiful part of a wife, I have to endure the laborious role of a doctor.'[99]

Unfortunately, the surviving sources do not let us solve with certainty many of the problems to do with either terminology or the exact extent of duties of the women active in medical professions in ancient Rome, leaving them in the realm of guesses and theories, even as they give rise to much scholarly discussion.[100] At the same time, it should be borne in mind that modern categories of medicine cannot be applied to describe the realities of the time. In theory, anybody could have claimed to be a physician in Rome. Often, the only way to verify a person's declaration as to their profession was to rely on the opinions of others.[101]

It would seem that despite classicists and historians debating this, sometimes very hotly, it is virtually impossible to distinguish between the requirements midwives and female physicians had to meet in ancient Rome, and what the scope of their work was, all the more because ultimately, there is little we are able to say about the range of professional specialization and education of *medicae*. Based on epigraphic analysis, A. Alonso Alonso determined the characteristic features which point to distinctions between *obstetrices* and *medicae*, not merely in terminology, but also in access to the profession and the skills involved. Those were social background (we do not know of a single freeborn *obstetrix*, but for *medicae* it was not unheard of) and education (no preserved inscription mentions a midwife's theoretical education,[102] but among *medicae*, cases are known of physicians who boasted of their thorough learning, such as Naevia Clara or Scantia Redempta).[103] Our knowledge could be expanded by inscriptions such as one published recently, where Publicia Procula refers to herself as both *physician* and *midwife* (*medica idem opstetrix*), and so draws a clear line between the two professions.[104]

Why not a man-physician?

In Rome, giving birth, a very intimate moment in a woman's life, occurred among women – something confirmed by Soranus' treatise. A male doctor only attended in the case of a so-called abnormal birth, but even then his first task was to interview the midwife and to gather as much information as possible.[105] Another task usually reserved for a male physician was making the genitals limp so as to make the examination more effective, allowing for decisions on how to proceed. Other than that, it seems the doctor only watched, instructing the midwife and her assistants on how to behave and what to do.[106] Soranus remarks that in principle, the male physician should only take the midwife's place – that is, sit in front of the parturient ('namely, so that his arms are aligned with her legs') – and get ready for surgical intervention if it is suspected that the baby died in the womb or got stuck in the birth canal. One of the women present was supposed to help him by holding the labia open to make it easier for him to insert the proper instruments safely.

In many places, surgical instruments (namely, specula) have been found which seem unambiguously related to women's ailments.[107] They were most likely the property of (male) physicians, but assuming the term *medica* meant a woman, we must allow that *medicae* could have used such instruments as well.

Soranus writes that (presumably male) physicians existed called 'women's doctors' (γυναικείους ἰατρούς), because they treated women's ailments, but he notes that in the case of typically feminine diseases and conditions, women still availed themselves of the services of midwives rather than consulting a doctor.[108]

What could have been the reason women did not want to employ the services of male doctors? Perhaps it was shame.[109] Both giving birth and gynaecological interventions could have been considered extremely embarrassing experiences for a woman. In iconography, one can see that even when the very moment of birth is depicted, any midwives present usually avert their eyes, looking away from the patient.[110] Soranus even exhorted the midwife to refrain from 'staring at the vulva lest the flesh should contract from shame'.[111] The presence of a male stranger may have been all the more embarrassing and discouraging. It is to Greek women, or to their sense of shame and embarrassment, that Roman women owed the possibility of consulting women trained in medical professions.

In a clearly aetiological story,[112] the Roman author Hyginus mentions Hagnodice, a maiden who could not look idly at the suffering and death of women who hid their ailments through fear of male physicians. In order to help them, Hagnodice resolved to become a physician herself. However, for that, she needed to resort to deception:

Nam Athenienses caverant ne quis servus aut femina artem medicam disceret. [H]agnodice quaedam puella virgo concupivit medicinam discere, quae cum concupisset, demptis capillis habitu virili se H[e]rophilo cuidam tradidit in disciplinam. Quae cum artem didicisset, et feminam laborantem audisset ab inferiore parte, veniebat ad eam, quae cum credere se noluisset, aestimans virum esse, illa tunica sublata ostendit se feminam esse, et ita eas curabat. Quod cum vidissent medici se ad feminas non admitti, [H]agnodicen accusare coeperunt, quod dicerent eum glabrum esse et corruptorem earum, et illas simulare imbecilitatem. Quo[d] cum Areopagitae consedissent, [H]agnodicen damnare coeperunt; quibus [H]agnodice tunicam allevavit et se ostendit feminam esse. Et validius Medici accusare coeperunt, quare tum feminae principes ad iudicium venerunt et dixerunt, Vos coniuges non estis sed hostes, quia quae salutem nobis invenit eam damnatis. Tunc Athenienses legem emendarunt, ut ingenuae artem medicinam discerent.

For the Athenians forbade slaves and women to learn the art of medicine. A certain girl, Hagnodice, a virgin desired to learn medicine, and since she desired it, she cut her hair, and in male attire came to a certain Herophilus[113] for training. When she had learned the art, and had heard that a woman was in labor, she came to her. And when the woman refused to trust herself to her, thinking that she was a man, she removed her garment to show that she was a woman, and in this way she treated women. When the doctors saw that they were not admitted to women, they began to accuse Hagnodice, saying that he was a seducer and corruptor of women, and that the women were pretending to be ill. The Areopagites, in session, started to condemn Hagnodice, but Hagnodice removed her garment for them and showed that she was a woman. Then the doctors began to accuse her more vigorously, and as a result the leading women came to the Court and said: You are not husbands, but enemies, because you condemn her who discovered safety for us. Then the Athenians amended the law, so that free-born women could learn the art of medicine.[114]

Hyginus stresses that through her ruse, Hagnodice made knowledge accessible to patients, providing them with healthcare in a form they could accept: that is, in the form of a physician who, as a woman, did not threaten their sense of sexual shame.[115]

Almost four centuries later, in the preface to his Latin translation of Soranus' Greek gynaecology handbook, Caelius Aurelianus wrote that the ancients had finally decided to establish female doctors so woman in need of medical assistance and examination did not have to endure a man's gaze.[116]

Thus it was allegedly shame that was behind granting women access to the profession of the physician, motivating authors to record gynaecological traditions and obstetric knowledge.[117]

4

Pregnancy and Its Course

'A long time is needed so that a child, once conceived, may come to be born'[1]

Symptoms of pregnancy

Soranus believes that although menstruation and pregnancy are beneficial in that they contribute to creating a human being, they are still not good for women. He notes that, while women who used to suffer from painful periods have rid themselves of the monthly problem by becoming pregnant, they only actually replace one hardship with another:

εἰ δὲ καὶ ὑπὸ τῆς συλλήψεως ἀπαλλάσσονται, βοήθημα γίνεται νόσων ἡ σύλληψις, οὐ τηρητικὸν τοῦ ὑγιαίνειν, ὥσπερ οὐδ' ἡ φλεβοτομία διὰ τοῦτο ὑγιειὸν γίνεται παράλημμα, διότι λύει νόσους.

Even granted that they are relieved by conception, conception is not a means of preserving health but an aid against disease; just as venesection does not become healthful because used as a treatment it resolves diseases.

Pregnancy, he claims, comes with other unfavourable ailments attached:

ὅτι δὲ τὴν ἀτροφίαν καὶ τὴν ἀτονίαν καὶ τὸ προωρότερον γῆρας αἱ κυήσεις ἀποτελοῦσι, πρόδηλον μὲν κἀκ τῶν ἐναργῶν.

And that pregnancies bring about atrophy, atony, and premature old age, is manifest from the obvious facts.[2]

Soranus thinks the first characteristic symptom of pregnancy is feeling ill. On the tenth day counting from conception, other symptoms usually appear, namely headaches, dizziness, blurred vision and loss of appetite.[3] Solinus lists similar symptoms:

Quod si natalis materia haeserit, decimus a conceptu dies dolore grauidas admonebit. Iam inde incipiet et capitis inquietudo, et caligine uisus hebetabitur; ciborum quoque fastidiis stomachi claudetur cupido.

The pregnant mother will be troubled by pain on the tenth day from conception. From this time she will become restless in mind, and her sight will dim with darkness. Also the desire of her stomach lessens and she begins to loathe food.[4]

Soranus believes it is only the man and his seed that are responsible for reproduction; the woman's role is purely that of a receptacle. Because of that, he sees conception as 'seed being retained in the uterus', where it ought to remain long enough that it can transform into an embryo and then a foetus (that is, six days). It is only once 'the contents of the uterus has taken shape, and no sperm remains' that he considers the term *foetus* applicable. He sums up his reflections on the subject by saying:

ἀνάληψις μὲν γάρ ἐστιν ἡ φορὰ τοῦ σπέρματος ἐπὶ τὸν πυθμένα τῆς ὑστέρας, σύλληψις δὲ ἡ μετὰ τὴν φορὰν κράτησίς τε καὶ συγκόλλησις· καὶ ἀνάληψις μὲν μόνου ἐστὶ σπέρματος, σύλληψις δὲ καὶ ἐμβρύου.

[There is also a difference between reception and conception.] For reception is the conveying of the seed to the fundus of the uterus, whereas conception is its retention and attachment after its conveyance; furthermore reception refers to the seed only, while conception refers to the embryo too.[5]

That moment leads to another symptom of pregnancy, clear also to other ancient authors: menstruation fails to occur at the expected time, because

τὴν δ᾽ ὑστέραν οἷον ἀρότῳ καὶ σπόρῳ γῆν ἐν φυτοῖς ὀργῶσαν ἐν καιρῷ παρέχειν. ὅταν δὲ τὴν γονὴν ἀναλάβῃ προσπεσοῦσαν ἡ ὑστέρα καὶ περιστείλῃ, ῥιζώσεως γενομένης· 'ὁ γὰρ ὀμφαλὸς πρῶτον ἐν μήτρῃσιν,' ὥς φησι Δημόκριτος, 'ἀγκυρηβόλιον σάλου καὶ πλάνης ἐμφύεται, πεῖσμα καὶ κλῆμα' τῷ γεννωμένῳ καρπῷ καὶ μέλλοντι· τοὺς μὲν ἐμμήνους καὶ καθαρσίους ἔκλεισεν ὀχετοὺς ἡ φύσις, τοῦ δ᾽ αἵματος ἀντιλαμβανομένη φερομένου τροφῇ χρῆται καὶ κατάρδει τὸ βρέφος ἤδη συνιστάμενον καὶ διαπλαττόμενον, ἄχρι οὗ τοὺς προσήκοντας ἀριθμοὺς τῇ ἐντὸς αὐξήσει κυηθὲν ἑτέρας ἀνατροφῆς καὶ χώρας δέηται.

when the womb receives the seed as it encounters it and enfolds it and it has taken root there ('for the umbilical cord grows at first in the womb,' as Democritus says, 'as an anchorage against the swell and drift, a cable and vine 'for the fruit now conceived that is to be'), Nature shuts the monthly canals of purification and, taking the drifting blood, uses it for nourishment and irrigates the embryo, which already is beginning to be formed and shaped, until, having been carried the number of months proper to its growth within the womb, it needs other nourishment and abiding-place.[6]

Other, somewhat secondary signs believed to portend pregnancy included heaviness in the pelvis, sore breasts and stomach problems. The ultimate proof was believed to be enlarged breasts.

> μετὰ δέ τινα χρόνον κἀκ τοῦ τὴν ἐπίμηνον κάθαρσιν ἐπέχεσθαι ἢ ἐπ' ὀλίγον φαίνεσθαι, βαρυτέραν δὲ γίνεσθαι τὴν ὀσφὺν καὶ λεληθότως ἐπαίρεσθαι τοὺς μαστοὺς μετά τινος ἐπιπόνου συναισθήσεως, ὑπανατρέπεσθαι δὲ τὸν στόμαχον καὶ τὰ ἐπὶ τοῦ στήθους ἀγγεῖα κυρτὰ καὶ πελιὰ φαίνεσθαι καὶ τὰ κύλα τῶν ὀφθαλμῶν ὑπόχλωρα, ποτὲ δὲ καὶ σπίλους μελανίζοντας ἐπιπολῆς ταῖς ὄψεσιν ἐπιτρέχειν καὶ τὴν λεγομένην ἔφηλιν γενέσθαι· μετὰ δὲ ταῦτα τήν τε κίσσαν ἐπιφαίνεσθαι καὶ πρὸς λόγον τῆς τοῦ χρόνου προκοπῆς διογκοῦσθαι τὸ ἐπιγάστριον, εἶτα καὶ κινήσεως τοῦ κατὰ γαστρὸς ἀντιλαμβάνεσθαι τὴν κυοφοροῦσαν.

Later on also from the facts: that the monthly catharsis is held back or appears only slightly, that the loins feel rather heavy, that imperceptibly the breasts swell, which is accompanied by a certain painful feeling, that the stomach is upset, that the vessels on the breast appear prominent and livid and the region below the eyes greenish, that sometimes darkish splotches spread over the region above the eyes and so-called freckles develop. And still later, from the appearance of the pica and from the swelling of the abdomen in proportion to the passage of time; and then from the fact that the gravida perceives the movement of the fetus.[7]

The pregnancy symptoms presented above, which are those ancient authors mention the most often, indicate that verifying pregnancy, or early pregnancy at any rate, depended on fairly arbitrary evaluation and interpretation. In many cases, it must have come down to the knowledge and, more importantly, the experience of the physician or midwife involved.

Boy or girl?

> Ἱλαρίωνα(*) Ἄλιτι τῆι ἀδελφῆι(*) πλεῖστα χαί-
> ρειν καὶ Βεροῦτι τῇ κυρίᾳ μου καὶ Ἀπολλω-
> ναριν(*). γίνωσκε ὡς ἔτι καὶ νῦν ἐν Ἀλεξαν-
> δρέᾳ(*) σμεν(*)· μὴ ἀγωνιᾷς ἐὰν ὅλως εἰσ-
> πορεύονται(*), ἐγὼ ἐν Ἀλεξανδρέᾳ(*) μενῶ(*).
> ἐρωτῶ σε καὶ παρακαλῶ σε ἐπιμελη-

θι(*) τῷ παιδίῳ καὶ ἐὰν εὐθὺς ὀψώνι-
ον λάβωμεν ἀποστελῶ σε(*) ἄνω. ἐὰν
πολλὰ πολλῶν τέκῃς ἐὰν ἦν ἄρσε-
νον ἄφες, ἐὰν ἦν θήλεα ἔκβαλε.
εἴρηκας \δὲ/ Ἀφροδισιάτι(*) ὅτι μή με
ἐπιλάθῃς· πῶς δύναμαί σε ἐπι-
λαθεῖν; ἐρωτῶ σε οὖν ἵνα μὴ ἀγω-
νιάσῃς.
(ἔτους) κθ Καίσαρος Παῦνι κγ.

Hilarion to his sister Alis, many greetings, also to my lady Berous and Apollonarion. Know that I am still in Alexandria; and do not worry if they wholly set out, I am staying in Alexandria. I ask you and entreat you, take care of the child, and if I receive my pay soon, I will send it up to you. Above all, if you bear a child and it is male, let it be; if it is female, cast it out. You have told Aphrodisias, 'Do not forget me.' But how can I forget you? Thus I'm asking you not to worry. The 29th year of Caesar, Pauni 23. (verso) Hilarion to Alis, deliver.[8]

This frequently quoted excerpt from a surviving letter from Roman Egypt, written by a man to his wife, contains a request (or command) for her to get rid of her baby if she gives birth to a girl. Exposing newborn children was not only accepted and legal, but also common in all the societies of the Mediterranean. In Rome, the *ius exponendi* was among the important rights which, combined, constituted the special status of the father of a family (*pater familias*). Female babies were abandoned more often than male, because according to the widespread belief, girls were weaker, required more attention, and, most importantly, needed to be provided with a dowry once they grew up.[9] Romans did their best to predict whether the pregnant woman would have a boy, long awaited by the family, or a girl, who was not necessarily welcome. The problem was discussed of a tendency to bear children of one gender. For Pliny, it is beyond all doubt that

> aliaeque feminas tantum generant aut mares, plerumque et alternant, sicut Gracchorum mater duodeciens et Agrippina Germanici noviens. aliis sterilis est iuventa, aliis semel in vita datur gignere;
>
> some women have only female or only male children, though usually the sexes come alternately—for instance in the case of the mother of the Gracchi this occurred twelve times, and in that of Germanicus's wife Agrippina nine times.[10]

Censorinus quotes in his work a theory of Alcmaeon, according to which the child's gender depends on which parent's seed was stronger. Hippo, in turn, thought women were born of weaker seed, and men of stronger. In Parmenides' opinion, boys and girls were created from sperm received by the right-hand and left-hand side of the uterus respectively,[11] although he was not able to prove it. Meanwhile, Soranus cites Hippocrates' claim regarding the possibility of determining the child's gender *in utero*. Supposedly, a boy would be born if the woman's right breast was larger than her left, her skin was clear and her vitality high during pregnancy; a girl was more likely if the pregnant woman's left breast was larger and she herself was generally pale.[12]

Pliny is another author quoting the popular opinion that women about to give birth to boys have healthier skin and an easier time during labour, with the first movement of a male child in the womb occurring around the fortieth day of the pregnancy. If, however, a girl is to be born, the pregnancy is more difficult: the woman is in pain, her thighs and genitals slightly swollen, and a female foetus begins to move around day ninety.[13] Those claims were later taken over by Solinus:

> Plane si corpusculum in marem figuretur, melior est color gravidis et pronior partitudo uteri, denique a quadragesimo die motus. alter sexus nonagesimo primum die palpitat et concepta femina gestantis uultum pallore inficit, crura quoque praepedit languida tarditate.

> Certainly, if the little body is being fashioned into a male child, the colour of the mother is better, and the birth is easier. Also the baby begins to stir from the 40th day. A female first quivers after the 96th day. The conception of a female dyes the countenance of the pregnant mother with pallor. Also it hinders her legs with a faint lethargy.[14]

Folk medicine supplied practical advice on increasing the chances that the baby born would be of the desired gender, since 'science-based' medicine had little to offer in that regard. For example, women were advised to eat artichokes,

> nam Glaucias scribit cibum cardui adiuvare ut masculos procreent;

> for Glaucius writes that artichokes help birth males.[15]

The course of a normal pregnancy: Advice given to the pregnant

However, during pregnancy, the child's gender became a secondary concern. The Romans were aware that women needed to be particularly careful during pregnancy if they wanted to go through it safely and bear healthy children.[16] One piece of evidence is the preserved correspondence of Pliny the Younger. In a letter to Fabatus, his wife's grandfather, Pliny recounts the tragic events which occurred in his home:[17]

> Quo magis cupis ex nobis pronepotes videre, hoc tristior audies neptem tuam abortum fecisse, dum se praegnantem esse puellariter nescit, ac per hoc quaedam custodienda praegnantibus omittit, facit omittenda.

> I know how anxious you are for us to give you a great-grandchild, so you will be all the more sorry to hear that your granddaughter has had a miscarriage. Being young and inexperienced she did not realize she was pregnant, failed to take proper precautions, and did several things which were better left undone.[18]

Unfortunately, Pliny does not go into details about his wife's actions nor list the precautions, but it was common knowledge that the conditions in which a pregnant woman lived could affect the baby's development. Although some of the beliefs popular then were more of a folk superstition than anything else, it cannot be ruled out they were universally held and influenced women greatly. It is a shame that information about the broadly understood pregnancy hygiene, such as advice on lifestyle, nutrition and potential threats to avoid while pregnant, is generally so scant in the surviving sources,[19] but it was emphasized that if a pregnant woman did not respect her health, failed to follow the recommendations mentioned above, and risked illness, she created, possibly unwittingly, conditions which could contribute to a miscarriage or premature birth, so women were strongly advised to obey their doctors' orders. Soranus advises that throughout pregnancy the woman should avoid excessive gain or loss of weight, shun strong emotions, control her medication use and consumption of spicy food, and avoid blood-letting. Even though he carefully remarks that it may of course happen that even women who do not observe all the recommendations have a safe pregnancy and give birth to healthy offspring, he also points out that the formation of new life is affected by so many factors that nobody can predict which of them might prove harmful.[20] Still, it remains Soranus' greatest merit that he systematized existing knowledge on healthcare to be provided to pregnant women. To that purpose, he divided process into three stages. During the first stage, the goal was for the woman to keep the pregnancy; during the second, the goal was to take care of the pregnancy; during the third, the midwife should focus on correct preparations for labour and delivery.[21] Thus Soranus' text displays a *sui generis* holistic approach to the pregnant woman: one should take care of both her well-being and any issues to do with her health in general. Unfortunately, we do not know how widely his work was known or how universally his advice was followed. Was it a compilation of observations made by professionals (physicians, midwives) or a collection of measures and prescriptions that were already fairly common knowledge? For example, as we analyse the diet suggested for the pregnant woman to follow (see below), we may well doubt if any woman from outside the *nobilitas* circles could afford the dishes and foodstuffs included in it.

The first stage of pregnancy

The list of activities to avoid early in the pregnancy, since they could cause one to lose the foetus, is very long.[22] Soranus believes one should avoid all shocks, as if they do happen,

ἐξίεται γὰρ τὸ σπέρμα καὶ διὰ φόβον καὶ διὰ λύπην καὶ χαρὰν αἰφνίδιον καὶ καθόλου διανοίας ἰσχυρὰν ταραχὴν καὶ γυμνασίαν σφοδρὰν καὶ βιαίους κατοχὰς πνεύματος, βῆχας, πταρμούς, πληγάς, πτώματα, καὶ μᾶλλον τὰ ἐπὶ τῶν ἰσχίων, βάρους ἄρσεις, πηδήματα, σκληρὰς καθέδρας, φαρμακείας. δριμέων καὶ πταρμικῶν προσφοράν, ἔνδειαν, ἀπεψίαν, μέθην, ἔμετον, κοιλιολυσίαν, ῥύσιν αἵματος διὰ ῥινῶν καὶ αἱμορροΐδος ἢ ἄλλου τόπου καὶ χαλασμὸν διά τινος τῶν θερμαίνειν δυναμένων καὶ διὰ πυρετὸν δὲ σφοδρὸν καὶ ῥῖγος καὶ σπασμὸν καὶ τὸ κοινότερον πᾶν τὸ βιαίαν κίνησιν ἐπάγον, δι' ὧν ἔκτρωσις ἀποτελεῖται.[23]

For the seed is evacuated through fright, sorrow, sudden joy and, generally, by severe mental upset; through vigorous exercise, forced detention of the breath coughing, sneezing, blows, and falls, especially those on the hips; by lifting heavy weights, leaping, sitting on hard sedan chairs, by the administration of drugs, by the application of pungent substances and sternutatives; through want indigestation, drunkenness, vomiting, diarrhea; by a flow of blood from the nose, from hemorrhoids or other places; through relaxation due to some heating agent, through marked fever, rigors, cramps and, in general everything inducing a forcible movement by which a misscariage may be produced.

He also advises the pregnant woman to avoid sex in that time, so as not to disturb 'the uterus, which needs quiet'.[24]

The second stage of pregnancy

Around day forty, the second stage of the pregnancy begins. In Soranus' opinion, this is characterized by pica, that is, unexpected craving for inedible and less edible things, such as coal, earth, or unripe fruit. He thinks that in some women, those cravings (and digestive problems) last until the fourth month, while some others have an upset stomach until they give birth, and others still, not at all, so he recommends that each case be considered individually.[25]

Should nausea be frequent, Soranus' advice is to soothe the stomach by eating dry wheat bread and taking baths daily. If a stronger remedy is needed because of vomiting, he says to rub the woman's belly with oils: rose, myrtle, or mastic oil, as all three fortify a weakened stomach.[26] One alternative is to make a poultice of dried dates soaked in sour wine or vinegar (figs could be used in place of dates).[27] The mixture was applied onto the woman's abdomen, which was then wrapped in linen bandages. If the poultice failed to help too, a large heated cup would be applied near the stomach.[28]

To avoid the risk of upsetting the digestive system, or at least to reduce it, Soranus advises that the diet during this stage should be light,[29] including soft-boiled eggs and barley flour congee. The best poultry species, he writes, are those whose meat is considered delicate, that is, hazel grouse, partridge, mallard, fieldfare, thrush and pigeon; the best game, roe deer and hare. The meals of pregnant women should also contain a lot of fish, with mullet regarded as the healthiest and most suitable. While today, pregnant women are generally discouraged from eating shellfish, Roman women were advised to eat crabs, small lobsters and snails.[30] Other recommended foods were cooked vegetables, preferably steamed; it was emphasized that raw vegetables would cause flatulence and be difficult to digest. The vegetables listed most often were chicory, parsnip, asparagus and olives.[31] Of fruit well tolerated by women at this stage of pregnancy, pears, medlars, quince and grapes are mentioned most often. Soranus also recommends almonds, which are great at alleviating nausea, should it occur.[32] However, if a light diet was not enough and a woman experienced indigestion or heartburn, she should eat melons, drink water with cucumber seeds, drink sweet Cretan wine, spikenard tincture, or dittany of Crete.[33]

So Soranus; meanwhile, Pliny the Elder advises that the aches and ailments of pregnancy can be efficiently remedied with powdered dung of swine, wild or tame, mixed in with drink,[34] and pregnant women's unrestrained appetite can be controlled by drinking water with lemon seeds added.[35]

Among the foodstuffs mentioned by both Soranus and other ancient doctors was the radish, which was very popular in the regular diet of the Romans but believed too heavy for pregnant women. It was emphasized that during this stage, symptoms might include not only heartburn, loss of appetite or hunger for unusual foodstuffs and unripe, sour fruit, but also cravings which could endanger the woman's health or even life, such as for earth or stones.[36] According to superstition, if the pregnant woman ate food with too much salt in it, the newborn baby would have no nails.[37] In such a case, her close family was advised to explain this, telling her that satisfying her whim could harm both herself and the child.[38]

Soranus observes multiple times that the pregnant woman's diet affects the child and their health, since a foetus nourished by a healthy mother, being part of her body, would not fall ill either.[39] It was also thought some nutrients in particular influenced the baby's physical and intellectual development. Pliny, for instance, quotes one of such recipes for the perfect baby:

> Hermesias ab eodem vocatur ad liberos generandos pulchros bonosque non herba, sed conpositio nucleis pineae nucis tritis cum melle, murra, croco, vino palmeo, postea admixto theombrotio et lacte. bibere generaturos iubet et a conceptu, puerperas partum nutrientes; ita fieri excellentes animi et formae bonis.

> The same authority gives the name *hermesias* to a means of procreating children who shall be handsome and good. It is not a plant, but a compound of ground kernels of pine nuts with honey, myrrh, saffron and palm wine, with the later addition of theombrotion[40] and milk. He prescribes a draught of it to those who are about to become parents, after conception, and to nursing mothers. This, he says, results in children exceeding fair in mind and body, as well as good.[41]

The third stage of pregnancy

The would-be mum was advised to engage in a variety of activities before the seventh month of pregnancy began: walking, massage, bathing, speaking loudly, reading and sleeping. It was believed that with exercise, the body fortified itself and prepared for the hardship of labour. It was even stressed that difficult births were frequent in women who 'lived an idle life' while pregnant.[42]

Ancient physicians, Soranus among them, admonished women to be particularly careful in the seventh and eighth month of pregnancy, when they should refrain from sudden movements, and especially avoid riding in a cart:

> κατὰ δὲ τὸν ἕβδομον μῆνα τὰς μὲν σφοδροτέρας κινήσεις ὑφαιρετέον καὶ μάλιστα τὰς διὰ τῶν ὑποζυγίων, ταῖς δὲ ἄλλαις προσεκτικώτερον χρηστέον.

> At the seventh month she should give up the more violent movements and especially those caused by draught animals, while she should indulge in the others more cautiously.[43]

At this stage in their pregnancy, women were also advised not to press their nipples when bathing and applying olive oil to their skin:

εἰ δὲ μή, τοῖς προδεδιδαγμένοις χρῆσθαι. φυλάττεσθαι δὲ κατὰ τὰς τρίψεις ὀγκουμένων πλεῖον τῶν μαστῶν θλίβειν τὰς ὑπεροχὰς αὐτῶν, εὐχερῶς γὰρ ἀγανακτοῦντες ἀπόστασιν ὑπομένουσιν· διὸ καὶ τὰς συνήθεις στηθοδεσμίας ἐπιχαλῶσιν εἰς παραδοχὴν τῆς ἐπιδιογκώσεως τῶν μερῶν.

If, however, the breasts are considerably enlarged, one must take care, in rubbing, not to squeeze the tips, for being easily irritated, they are apt to develop an abscess; and for this reason women also slacken the customary breastbands to accommodate the enlarged parts.[44]

Another piece of advice was to protect (that is, support) the belly with a wide girdle or belt:

περιαλειπτέον δὲ καὶ κηρωτῇ τὸν ὄγκον δι᾽ ὀμφακίνου ἐλαίου καὶ μυρσίνου· τονουμένου γὰρ τοῦ δέρματος ῥήξεις οὐχ ὑπομένει, τηρεῖται δὲ ἀρρυτίδωτον.

One should also anoint the enlarged abdomen all over with a create containing oil made from unripe olives and myrtle, for if the skin is toned up it does not break, but is kept unwrinkled.[45]

The mixture so prepared strengthened the skin and was the most popular ancient way to avoid pregnancy stretch marks.[46]

Many doctors had a specific approach to women in their eighth month. The point was, on the one hand, to alleviate their various complaints at that stage, and on the other, to prevent premature birth, which was considered particularly risky for the child if it occurred then.[47] Thus the recommendations included little exercise, no long baths, and no intercourse.

However, with the eighth month coming to an end and the birth approaching, the woman was expected to untie the girdle supporting her belly, so that its weight could help induce labour, and warm baths became advisable so that 'the genital parts softened'. Other recommended ways of softening them were steam baths and hip-baths using a decoction of linseed, fenugreek, or mallow, as well as rinses with sweet olive oil or goose fat. Presumably the woman had to be in the care of a midwife by then, because the advice addressed at the midwife is common to 'anoint and widen with her finger the entrance to the uterus' even before delivery.[48] It was the midwife who examined the pregnant woman, diagnosed any abnormalities and decided if there was need to call for a doctor.[49]

Unusual pregnancies

Multiple pregnancy

As giving birth to more than one child at once – be it two, three, or four – was fairly rare and unexpected, reactions to it were sometimes ambivalent. Children from such births were seen as an excess, which could be interpreted as connected to abundance, fertility and welfare, or the other way round, to transgression, chaos, or even death.[50] It all depended on the circumstances of their birth and their numbers. Twins were usually welcome and seen as a sign of divine favour.[51] Plutarch praises the wisdom of nature, which has given women two breasts, so that if twins are born, there is a double source of nourishment. It was believed to be nature's way of defining the optimum number of children. Traces of such reasoning can be found in a series of terracotta images of breastfeeding mothers, symbols not just of motherhood but also of perfect fertility.[52]

Joy following the birth of twins was common to all social strata. As Tacitus wrote:

> Ceterum recenti adhuc maestitia soror Germanici Livia, nupta Druso, duos virilis sexus simul enixa est. Quod rarum laetumque etiam modicis penatibus tanto gaudio principem adfecit, ut non temperaverit quin iactaret apud patres nulli ante Romanorum eiusdem fastigii viro geminam stirpem editam: nam cuncta, etiam fortuita, ad gloriam vertebat.
>
> Germanicus' sister, Livia, who had married Drusus, was delivered of twin sons. The event, a rare felicity even in modest households, affected the emperor with so much pleasure that he could not refrain from boasting to the Fathers that never before had twins been born to a Roman of the same eminence: for he converted everything, accidents included, into material for self-praise.[53]

At times, that attitude was also present when more than two children were born. When it was triplets, references were made to the legendary, heroic Horatii who had fought the Curiatii from Alba, likewise triplets.[54] Dionysius of Halicarnassus explains that the two sets of triplets were born of twin sisters, daughters of the king of Alba, one of whom had married the Roman Horatius, while the other had become the wife of the Alban Curiatius. The sisters gave birth to their respective triplets on the same day and both communities took the event as an auspicious sign.[55] Another author, Aulus Gellius, recounts the birth of quintuplets – children of a servant to emperor Augustus – as something heroic, but also tragic, as the children died soon after birth. He reports that 'a monument was erected to her by order of Augustus on the via Laurentina, and on it was inscribed the number of her children'.[56] Strabo wrote that in Egypt, believed to be a land of exceptionally fertile women, one woman had given birth to septuplets, a story repeated in Pliny the Elder, although he only quoted the dry fact without specifying whether the children had been born alive and if so, whether they had lived through infancy.[57]

Still, in many cases simultaneous birth of three, four or more children was regarded as ominous. Although few sources present the attitudes of the public to the matter, some texts do cast multiple pregnancies in a bad light. In the *Liber prodigiorum*, Julius Obsequens lists triplets being born among the sinister phenomena that happened in 163 BCE: 'At Tarracina, male triplets were born ... At Privernum a girl was born without any hands ... At Caere a pig was born with human hands and feet, and children were born with four feet and four hands.'[58] The author does not specify if the triplets were born live and physically normal, but their birth was in a sense treated on par with the birth of deformed children.[59] In the *Historia Augusta*, too, the birth of quintuplets comes up on a similar list of alarming events which disturb the natural order:

> Adversa eius temporibus haec provenerunt: fames, de qua diximus, Circi ruina, terrae motus, quo Rhodiorum et Asiae oppida conciderunt ... et Romae incendium, quod trecentas quadraginta insulas vel domos absumpsit. ... fuit et inundatio Tiberis, apparuit et stella crinita, natus estet biceps puer, et uno partu mulieris quinque pueri editi sunt.

> The following misfortunes and prodigies occurred in his reign: the famine, which we have just mentioned, the collapse of the Circus, an earthquake whereby towns of Rhodes and of Asia were destroyed ... and a fire at Rome which consumed three hundred and forty tenements and dwellings ... Besides, the Tiber flooded its banks, a comet was seen, a two-headed child was born, and a woman gave birth to quintuplets.[60]

Pliny adds that towards the end of Augustus' reign, a woman by name of

> Fausta quaedam e plebe Ostiae duos mares, totidemque feminas enixa famem, quae consecuta est, portendit haud dubie.

> Fausta at Ostia was delivered of two male and two female infants, which unquestionably portended the food shortage that followed.[61]

There is no mention of whether the children lived, but Pliny does say such unusual births tended to herald famine. Disquieting accounts of multiple births are also to be found in Artemidorus' *Oneirocritica*. One of them recounts:

Ἔδοξέ τις γυνὴ ἐν τῇ σελήνῃ τρεῖς ὁρᾶν εἰκόνας ἰδίας. ἐγέννησε τρίδυμα θηλυκά, καὶ τὰ τρία τοῦ αὐτοῦ μηνὸς ἀπέθανεν. ἦσαν γὰρ αἱ εἰκόνες τὰ τέκνα, εἷς δὲ περιεῖχεν αὐτὰς κύκλος. τοιγάρτοι ἑνὶ χορίῳ, ὥς λέγουσιν ἰατρῶν παῖδες, περιείχετο τὰ βρέφη. ἔζησε δὲ οὐ πλείονα [χρόνον] διὰ τὴν σελήνην.

A woman dreamt that she saw three likenesses of herself on the moon. She gave birth to femat triplets and all three died in the same month. For the likenesses were the children, and a single circle surrounded them. Accordingly, then, the babies were enclosed within a single foetal envelope, as a doctors maintain. They did not live longer because of the moon.[62]

Even though our sources are few, it is likely that multiple pregnancies and births were very dangerous to the women.[63] Pliny remarks that even with twins, 'It is said that at the birth of twins neither the mother nor more than one of the two children usually lives'.[64]

Molar pregnancy

Not every time a woman's belly was enlarged, her period stopped, and her breasts were swollen could a baby be expected. Sometimes those symptoms indicated illness. Molar pregnancy is a form of apparent pregnancy, recognized in Graeco-Roman medical literature. It was usually seen as a kind of tumour. In Festus, in his extracts from Valerius Flaccus' *De verborum significatione*, one finds this explanation:

> Molucrum non solum quo molae verruntur dicitur, id quod Graeci μυλήκορον appellant, sed etiam tumor ventris, qui etiam virginibus incidere solet: cuius meminit Afranius in Virgine.
>
> *Molucrum* means not only the broom with which the mill is swept, which the Greeks call *mylékoron*, but also an abdominal tumor which tends to occur even in virgins, as mentioned by Afranius in his play *Virgo*.[65]

There is also a mention of apparent pregnancy in Soranus, who calls it *myle* or *mylos* and describes it as a hardening of the uterus caused by inflammation or sometimes a tumour growth. *Mylos* means *millstone*, a name reflective of the nature of the tumour, which is hard, heavy, and occasionally located at one point in the uterus, but much more often filling all of it, resulting in significant swelling of the abdomen. At the same time, periods cease, the breasts swell, the stomach is upset, the loins become heavy and the lower abdomen expands. As demonstrated above, all those symptoms could, in the opinion of ancient people, indicate pregnancy, but over tine, a clear distinction becomes observable: sharp pangs appear and no movement of a baby can be felt, unlike in pregnant women.

Soranus goes so far as to describe treatment for the disease, consisting in blood-letting, rinses, exercise and bathing in the sea. Pliny, in turn, describes the mole as a curiosity. He calls it a shapeless, lifeless growth, which cannot be either cut or punctured with iron. The mole moves around and stops menstrual bleeding just like a foetus would; it results in death sometimes, while on other occasions it grows old with the woman or is removed by acute diarrhoea.[66] Plutarch writes that while no woman ever has conceived without the help of a man, misshapen fleshy growths on the uterus exist, called μύλαι, which he believes to result from infection. Those grow to become hard and homogeneous.[67]

It was *molucrum* that the heroine invoked in Afranius' *Virgo*. With her belly growing, suspected by all of being pregnant and so of loose conduct, she wants to deny the suspicions and claims that it is in fact a mole, not a pregnancy.[68]

Miscarriage

Pliny really wanted to have children and so extend his family line. Before marrying Calpurnia, he had had two other wives, but no children were born of them.[69] In *Epistulae* 8.10, a letter I have already referred to above (dated by Sherwin-White[70] to 107 CE), he informs his young wife's family of her miscarriage. He presumably knew the news would make her grandfather Fabatus upset and disappointed; Calpurnia, too, was her family's only chance at descendants. There is no agreement among researchers on whether the marriage was made in 97 CE or 104 CE, but regardless, they had waited for that first pregnancy for either three or even ten years.[71] Pliny may have suspected Fabatus would regret marrying his granddaughter to a man who had no offspring from his previous marriages, and it is worth noting the letter contains nothing to reassure the family Calpurnia is feeling better, but its author does emphasize that the miscarriage proves her fertility with the very fact his young wife has conceived, indicating that 'the future looks hopeful'.[72] Clearly, he was afraid of Fabatus' reaction. He also stresses the miscarriage was not his wife's fault and instead happened by accident, although Calpurnia could hardly have had a deliberate abortion, since she knew how impatiently the whole family awaited her child. The pressure from both their families must have been enormous.[73]

Similar pressure must have been felt by many young wives who lost pregnancies. If an early pregnancy was lost, doctors usually advised them to try again, suggesting quiet and taking care of oneself, in terms of both general health and genital health in particular. Besides medical advice, sources contain some other information: advice, myths and superstitions, probably quite widespread and popular, on potential threats and avoiding them. For example Pliny, in his advice on preventing miscarriage, points to the beneficial effects of smoking (or curing) a lizard: 'Afterwards they fasten the lizard to a reed and hang it in smoke, and they say that as it dies the baby recovers.'[74] Amulets made from 'Samian stone' were liked by many; they supposedly protected pregnant women and reduced the risk of miscarriage.[75] Similar properties were attributed to aetites, which 'protects a foetus from all plots to cause abortion'.[76] Excessive bleeding after a miscarriage was thought to be treatable with a drink made of leeks. Dioscorides believed that in case of such haemorrhage a potion should be served containing seven scruples of leek seeds and the same amount of myrtle berries.[77]

Some women miscarried often, which did not mean they would never become mothers. Pliny writes that there are women who cannot carry to term (read, miscarry often), but 'if ever they succeed in overcoming this tendency by the use of drugs, usually bear a female child'.[78] Still, in his own case, Calpurnia's loss of pregnancy was a dark moment in their marriage, and the couple would never have a child.[79] Miscarriage would sometimes (especially later into the pregnancy) result in the mother dying as well. A sepulchral inscription is known for Tineia Hieropis, a married woman, her body buried (by her father) alongside that of her premature (or actually, miscarried) baby.[80]

Soranus underlines that occasionally miscarriage or death of the foetus are spontaneous, and lists symptoms which could point to imminent miscarriage:

Μελλούσης δὲ γίνεσθαι τῆς τοῦ ἐμβρύου φθορᾶς ταῖς φθειρούσαις παρακολουθεῖ κένωσις ὑδατώδης, εἶτα ἰχωρώδης ἢ ὕφαιμον ὑγρὸν καὶ οἷον ἀποπλύματα κρεῶν, ὅταν δὲ καιρὸς τῆς ἀπολύσεως ὑπάρχῃ, αἷμα καθαρόν, ἐπὶ τέλει δὲ θρόμβος αἵματος ἢ [τι] σαρκὸς ἀδιατύπωτον ἢ διατετυπωμένον παρὰ τὴν τοῦ χρόνου διαφοράν· ταῖς δὲ πλείσταις βάρος καὶ πόνος ὀσφύος καὶ ἰσχίων καὶ ἤτρου, βουβώνων. κεφαλῆς, ὀφθαλμῶν, ἄρθρων, στομάχου δῆξις, περίψυξις, περιίδρωσις, λειποθυμία, ποτὲ δὲ καὶ φρικώδης πυρετός, ταῖς δὲ καὶ λυγμὸς ἢ σπασμὸς ἢ ἀφωνία.

Besides, in most aborting women there is heaviness and pain of the loins, hips, and lower abdomen, of the groins, head, eyes, joints; a gnawing in the stomach, shivering and profuse perspiration, fainting, sometimes also a fever with chills, and in some cases hiccup or cramps or loss of voice.[81]

As Hippocrates says, in people about to miscarry those symptoms are preceded by breasts sagging, a sign confirmed also in Celsus.[82]

Thus the symptoms of the foetus dying include an outflow of the waters and suppurating fluid followed by bleeding, blood clots, or the foetus (depending on how advanced the pregnancy was). That is preceded by pains in the abdomen, hips and back, although Diocles adds headache, stomach ache, nausea, cold or hot flashes and cramps to the list.[83]

As for when it is possible for a woman to miscarry, Pliny maintains it happens to

> gravidis autem quarto et octavo mense, letalesque in iis abortus,
>
> mothers in the fourth and eighth months of pregnancy; and abortions in these cases are fatal,[84]

while Celsus believes miscarriage may also depend on weather and the season.[85]

Other factors believed to cause miscarriage included illness (such as gastroenteritis)[86] and eating various plants and herbs. For instance, Pliny warns pregnant women not to eat fern, as it may cause miscarriage (or, in women who are not pregnant, infertility).[87] In such cases, the procedure was to induce labour and remove the dead foetus to prevent intrauterine infection, relying on the help of various drugs, such as thyme.[88] Similar properties were attributed to powder made from 'the ashes of a mare's hoof'[89] and 'a pessary made from hare's gall mixed with leek sap and iris ointment'.[90] A dead foetus could also be removed with a 'pessary soaked in [bull's] gall with marjoram oil and hellebore oil',[91] 'the growth found on the knees of mules, drunk in honey',[92] 'savory, ground and applied to the skin of the belly',[93] or '[cabbage] eaten raw with vinegar'.[94]

The pregnant Marcia and the thunderbolt

At times, death of the foetus was attributed to unusual phenomena. One such case was the last pregnancy of Cato's wife Marcia. In book two of his *Natural History*, Pliny presents a short dissertation on lightning, and while he is at it, he mentions this event:

> Marcia ... princeps Romanarum, icta gravida partu exanimato ipsa citra ullum aliud incommodum vixit.
>
> Marcia, a lady of high station at Rome, was struck by lightning when enceinte, and though the child was killed, she herself survived without being otherwise injured.[95]

The story, seemingly dealing with weather phenomena, indicates that the lightning did Marcia no harm, but she did not know the same strike killed her baby. She is known as the mother of Cato's three children, two daughters and a son, but the unborn child whose death is recounted here was presumably her fourth pregnancy, as no other source mentions it[96]. Its omission from the biography by Plutarch becomes less of a surprise if one remembers that sources in general tend to ignore dead infants and toddlers.

Not all miscarriages ended as harmlessly for the women as in the cases of Pliny's wife Calpurnia or Cato's wife Marcia. Many must have died as they miscarried, as did Grata, honoured with an epitaph by her despairing husband, left alone with three young children:

> Veturia Grata // Vel nunc morando resta qui perges iter / etiam dolentis casus adversos lege / Trebius Basileus coniunx quae scripsi dolens / ut scire possis infra scripta pectoris / rerum bonarum fuit haec ornata suis / innocua simplex quae numquam servavit dolum / annos quae vixit XXI et mensibus(!) VII / genuitque ex me tres natos quos reliquit parvulos / repleta quartum utero mense octavo obit / attonitus capita nunc versorum inspice / titulum merentis oro perlegas libens / agnosces nomen coniugis Gratae meae
>
> Veturia Grata. Stop now and pay attention (and continue your journey later) and read about this untimely misfortune. Read what I, Trebius Basileus, her husband, have written in my grief, so that you may be able to preserve deep in your heart what is written below. To her own she was blessed with good qualities. She was blameless, artless and never a slave to deceit. She lived twenty-one years and seven months and produced with my help three children whom she left behind when they were still small. Her womb filled for a fourth time; in her eighth month she died. Now look in wonder at the first letters of these verses. I beseech you, read all the way through the epitaph of this deserving woman. Thus you shall learn the name of my wife, Grata.[97]

Male violence and the death of pregnant women

Unfortunately, occasionally the death of pregnant women was caused by violence from those closest to them.[98] One such woman was apparently Regilla, the wife of Herodes Atticus:

> ἦλθεν ἐπὶ τὸν Ἡρώδην καὶ φόνου δίκη ὧδε ξυντεθεῖσα· κύειν μὲν αὐτῷ τὴν γυναῖκα Ῥήγιλλαν ὄγδοόν που μῆνα, τὸν δὲ Ἡρώδην οὐχ ὑπὲρ μεγάλων

Ἀλκιμέδοντι ἀπελευθέρῳ προστάξαι τυπτῆσαι αὐτήν, πληγεῖσαν δὲ ἐς τὴν γαστέρα τὴν γυναῖκα ἀποθανεῖν ἐν ὠμῷ τῷ τόκῳ.

> A charge of murder was also brought against Herodes, and it was made up in this way. His wife Regilla, it was said, was in the eighth month of her pregnancy, and Herodes ordered his freedman Alcimedon to beat her for some slight fault, and the woman died in premature childbirth from a blow in the belly.[99]

Of course, similarities come to mind between that and the actions of emperor Nero, who kicked the pregnant Poppaea in his anger and as a result she died.[100] S. Pomeroy thinks violence was common in Herodes' marriage, as indicated by mentions of his explosive personality, but why would he have had his pregnant wife whipped? Philostratus only writes the reason was trivial. Later in his discussion he even goes so far as to express the opinion that saying Herodes issued any such orders is slander, seeing evidence for his innocence in how he mourned. Regilla's brother sued. According to Pomeroy, the senators acquiesced to the will of emperor Antoninus Pius and found the charges baseless.[101] Ultimately neither Herodes nor the freedman who allegedly did the whipping suffered any punishment. As M. Pawlak thinks, Herodes may have ordered Regilla punished for some reason or other, but he certainly did not want her dead.[102] We will likely never know the actual cause, but the event is a good opportunity to take a look at research into violence against women. Susan Deacy emphasizes that studies of ancient Greek cases of pregnant women being killed imply that abuse of power and violence resulted from the patriarchal character of ancient societies. However, applying evolutionary psychology analysis can also lead to the conclusion that violence during pregnancy should also be seen as connected with sexual jealousy and uncertainty regarding presumed paternity.[103]

Although Philostratus does not say what Regilla's punishment was for, he tells the reader not only that she was pregnant, but also how far along. Pomeroy considers that a deliberate move intended to speak in Herodes' favour during the trial,[104] all because of the then widespread belief that children born in the eighth month of the pregnancy are unlikely to live. Philostratus recounts that due to the whipping, Regilla gave birth prematurely first, and only died later,[105] and there are some reasons to believe the child did survive a short while.[106] Pawlak writes that in 1866 in Kifisii (Κηφισιά), next to a tomb then discovered, an epigrammatic epitaph was found dedicated to a child named Herodes, whose father was Herodes Atticus. The text implies Herodes was already in mourning for someone close to him (possibly his wife) when his son died, so it is possible the deceased

Herodes, who the epigram says lived three months, was Regilla's final child and a victim of his father's violence.[107]

'The lucky have children in three months'[108]

Reportedly, this was the saying which went around in Rome when Livia gave birth to a son, Drusus, three months after her marriage to Octavian, but Drusus was actually a child of Tiberius Claudius, whom Livia had just divorced. And while Octavian sent the boy off to his father, there were still sarcastic rumours in Rome. The anecdote, found in Cassius Dio, led to the question of how the Romans determined how many months pregnant a woman was, if they even did. There are in fact many mentions in the sources of when many famous people were born, which raises the same question. Was the prospective date of birth calculated in advance and if so, how?

Unfortunately, due to unfamiliarity with the menstrual cycle and there being no methods with which to determine early stages of pregnancy, both telling which month it was and calculating the date of the birth in advance must have relied on a collection of many observations and experiences, often quite imprecise. Still, for legal reasons (usually to do with inheritance or establishing paternity), attempts were made to determine the month of the pregnancy. The general principle was that the father was the mother's husband if the child was born no earlier than in the seventh month after the marriage began and no later than the tenth after it ended, provided however that the marriage was a *iustum matrimonium*.[109] Generally speaking, though, doctors estimated gestational age based on their experiences, observations, the accounts of others, and their own philosophical theories.[110] In Pliny's opinion, there is no such thing as a clearly defined duration of pregnancy. A human being 'is born throughout the year and after an uncertain time, one in the seventh month, another in the eighth, and so on until the tenth and early eleventh. No person born before the seventh month will live'. However, even being born in that month was considered rare, with children born then regarded as unlikely to survive. In a letter to Atticus, Cicero announces the birth of a grandson he had looked forward to:

> Tullia mea peperit xiiii Kal. Iun. puerum ἑπταμηνιαῖον. quod ηὐτόκησεν gaudeam; quod quidem est natum perimbecillum est.
>
> My Tullia has given birth to a seven months' child, a boy, on 19 May. For her safe delivery let me be thankful. As for the baby, it is very weakly.[111]

It is widely accepted that the question of the so-called conception period was already regulated by the Law of the Twelve Tables. The specific regulation, reconstructed based on Aulus Gellius' *Attic Nights*, where it comes up in the chapter on ancient physicians and philosophers debating the length of pregnancy, may have gone as follows: *Si qui ei in x. mensibus proximis postumus natus escit, iustus esto*.[112] A similar opinion was expressed by Plautus in his comedy *Aulularia*:

> quem ego auom feci iam ut esses filiai nuptiis? nam tua gnata peperit, decumo mense post: numerum cape;
>
> I've made you a grandfather on your daughter's wedding: your daughter's given birth, nine months later. Calculate for yourself.[113]

There is already something in Gellius about the formation of the foetus, and so indirectly about the predicted length of pregnancy, a few chapters earlier. The author notes there that seven days from fertilization, the embryo becomes able to 'take form'. Four weeks from the beginning, gender is defined, and forty-nine (seven times seven) days into the pregnancy, the human being is already fully formed. The power and influence of the number seven goes even farther, since before the seventh month is over, no viable birth is possible, either of a boy or a girl.[114] Thus if the pregnancy progressed normally, birth should occur 273 days after conception, that is, at the onset of week forty.[115] Still, premature births did happen, as did post-term pregnancies, and it is those that are discussed in chapter 16 of book three of the *Attic Nights*. Introducing the discussion, the author tells the reader he is presenting the opinions of ancient physicians, philosophers, poets, and other information of note.

According to Gellius, children are only rarely born in the seventh month, and Pliny adds that if they are, then they were conceived the day before the full moon, the day after the full moon, or on the day of the new moon.[116]

Invoking his 'philosophers and physicians', without specifying any names, Gellius writes that children are rarely born in the seventh month, never in the eighth, often in the ninth and most often in the tenth. That was also the common belief. It was traditionally accepted that children were born in the ninth or tenth month, as reflected, in the opinion of ancient Romans, in the names of the Parcae Nona and Decima.[117] Importantly, when referring to the tenth month, Gellius clarifies that ten full months are meant, not nine months and the tenth underway.[118] Censorinus is another author who believes there is no consensus regarding the length of pregnancy and emphasizes that although scholars have long debated in which month since conception babies are usually born, they have not been able to reach unambiguous conclusions. In his opinion, Hippo of Metapontum estimated that birth could occur between the seventh and tenth month of the pregnancy, since the foetus is already mature by the seventh, and the number seven is the most important in all things in general.[119] His opinion was shared by the Pythagorean Theano, Aristotle, Diocles, Euenor, Strato, Empedocles and Epigenes. Euryphon of Cnidus, meanwhile, consistently disagreed that birth in the seventh month was even possible, although he did think, unlike many others, that an eighth-month normal birth could happen.[120]

The eighth month

Another quote Gellius has about birth in the eighth month is the enigmatically worded claim of Hippocrates that any baby born then 'simultaneously does and does not exist'. Apparently another physician, Sabinus, explained that mysterious utterance by saying the baby does exist in that it seems to be alive, but also does not, because it dies immediately. Born alive, the child has no chance to stay that way.[121] It was quite widely accepted that eighth-month births are not viable, although Censorinus' opinions tended to follow from the mathematical theories he professed rather than medical knowledge, observation and experience.[122]

Eighth-month birth, should it happen, could lead to many legal problems. Gellius cites another story, this one centred on verifying that the *ius trium liberorum* has been acquired.[123] There was some debate as to whether a child born in the eighth month of the pregnancy, dead soon after birth, could be taken into account when granting that privilege. From Gellius it would seem not, as lawyers believed an eighth-month birth should be seen as a miscarriage. Still, the question arises in the case under discussion of whether the birth should not be counted because of occurring in the eighth month or because the child died soon after. Perhaps Gellius did think that only miscarriage was possible in the eighth month, but he could hardly have not known that for the right of three children to apply, the baby needed to live at least until the *dies nominum*, even if the birth happened in the ninth or tenth month.[124]

In Pliny's opinion, eighth-month births are common in Egypt, and in Italy, too; contrary to what the ancients used to think, children born in the eighth month often survive. He quotes examples, one of them being Caesonia, daughter of Pomponius and wife of emperor Caligula. However, the life of those born in the eighth month is in danger until day forty, although unfortunately Pliny does not explain why.[125]

Post-term pregnancy

Due to legal consequences, discussions of maximum pregnancy length were more important than those on eighth-month birth, especially if the child was born *postumus*.[126] The Law of the Twelve Tables ruled that a posthumous child inherits if the birth is live and occurs before ten months pass from conception. However, it must have been a common problem for children to be born later than that, because the matter comes up in Varro too. He writes that in that case children born in the eleventh month counting from the death of the testator should be included as well as children born in the tenth, as their rights are the same.[127] Gellius' support for this is actually Homer, in whose work Poseidon, leaving the girl he had just had sex with, told her to rejoice, as she would give birth after a year passed.[128] Gellius himself relied on the philosopher Favorinus for his interpretation of the passage.[129]

Another example in the *Attic Nights* is one of a woman of immaculate reputation who had a child in the eleventh month since her husband's death, resulting in a debate on whether the child should be considered posthumous or illegitimate. Invoking the Law of the Twelve Tables, her opponents claimed the child could not be regarded as the dead man's, because it were born later than ten months after his death. The matter reached the emperor. Having inquired, Hadrian ruled that it was possible for a baby to be born as late as the eleventh month of the pregnancy, supporting his verdict with the opinions of ancient physicians and philosophers.[130]

Gellius also remarked that when listing examples of post-term pregnancies, one must not omit one hardly credible piece of information recounted by Pliny in book seven of his *Natural History*.[131] Quoting Masurius Sabinus, a lawyer contemporary with Tiberius, Pliny wrote of a ruling issued by praetor Lucius Papirius, who denied a remote inheritor, because he believed the inheritance should fall to a posthumous child. The context indicates that the man trying to claim the inheritance believed himself in the right, because the child was born in the thirteenth month counting from the death of the mother's husband. The woman insisted she had in fact carried the foetus for thirteen months. The praetor believed her, and justified his decision with the explanation that the law did not clearly define the maximum possible length of pregnancy.[132]

Pregnancy in the light of visual sources

In his *De consolatione ad Helviam matrem*, Seneca writes of his mother thus:

numquam te fecunditatis tuae, quasi exprobraret aetatem, puduit, numquam more aliarum, quibus omnis commendatio ex forma petitur, tumescentem uterum abscondisti quasi indecens onus, nec intra viscera tua conceptas spes liberorum elisisti.

you have never blushed for the number of your children, as if it taunted you with your years, never have you, in the manner of other women whose only recommendation lies in their beauty, tried to conceal your pregnancy as if an unseemly burden, nor have you ever crushed the hope of children that were being nurtured in your body.[133]

However, this is unfortunately an isolated case; descriptions of pregnant women are extremely rare in Roman sources, so it is not clear to us today what Seneca meant by 'you have never ... tried to conceal your pregnancy'. Could he have meant some custom of Roman women hiding their pregnancy from view, or was it just about some specific pregnancy clothing? Perhaps flaunting a pregnancy belly was not a done thing. While we have hundreds of terracotta figurines of mothers with infants and toddlers, images of pregnant women are much less common.[134] One such preserved image is a headless statue of a pregnant woman, probably left as a votive offering in a temple at Halatte.[135]

Another, much more primitive image in soft limestone, also a votive offering,[136] likewise depicts a pregnant woman (?). The belly, represented by a clearly protruding sphere, sits in the centre of an armless body.

In the Wellcome Collection, there is another sculpture, a terracotta figure of a woman, unfortunately lacking the head and arms. It is a votive offering, perhaps an expression of hope or gratitude for a lucky birth (Photograph 5). Then there is the image shown in Photograph 6, also a depiction of a pregnant woman.[137]

The figurines of naked pregnant women found during archaeological excavations in Caura and other places in Spain are much more schematic and less elaborate. M. Oria Segura believes they may have been votive offerings and gifts left in temples of Dea Caelestis by worshippers praying for pregnancy or for safe delivery.[138]

Moreover it needs to be strongly emphasized that visual sources warrant great caution, especially if the exact place they were discovered is unknown or unconfirmed.[139]

The dearth of visual sources for pregnancy in Roman culture goes hand in hand with the frankly astonishing lack of discussion on pregnant women, their looks, moods and states of mind. Of course, that is largely a result of the fact that culture was the work of men, for whom the product (that is, offspring) was much

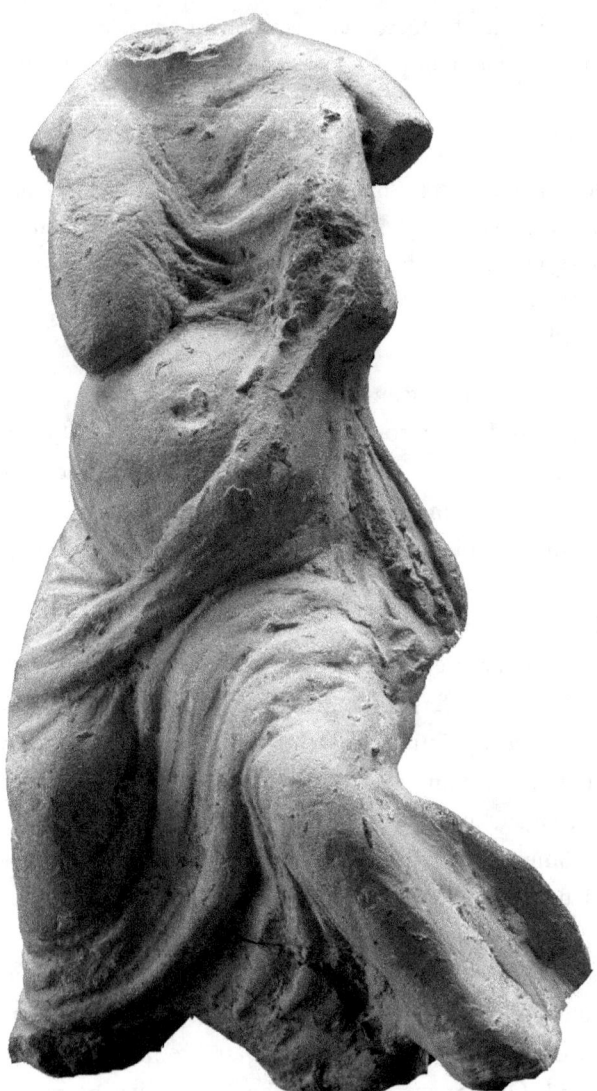

Figure 5 Pregnant woman (a votive offering?) © Wellcome Collection (CC BY 4.0).
Source: https://wellcomecollection.org/works/pq2ng4qh

more interesting than the process (that is, pregnancy). As N. Kampen writes, 'children born and alive, children miscarried, born dead, dead in infancy, worries about the lack of children: these signal patriarchal concerns among elite men for whom heirs mattered at least as much as did affective relationships'.[140] But there are no debates over pregnancy and hardly any depictions of it. Kampen wonders

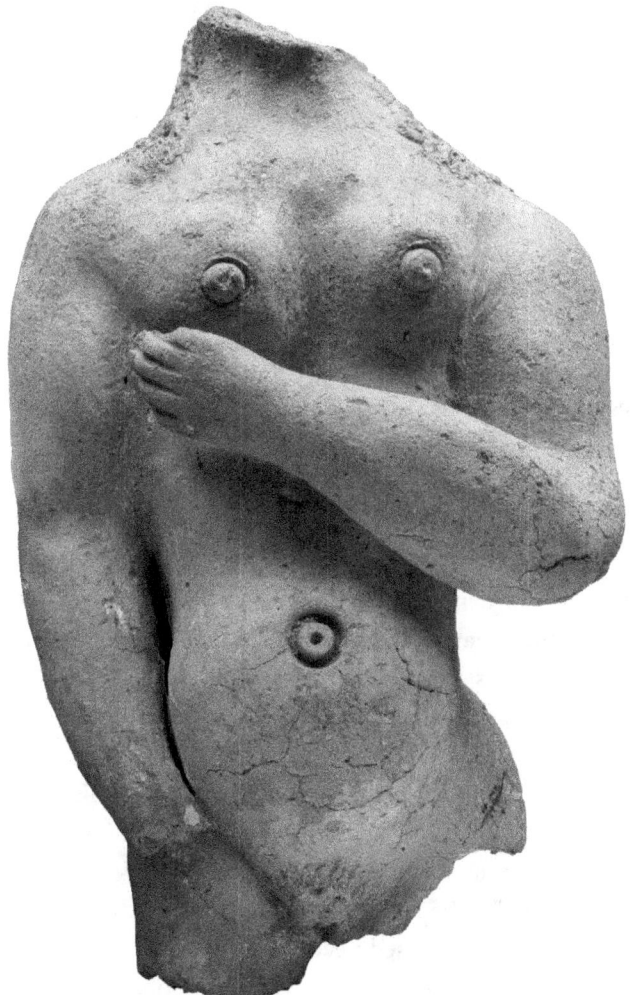

Figure 6 Pregnant woman. A votive offering found in Suffolk © Wellcome Collection (CC BY 4.0).
Source: https://wellcomecollection.org/works/mdncfvbn

if the reticence in describing that period, so important in a person's life, stems from modesty. Or was pregnancy not highlighted because it was seen as unclean or overly sexual? Or was there a connection to fear of investing one's emotions and attention in a person who might simply die in childbirth? She emphasizes that in a culture where women's voice is virtually unknown to us, and images of women were created by men, there is little those images can tell us of women's relationships to their bodies, and so of pregnancy,[141] a subject on which the men are unwilling to speak up.

5

Parturition

'But let her who is with child unbind her hair before she prays, in order that the goddess may gently unbind her teeming womb'[1]

Symptoms of the onset of labour

Birth is one of the few experiences that are, beyond any doubt, common to all people. It is no wonder that the moment a child is born, often called a miracle in spite of medical progress, fascinates not just biologists and physicians, but also historians, anthropologists and ethnographers.

In the opinion of ancient authors, symptoms of imminent labour include a feeling of heaviness in the abdomen, an ache around the hips, and the uterus descending characteristically. Under examination, a midwife would feel a softened cervix and the appearance of mucus. Soranus observes that right before the onset of labour the by then large foetus puts pressure the urinary bladder, so that the woman feels an increased need to urinate. Also before birth, a mucus plug appears, either clear or coloured with the blood from bursting blood vessels.[2]

Normal labour

Births took place in rooms which people tried to specially arrange for the occasion. If possible, a midwife was called, who should prepare olive oil, warm water, a soft natural sponge, several pieces of woollen fabric, a head pillow, bandages with which to swaddle the newborn child, a pillow on which to place the child until the placenta was passed, and finally a birthing stool or chair.[3] In the house, two beds ought to be made ready, one hard for use during delivery, and one soft for the woman to rest on after.[4]

The first stage of labour

During the first stage of labour, the woman giving birth would lie on a low bed with her hips supported, her feet placed together and her thighs spread apart. As the birth progressed, the midwife could try to speed up the process by massaging the cervix with the oiled index finger of her left hand.[5] When the dilatation reached the size of a chicken egg, the woman was moved to a birthing chair, provided she was strong enough and it looked like the birth would be easy.[6]

The second stage of labour

The second stage took place on the birthing chair.[7] Obese women and women with spine problems were, however, advised to remain on the bed on their knees and elbows so that the uterus would drop and line up with the cervix, which was supposed to facilitate the delivery. The same was recommended if the people accompanying the woman giving birth realized it would be multiple.[8] Still, it was generally believed labour would be easier if the woman were sitting up, that is, preferably on the birthing chair.

Soranus describes such a chair in detail. In the seat, there was a semicircular opening, which

> δεῖ δὲ κατὰ τὴν μεσότητα τοῦ δίφρου καὶ καθ' ὃ μέρος ἐπικουφίζουσιν, μηνοειδῶς σύμμετρον εὐρυχωρίαν ἐκκεκόφθαι πρὸς τὸ μήτε μείζονος αὐτῆς ὑπαρχούσης [μήτε μικροτέρας] μέχρι τῶν ἰσχίων καταφέρεσθαι, μήτε τοὐναντίον στενῆς [εἰς τὸ μὴ] πιέζεσθαι τὸ γυναικεῖον αἰδοῖον, ὅπερ χαλεπώτερον, τὴν γὰρ πλατυτέραν ἔκτρησιν ἐνδέχεται προσεκπληροῦν ῥάκη παραβάλλουσαν. τοῦ δὲ ὅλου δίφρου τὸ σύμπαν πλάτος ἱκανὸν ἔστω πρὸς τὸ καὶ τὰς εὐσαρκοτέρας χωρεῖν γυναῖκας, σύμμετρον δὲ καὶ τὸ ὕψος, ταῖς γὰρ μικρομεγέθεσιν ὑποπόδιον ὑποτιθέμενον ἀναπληροῖ τὸ ἐλλεῖπον. τῶν δὲ ὑπὸ τῆς ἕδρας πλευρῶν τὰ μὲν ἐκ πλαγίων ὅλα σανίσιν ἐσκεπάσθω, τὸ δὲ ἔμπροσθεν καὶ τὸ ὄπισθεν ἀνεῴχθω πρὸς τὴν λεχθησομένην ἐν ταῖς μαιώσεσιν χρείαν. ἐκ δὲ τῶν ἄνω πλευρῶν κατὰ μὲν τὰ πλάγια μέρη δύο πιοειδῆ τυγχανέτω τῷ διαπήγματι πρὸς τὸ κατὰ τὰς ἐντάσεις ἐπ' αὐτὰ τὰς χεῖρας ἐνστηρίζειν, ἐξόπισθεν δὲ ἀνάκλιτον, ὥστε καὶ τὴν ὀσφὺν καὶ τὰ ἰσχία τὸ ἀντιβαῖνον ταῖς ὑπαναχωρήσεσιν ἔχειν· εἰ γὰρ καὶ γυναικὸς ἐξόπισθεν ἑστώσης ἀνακλιθεῖεν, τῷ ἀνωμάλῳ σχηματισμῷ παραποδίζουσιν τὴν ἐπ' εὐθεῖαν τοῦ ἐμβρύου φοράν. ἔνιοι δὲ κατὰ τὰ κάτω μέρη τοῦ δίφρου ἔκθετον ἄξονα προσβάλλουσιν ἐξ ἑκατέρου μέρους περιαγωγίδας ἔχοντα καὶ τύλον, ἵνα ἐν ταῖς ἐμβρυουλκίαις περιτιθέντες βρόχους ἢ σπάρτα κυκλοτερῶς τοῖς βραχίοσιν ἢ ἄλλοις μέρεσιν

τοῦ ἐμβρύου καὶ τὰς ἀρχὰς ἀποδήσαντες πρὸς τὸν τύλον [διὰ] τῆς περιαγωγῆς τὴν ὁλκὴν ποιήσωνται, μὴ συνιέντες τὸ κοινόν, ὅτι τὴν ἐμβρυουλκίαν ἐπὶ κατακειμένης δεῖ γίνεσθαι τῆς δυστοκούσης. δεῖ δὴ τοιοῦτον εἶναι δίφρον οἷον εἰρήκαμεν, ἢ καθέδραν ἔμπροσθεν ἢ καὶ ὄπισθεν ἐκτετμημένην. †ἐκ κοιλοῦ δὲ γενομένης ἡ γεγονεῖσα ἔτι ἐξόπισθεν προστίθεταί τι ὡς συνήθως τοῖς δέρμασιν κατερραμμένης.

A midwife's stool, in order that the laboring woman may be placed in position upon it. In the middle of the stool and in the part where they give support one must have cut out a crescent-shaped cavity of medium size, neither too big so that the woman sinks down to the hips, nor, on the contrary, narrow so that the vagina is compressed. The latter is the more troublesome, for the excessively wide hole can be filled up, if she puts pieces of cloth between. And the entire width of the whole stool must be sufficient to accommodate relatively fleshy women too; and its height medium, for in women of small size a footstool placed beneath makes up the deficiency. Concerning the area below the seat, the sides should be completely closed in with boards, whereas the front and the rear should be open for use in midwifery, as will be related. Concerning the area above, on the sides there should be two parts shaped like the letter I for the crossbar on which to press the hands in straining. And behind there should be a back, so that both the loins and hips may meet with resistance to any gradual slipping; for if they reclined even with a woman standing behind, by the crooked position they would hinder the movement of the fetus in a straight line. To the lower parts of the stool some people, however, affix a projecting axle which has windlasses on each side and a knob, so that in extractions of the fetus they may place nooses or ropes circularly round the arms or other parts of the fetus, attach the ends to the knob and effect the extraction [by] rotation-not knowing the general rule that extraction of the fetus in difficult labor must take place with the woman lying down. The stool then must be such as we have said, or it must be a chair, cut out in front or also in back.[9]

If there was no backrest, a strong person should stand behind the woman giving birth, supporting her. Beneath the seat, the sides of the chair were to be solid, but the front and back were supposed to be open to give the midwife easy access and make her work easier. Of course, if such an elaborate device was not available, any chair could be used as the birthing chair, although then it was best to cut openings in it.[10]

Usually, the midwife did not deliver the baby on her own. Other women assisted her, standing to the sides of and behind the woman giving birth.[11] The one in position behind her back had to be strong enough to hold her up if needed. The midwife herself sat in front on a low stool, watching over the correct course of the birth from there.¹² Just such a depiction of delivery, considered iconic by many, was found at Isola Sacra in Ostia.¹³ Although the style and execution of the relief sculpture are very primitive and schematic, the relationship between the three figures pictured, and their roles, are clear enough, believes N. Kampen.¹⁴ Still, one must not forget that images of women in childbirth or right after it are fairly rare in visual sources, the same as with pregnant women.¹⁵ Naturally those images do not contain all the details described in a textbook of medicine, and usually they do not depict all the actions undertaken. Their role was different, as most of the images that fall into this category are a response to a desire to have a baby and the hope for a happy birth (magic engraved gems), a documentation of happy or dramatic events (relief sculptures, usually sepulchral ones), or they focus not so much on the birth itself as on the midwife present.

It is just such a scene that can be seen on a small ivory tablet, now in the Archaeological Museum in Naples.¹⁶ The relief sculpture shows four women. The one giving birth wears a tunic and sits on a chair. One of her hands rests on a long stick or pole; with the other, she leans against the woman standing behind her, presumably an assistant of the midwife. Her feet rest on a low stool, a position which was probably supposed to help her push.¹⁷ The midwife sits facing her on another low stool. She seems to already hold a newborn infant's head in her hands. Another assistant stands behind her, holding her hands out as if she were the one about to receive the child.

The right kind of interaction between the parturient and the doctor or midwife was important during delivery. It was understood that women giving birth for the first time should be advised on how to breathe to make the process easier. They were also told not to eat too much, but if the birth took too long and the woman was weak, the recommendation was for her to eat a little bread, some barley gruel or a piece of an apple.¹⁸ The midwife should ideally look into the face of the woman giving birth, comfort her and foretell a smooth delivery.¹⁹

When the moment of delivery was near, Soranus advised the midwife to carefully insert her fingers and lightly pull the child in the pause between contractions, as pulling during a contraction could cause inflammation, haemorrhage, or uncontrollable uterine cramps. At the same time, the assistants were to press downwards on the belly, rubbing it.²⁰ Immediately before the grand finale the midwife would wrap her hands in fabric or thin papyrus, which was on the one hand supposed to stop the baby from slipping out of her hands, and on the other to prevent her from inadvertently squeezing the baby too hard.²¹

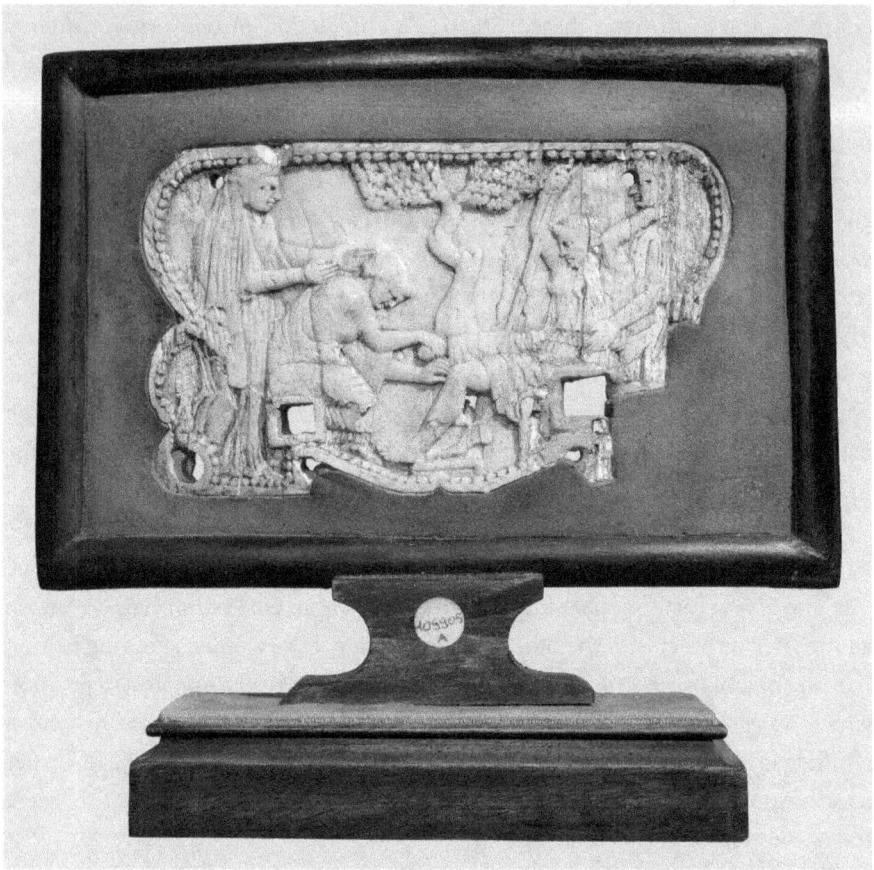

Figure 7 Birth scene © Museo Archeologico Nazionale di Napoli. Photo by Giorgio Albano.
Source: Ministero della Cultura. Museo Archeologico Nazionale di Napoli.

The third stage of labour

This stage was seen as crucial for the woman's chance to live, which is probably why Soranus had a whole chapter on it, presenting both his own and other doctors' opinions on how to make sure the placenta was passed safely and what to do should problems occur, as it was already known by then that both extracting the placenta by force and leaving it in the womb were a danger to the woman's health and life. The inflammation, or even suppuration, caused that way could lead to generalized infection of the whole body and death during the postpartum period.[22] Soranus recommends that immediately after the delivery, when the placenta is still connected to the navel, the midwife should hand over the child, covered in linens, to an assistant, insert her hand by moving it along the umbilical cord, and pull the whole placenta out through gentle movements in time with the uterine contractions, never jerking or tearing it off. Of course, the woman giving birth ought to help her too.[23] Only if passing the placenta took a long time was she advised to cut the cord first and only later follow the instructions just listed. If no part of the umbilical cord protrudes (for example, because it has been torn during a necessary intervention if the birth is difficult),[24] the Greek physician recommends lubricating one's hand with olive oil and extracting the placenta. Should the placenta remain attached to the uterus, the midwife must slowly and carefully try to get it unstuck, and if that fails, Soranus recommends douching and poultices on the genitals to induce contractions and, as a result, detachment.[25]

While discussing the matter, Soranus also lists other physicians' advice on how to remove the placenta, emphasizing, however, that he disagrees, because most of the time the actions recommended by them could be excessively irritating, and so lead to complications and inflammation. For example, he reports Hippocrates as recommending using sneeze-inducing drugs while holding the nostrils closed; Euryphon of Cnidus as advocating diuretic potions made of dittany and sage, suppositories of soapwort, Illyrian iris, cantharidin and honey, as well as being shaken around; Dion as prescribing potions of 'elelisphacus',[26] myrtle and parsley seeds. Another physician, Strato, apparently poured into a silver or copper vessel plated with tin the aromatic spikenard root, cinnamon, artemisia, dittany, lily oil or rose oil, and honey.

> καὶ κρατήσας τὸ πωμάτιον αὐλίσκον περιτίθησιν, οὗ τὸ ἕτερον πέρας εἰς τὸ γυναικεῖον ἁρμόζει αἰδοῖον καὶ πυριᾷ τοὺς τόπους δι' ὀλίγου πυρὸς ἀναθερμαίνων τὰ ἀγγεῖα.
>
> Then he takes hold of the lid, puts a pipe around, the other end of which he fits into the vagina, and foments the region by warming the vessel over a small fire.[27]

Mantias, in turn, said to place the newborn in between the mother's thighs so that the child could pull the placenta out with its own movements and strength. Should that fail, he attached a lead weight to the part of the placenta already protruding so it would be extracted by its pull.[28]

Pliny, Gargilius and the *Cyranides* also list many folk recommendations to use drugs made of plants and animals. Those were apparently in widespread use when the placenta failed to detach itself smoothly. One such universal plant mentioned in Gargilius is thyme.[29]

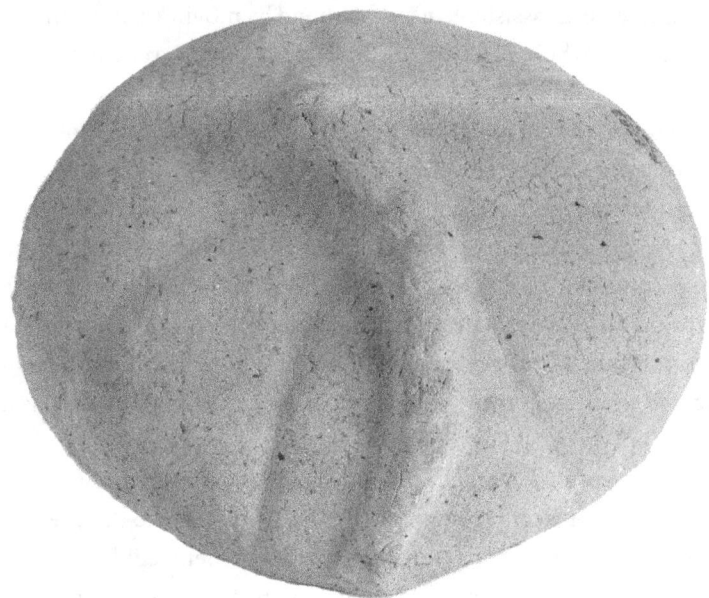

Figure 8 Terracotta image of a placenta with the umbilical cord © Wellcome Collection (CC BY 4.0).
Source: https://wellcomecollection.org/works/kgnzk9je

Once the delivery was successfully over, the young mother was moved to the soft bed to rest, and care was given the newborn.[30] A scene depicting just that – a woman resting, happy with her new baby – is shown on a small stele (15 centimetres in height) in the museum of the Abbey of Saint-Germain d'Auxerre, Yonne.[31] Below the main body of the relief sculpture, which shows a man standing in a shrine, there is a birth scene. A naked woman reclines, perhaps on a bed, lifting the child she seems to have just given birth to. Before her, another person kneels, supporting the baby's legs. This is probably the midwife. Unfortunately, the image is small and, worse, not too well preserved, which makes it hard to interpret. The newborn child is quite distinct, with a well discernible head, nose and eyes.[32]

Closely monitored labour

When describing the conditions under which delivery ought to happen, Soranus emphasizes that the woman giving birth should be comfortable, but comfort may have been unobtainable for those women whose pregnancy caused extra excitement for legal reasons, so they were in the 'special care' of a praetor. One type of such a situation was when a posthumous child was to be born, and the other inheritors did not want their part, which may have been considerable, to be reduced.

A legitimate posthumous child had the right to inherit the same way as their older siblings. In the *Digest* there are regulations prescribing how it should be determined when the child was conceived and whether the mother's deceased husband can be considered the child's father.[33] Since he could no longer declare if he acknowledged the baby or not, the widow's pregnancy had to be monitored closely, and the security during the delivery itself was frankly grotesque, seen from the perspective of our times. The goal was to prevent any kind of deception.

There is an allusion to such deception in a passage in one of Catullus' poems. At the end of Carmen 67 (*O door* ...), where the door is a witness to a young wife's immoral actions, a 'mysterious stranger' appears:

> praeterea addebat quendam, quem dicere nolo
> nomine, ne tollat rubra supercilia.
> longus homo est, magnas cui lites intulit olim
> falsum mendaci ventre puerperium.
>
> I spoke; she thought, no doubt, that I had neither tongue nor ear. She added besides one whom I do not choose to mention by name, lest he should arch his red brows. He is a tall man, and was once troubled with a great lawsuit, from a falsely imputed childbirth.[34]

As A. Klęczar notes, the poem does not reveal the identity of the lover, the mysterious man with red eyebrows; there is only a veiled reference to a lawsuit concerning a 'false' childbirth. It all sounds rather enigmatic. Perhaps the point of the lawsuit was that a woman tried to pretend she was pregnant in order to accuse the redhead of seduction or rape, but considering the Roman inheritance law, the pretend pregnancy may have been part of an attempt at fraud.[35]

When a woman whose pregnancy was monitored by a praetor went into labour, she was to notify all those concerned with the matter of the potential inheritance or their representatives, in case they wanted to send someone to witness the birth. Of course, it was the members of the deceased husband's family who cared the most, since they stood to inherit. It was mostly them who were interested in an examination to verify if the woman had in fact been pregnant, if the child was born alive and had not been smuggled in from the outside, resulting in a clear recommendation that the delivery room have only one entrance, and if there were more, that they be boarded up on both sides. Nor could the woman give birth in her own home; rather, the praetor monitoring her would indicate the house of some woman of immaculate reputation for the purpose. The door to the room was guarded by three freeborn men and three freeborn women, often accompanied by two more people, who had the right to search anybody who entered the house, and every room in the house that the new mother wished to enter. Any party with interest in the inheritance could pick and send over as many as five free women as witnesses, but in the room where the baby was to be delivered, there could be at most two midwives, ten free female witnesses and six female slaves. Th room was also supposed to contain at least three light sources, as darkness favoured deception, such as smuggling a child in. Breaking those regulations could end in being excluded from the *bonorum possessio*, but the law did allow for a departure from such a strict application 'if the woman's actions which made impossible either the examination to confirm pregnancy or the supervision of the pregnancy and birth, stemmed, not from ill intentions, but from ignorance of the rules'.[36]

Unfortunately, it is not known how often that procedure, so complicated organizationally, was implemented, but the description is so detailed that it may have been necessary occasionally.

Fears that a child might be smuggled in for the sake of undeserved inheritance cannot have been rare. A case of such smuggling was decided by one of the most famous trials of the time (moral in appearance, but actually political), recounted in Tacitus.[37] The Roman aristocrat Aemilia Lepida was accused of trying to extort the fortune left by her ex-husband Publius Sulpicius Quirinius by (among other means) supplying a spurious infant (defertur simulavisse partum ex P. Quirinio, divite atque orbo) to be a potential heir so she could take over the assets.[38]

Inducing labour and pain relief

Inducing labour

Should the dilatation be insufficient, Soranus recommended massage and irrigation with warm olive oil or an infusion of fenugreek, mallow and egg white. 'For thus pressure is relieved while the difficult passages are moistened to slipperiness.'[39] Those two are essentially the only methods he believed effective and, more importantly, safe for the mother and child, but much more advice on how to induce and facilitate labour can be found in non-medical texts, which were based on folk beliefs. For example, Pliny lists quite a few ideas, which were likely put into practice as well. From reading his work, one learns, for instance, that labour is immediately started by the vapours of hyaena fat, which must have been a highly esteemed form of treatment. The efficacy of the same animal's fat is extolled by the *Cyranides*: 'fumigation with the smoke of burnt [hyaena] fat from its lumbar bones is the best parturient agent in women who cannot give birth'.[40] At the same time, placing a hyaena's right paw on an expectant woman would make the birth easier. But it was crucial not to make a mistake, as using a left paw could cause the woman to die in childbirth.[41]

Aromatherapy, so to speak, was in fact among the most common methods of inducing labour. According to the Cyranides, smoking

ἡ δὲ κόπρος καπνιζομένη ὑπὸ τὸν δίφρον τῆς κυούσης ὠκυτόκιός ἐστιν,

[cow] manure placed under the bed of a woman in labour speeds it up and causes the placenta and the sac to be passed.[42]

Burnt vulture dung 'cures uterine contractions and helps the foetus emerge.'[43] Apparently, a similar effect could be obtained through fumigation with the smoke from a burnt hoof of a mare,[44] and even spiders' eggs[45] were believed to help women by inducing labour when made into an amulet or used for fumigation.[46] Partridge eggs had similar effects, although the method of application was not listed.[47] Unusual properties of this sort were also attributed to eagle feathers (but only ones taken from the left wing); if one soaked them in olive oil and used them to anoint the woman in difficult labour 'from her feet all the way up to the os sacrum', she would give birth immediately.[48] An eagle feather placed under a woman's feet was thought to work that way too, and one should have some aetites at hand: 'when split, it is beautiful, fiery in colour, and worn as an amulet, it protects the foetus in the womb as well as preventing miscarriage. It also makes birth easier.'[49] In the *Cyranides* one reads that if there is a person 'holding a [seagull's] heart in their hand' anywhere near a woman in labour, they should 'approach, and she will give birth at once'.[50] 'Wing feathers [of a swallow] combined with basil root and hung on the woman's body as an amulet will speed up delivery if there are complications,'[51] but some things should not be given a woman in labour to eat or even kept around her. Such was the case with pears and apples, which should be

aiunt et ipsa poma removenda cum feminae partus incubuit: si in eodem loco fuerint, difficulter uteri claustra reserari

kept far from the woman when her time comes to give birth, since if they remain in the same place where she is, the locks of the womb will not open easily.[52]

Still, Soranus warns his readers thus:

> τὸ δὲ ὠκυτόκια προσαναγράφειν, ὡς ἄλλοι καὶ οἱ περὶ τὸν Ἱπποκράτην ἐποίησαν, σχεδιάζοντός ἐστιν. οὔτε γὰρ δάφνης φύλλα ξηρὰ μετὰ θερμοῦ ὕδατος οὔτε δίκταμνον ἢ ἀβρότονον καὶ κεδρία καὶ ἄνισον μετὰ γλυκέος καὶ παλαιοῦ ἐλαίου οὔτε καρπὸς ἀγρίου σικύου κηρωτῇ προσπλασσόμενος φοινικίνῃ καὶ ὀσφύι περιαπτόμενος ὠκυτοκίαν παρασκευάζει.

> But to prescribe in addition drugs promoting quick birth, as did the followers of Hippocrates among others, is without foundation. For neither dried leaves of sweet bay in warm water, nor dittany or southernwood and cedar resin, and anise with sweet old olive oil, nor the fruit of the wild cucumber added to a date salve and fastened upon the loins effect quick birth. Whereas the above-mentioned treatment removes the morbid condition and thus also removes the resulting ill effect.[53]

Pain relief

People in antiquity had very few options when it came to alleviating labour pains, but the sources provide doctors' advice, folk remedies and prayers for the suffering to ease in that moment, so important to women.[54]

Soranus takes the opportunity to point to the psychological aspect of delivery. He believes that the physician or midwife should in every case comfort and reassure the woman rather than frighten her, as well as emphasize correct breathing, seeing to it that she 'holds her breath as much as possible, driving it inside'.[55] In his opinion, pain treatment must be similar in normal and abnormal births. When the birth goes right, he writes,

> *** τοὺς δὲ πόνους τὸ μὲν πρῶτον τῇ διὰ θερμῶν τῶν χειρῶν προσαφῇ πραΰνειν, τὸ δὲ μετὰ ταῦτα βρέχειν ῥάκη ἐλαίῳ γλυκεῖ καὶ θερμῷ καὶ ἄνωθεν ἐπιρρίπτειν κατ' ἐπιγαστρίου τε καὶ πτερυγωμάτων καὶ συνεχέστερον τῷ θερμῷ καταβρέχειν ἐλαίῳ, τιθέναι δὲ καὶ κύστεις ἐλαίου πεπληρωμένας θερμοῦ.

> one must first soothe the pains by touching with warm hands, and afterwards drench pieces of cloth with warm, sweet oil and punt them aer the abdomen as well as labia and keep them saturated with the warm oil for a time, and one must also place bladders filled with warm oil alongside.[56]

He repeats the same advice when describing abnormal birth:

> ταῖς δὲ ἐν ὀδύνῃ καὶ κύστεις ἐπιβάλλειν ἐλαίου θερμοῦ [πλήρεις] ἢ μαρσίπους ὠμὴν λύσιν θερμὴν ἔχοντας· εἰ δὲ μή, καὶ διὰ φορείου κινεῖν ἐν ἀέρι συμμέτρως θερμῷ μετεωροτέραν τὴν κεφαλὴν ποιήσαντες τῆς καμνούσης.

Then one should also spread linseed or fenugreek in olive oil and hydromel over the pubes, the abdomen and loins, and should administer an oily sitz bath or fomentation with sea sponges, quickly wiping the moisture off with pieces of cloth. If patients are in pain, bladders (full) of warm olive oil should be applied or bags containing warm ground grain. Otherwise one may move them about on a litter in moderately warm air.[57]

The excerpts quoted above indicate it was the midwife who massaged the woman giving birth with a warmed hand and laid on her belly pieces of cloth soaked in warm olive oil or an animal bladder filled with it. Poultices were sometimes made of bags filled with coarse flour, or the woman was simply moved to a cooler room. The importance of correct breathing for reducing pain and for increasing the chances of a smooth birth was well understood.[58]

Pliny's advice on the subject probably comes from folk medicine sources. One drug worth administering is a potion with an admixture of a sow's dung, which will soothe the pain just like 'a sow's milk added to honey', and another effective remedy, in his opinion, was anise, which can be made into a poultice or a drink with dill.[59]

Abnormal labour

Labour that took longer than normal or was more painful than average caused fear and could have indicated serious complications were imminent. We must remember that abnormal birth sharply increased the risk of death for the child, the mother, or both.

An epitaph from Salona mentions Candida, a good wife who lived around thirty years. It was set up by her husband Iustus. Remembering the death of his beloved, he recounted the circumstances of that tragedy in some detail. Thanks to him, we know Candida was four days dying as she tried to give birth. Unfortunately, she failed and died.[60]

Abnormal birth was, alongside childbed fever (caused by injury or, more often, the placenta being passed incorrectly), one of two most common cases of women's death.

Causes of abnormal labour

The high mortality of mothers and newborn children during delivery meant physicians had a lot of interest in the issue.[61] They tried to understand and learn to predict problematic births, looking for the reasons why some women gave birth more easily than others. They attempted to intervene suitably and save both the mother and the child. Finally, they looked for ways of acting in borderline situations, when it was understood that it would be virtually impossible to keep the baby alive.

Difficult labour as the woman's fault

The most general definition of a difficult birth (or difficult labour) is to be found in Soranus: 'it is a difficult birth when there is difficulty for any reason'.[62] While usually it was enough for a midwife to be present, when the birth was difficult a doctor was called in too. Before examining the woman in labour and deciding on any steps to take next, he should listen to what the midwife had to say about the condition of the patient.[63]

It was thought the birth might be difficult if the woman was emotionally unstable, or suffered from excessive 'sadness, joy, anger or indulgence'. Soranus adds that inexperienced women tend to cause more problems and have a harder time giving birth than women who have done it before. Obesity is also listed among the causes of difficult birth,[64] as is the woman not believing she is pregnant (that is, repressing the fact).[65]

Next, Soranus reports other physicians' views on the causes of difficult births. He says that Diocles of Carystus believed *primiparae* to have more difficulty than *multiparae*, and birth to be hard when the foetus is large, not fully formed, or dead. Cleophantus, as quoted by Soranus, also points out the problems *primiparae* have, especially if their hips are narrow, and sees an abnormal presentation of the child as another source of problems. Apparently he also mentioned that birth came more easily to women who had been active during their pregnancy than to those who had moved about little and led 'an idle life'. Herophilus, in turn, thinks that '*multiparae*, too, can have difficulty giving birth'.[66]

Another physician to see the causes of difficult birth in the woman's body type (but also in the child) was Demetrius, a student of Herophilus.[67] He lists lumbar spine problems, the pubic symphysis being too narrow, the hips being too narrow, the cervix dilating too slowly, and past inflammations, tumours and abscesses.

Reportedly Cornelia, mother of the Gracchi, had an anatomical anomaly, even though she had twelve children. It is mentioned in Solinus:

> Feminis perinde est infausta nativitas, si concretum virginal fuerit, quo pacto genitalia fuere Corneliae, quae editis Gracchis ostentum hoc piavit sinistro exitu liberorum.

For female babies, there is another unpropitious manner of birth. This is when the child is born with the vulva grown together. In this way were the genitalia of Cornelia, mother of the Gracchi – she atoned for the portent by the unlucky death of her children.[68]

Demetrius thinks trouble giving birth can happen to both older and young women, those afraid of giving birth and those who cannot assume the correct position during delivery. He also attributes importance to mental weaknesses (infirmity, fear, or 'lack of awareness'). Soranus agrees with him on all those counts.[69] He seems to be aware of psychosomatic connections and is interested in both the physical and the mental well-being of his patients. He also values the midwife's opinion, which helps him understand the case.

Among the causes of difficult birth mentioned most often is the size of the foetus, which the author advises to estimate 'from the size of the belly', although if that does not change as expected during delivery, one should assume there are more foetuses, which is a threat to the woman as well.[70]

Even though few sources touch upon the subject, we can guess multiple pregnancy and birth were very dangerous to the woman. Pliny remarks that already

> editis geminis raram esse aut puerperae aut puerperio praeterquam alteri vitam. si vero utriusque sexus editi sint gemini, rariorem utrique salutem.
>
> at the birth of twins neither the mother nor more than one of the two children usually lives, but that if twins are born that are of different sex it is even more unusual for either to be saved.[71]

Another reason why birth might be problematic or carrying to term hard could be the mother's young age:

> κίνδυνος [γὰρ] τὸ καταβληθὲν σπέρμα συλληφθῆναι μικρομεγέθους ἔτι τῆς μήτρας ὑπαρχούσης καὶ διὰ τοῦτο θλιβησομένου μετὰ τὴν ὄγκωσιν τοῦ ἐμβρύου καὶ οὕτως ἤτοι φθαρησομένου παντελῶς ἢ τοὺς χαρακτῆρας ἀπολέσαντος ἢ πάντως ἐν τῷ καιρῷ τῆς ἀποτέξεως κίνδυνον παρεξομένου τῇ κυοφορούσῃ τῷ διὰ στενῶν ἔτι καὶ ἀτελειώτων ἀκμὴν τῶν περὶ τὸ στόμιον τῆς ὑστέρας μερῶν διέρχεσθαι. συμβαίνει δὲ οὕτως καὶ ἀτροφεῖν ἔνια τῷ μήπω τὴν ὑστέραν μεγάλοις ἀγγείοις καταπεπλέχθαι, λεπτοῖς δὲ καὶ οὐχ ἱκανοῖς τοσοῦτον αἷμα παρακομίζειν, ὅσον ἱκανόν ἐστιν τὸ κατὰ γαστρὸς διαθρέψαι.
>
> danger arises when the injected seed is conceived while the uterus is still small in size. The embryo, in consequence, is subject to pressure after its enlargement and will therefore either be entirely destroyed or lose its characteristics. Or, in

any event, at the time of parturition it will endanger the gravida by passing through the parts around the orifice of the uterus which are still narrow and as yet imperfect. Thus it also happens that some embryos atrophy because the uterus has not yet been entwined with big vessels but only with small ones incapable of conducting sufficient blood to nourish the fetus.[72]

For that reason, Soranus believed it dangerous to marry to early.[73]

Difficulties due to the presentation of the baby

As I have indicated above, the danger grew if the pregnancy was multiple or the child was positioned abnormally. The presentation considered normal or correct was head first, with the arms held straight along the body and the foetus moving in a straight line.[74] Other positions were considered abnormal, but depending on the type, more and less perilous ones were still distinguished. Abnormal ones which, however, still made it easy to intervene included the breech presentation, especially if the baby moved in a straight line, with arms also straight and parallel to the legs. Such births are also mentioned in Pliny, who suggests that the way of being born can influence a person's whole life. His opinion is repeated by Solinus, who writes:

> Contra naturam est, in pedes procedere nascentes: quapropter velut aegre parti appellantur Agrippae. Ita editi minus prospere vivunt, et de vita aevo brevi cedunt. Denique in uno M. Agrippa felicitatis exemplum est, nec tamen usque eo inoffensae, ut non plura adversa pertulerit, quam secunda; namque misera pedum valetudine et aperto coniugis adulterio, et aliquot infelicitatis notis praeposteri ortus omen luit.

> It is against nature for children to be born feet first. Just like other children brought forth with difficulty, those who are born thus are called 'Agrippa'. These same mostly lead unfortunate lives, and die young; only in one man, Marcus Agrippa, was it a sign of felicity. Nevertheless, one could hardly say he was completely untouched by hardship. It is rather that he had less of adversity than of good fortune. By the wretched pain of his feet, by the open adultery of his wife and by several other unhappinesses he paid for the foretoken of his inverted birth.[75]

Oblique lie was also regarded as common, and Soranus notes that it comes in three forms 'depending on whether the body part presenting first is a side, a hip, or the belly'. Of those, he thinks a side presenting is better, since it leaves room for the midwife's hands so she can turn the baby. An intervention is also necessary when the child's head rests against one side of the uterus, or when the arms or legs slip out. However, it is 'the folded position that is the worst of all, particularly if the hips present first. This position comes in three types as well. The parts presenting first are either the thighs and head, or the belly, or the hips'.[76]

In each of the cases just listed, the midwife should insert her oiled left hand, having first cut her nails so as not to injure the parturient, and on the dilation, try to grasp the foetus firmly and position it facing the exit, which should be done simultaneously with the patient assuming the correct position. Namely, she ought to lie on her other side:

παρὰ φύσιν δὲ ἐσχηματισμένου τοῦ ἐμβρύου τὸν κατὰ φύσιν ἀποδιδόναι σχηματισμόν. καὶ εἰ μὲν ἐπὶ κεφαλὴν ἐνεχθὲν παρεγκέκλιται, καθεῖναι τὴν εὐώνυμον χεῖρα λελιπασμένην (ὠνυχισμένων τῶν ἄκρων εἰς τὸ μὴ νύσσειν ἐκτεταμένων τῶν δακτύλων [καὶ] κατὰ τὰς ῥᾶγας συμβεβλημένων ἀλλήλοις μειούρου χάριν σχηματισμοῦ εἰς τὸ ἀσκυλτότερον τῆς καθέσεως) [καὶ] καθ' ὃν καιρὸν φυσικῶς τὸ τῆς ὑστέρας διαστέλλεται στόμιον (εἰς τὸ μὴ συνιόντος αὐτοῦ καὶ συστελλομένου μετὰ σκληρᾶς ἀντιβάσεως γίνεσθαι τὴν ἔνθεσιν), τοῦ ἐμβρύου λαβόμενον κατ' εὐθὺ τοῦ στόματος τῆς ὑστρέρας παράγειν αὐτο συνεργοῦντα τῇ μεταθέσει καὶ διὰ τῆς ἀκολούθου κατακλίσεως. ἐπὶ γὰρ τὸ ἀντικείμενον μέρος ἐσχηματίσθαι δεῖ τὴν κάμνουσαν, ἐπὶ δεξιὰν μὲν, εἰ τύχοι, πλευρὰν εἰς τὰ εὐώνυμα τοῦ ἐμβρύου παρεγκεκλικότος.

assisting the change by making the parturient lie in the respective positions. For the patient must be placed on the opposite side: on the right side in those cases where the fetus is deviated to the left, but on the left side if the fetus has wandered to the right. She should lie back in a sloping position if the fetus has deviated forward as if against the abdominal wall, but should kneel forward with her face lowermost if the embryo has deviated inward as if against the loins.[77]

Soranus emphasizes that all those procedures should be carried out decisively, but calmly, so the patient is not hurt and the child is not 'crippled'. He further stresses that many children whose delivery was difficult survived.[78]

In circumstances when there seemed no chance of saving the baby, then the utmost efforts were made to save the parturient. It was known that difficulties giving birth could be due to a bone of the dead foetus denuded of all soft flesh puncturing the uterus:

γίνεται δυστοκία καὶ παρὰ τὸ τερατῶδες κυΐσκεσθαι, καὶ παρὰ τὸ γεγυμνῶσθαι δὲ τὸ ἔμβρυον καὶ νυσσομένης τῆς μήτρας ὑπὸ τοῦ ὀστέου·· γυμνοῦται δὲ τοῦ ἐμβρύου τὸ ὀστέον μυδώσης τῆς σαρκός (τοῦτο δὲ σπανίως γίνεται), ἢ πολλάκις ἀπείρως ἐμβρυουλκουμένου τοῦ ἐμβρύου ἀποσπῶνται σάρκες καὶ τὰ γυμνούμενα ὀστέα νύσσει τὴν μήτραν,

furthermore, if the fetus has become denuded and the uterus is injured by the skeleton. The skeleton of the fetus is denuded if the flesh has rotted (which happens rarely), or often when the fetus is being inexpertly extracted, the flesh is torn off, and the bare bones injure the uterus.[79]

Saving the mother

Sometimes, however, none of the above helped and the doctor decided to try surgery:

> διὰ χειρουργίας ἐκκόπτειν, εἴτε θύμος ἐστὶν εἴτε κόνδυλος ἀπὸ ἐπαναστάσεως εἴτε διαφράττων ὑμὴν ἢ σαρκὸς περίφυσις ἢ ἄλλο τι τῶν τοιούτων ἐμποδίζον.

> One should push aside a tumor with ointment if it lies close by. If not, one should cut it out surgically whether it be a warty excrescence, or a calloused swelling, or a dividing membrane, or a growth of flesh, or any other such obstacle.[80]

Among additional circumstances which forced a quick intervention were inflammation and infection combined with loss of consciousness, shivering, a weakening pulse, fever and convulsions.[81] If the child was also found to be dead or the foetus got stuck and the labour made no progress, Soranus believed that one must 'resort to more vigorous measures, that is disembowelment, debraining, or extracting the child from the mother's womb in order to save her'.[82]

Thus the first step was to estimate if the child was alive. Soranus has this to say:

> ἐὰν γὰρ ζῳόν, ὠδίνει ἡ κύουσα καὶ ἐντείνεται, θερμόν τε αὐτῆς [τὸ ἐπιγάστριον εὑρίσκεται, τῇ δὲ καθέσει] τῶν δακτύλων καὶ αὐτὸ τὸ ἔμβρυον εὐανθὲς ὁρᾶται, ἐὰν δὲ ᾖ νεκρόν, οὐχ οὕτως ὠδίνει ἡ κύουσα τό τε ἐπιγάστριον αὐτῆς ψυχρὸν γίνεται, τῇ [δὲ] καθέσει τῶν δακτύλων οὔτε θερμὸν ὑποπίπτει τὸ ἔμβρυον οὔτε ἀσθμαῖνον, ἐάν τε καὶ προπέσῃ τι μέρος, τοῦτο μέλαν καὶ νεκρῶδες εὑρίσκεται.

> For if it is alive, the parturient has labor pains and strains down, her [abdomen is found] warm [and on insertion of] the fingers the fetus itself is seen to be flushed. But if it is dead, the parturient does not have pains in this manner and her abdomen is cold; [and] upon inserting the fingers the fetus appears to be neither warm nor gasping for breath; moreover, if a part has prolapsed it is found black and necrotic.[83]

If the child was still alive, one should kill it as fast as possible so it did not suffer when extracted live. We know something about the circumstances when the procedure was performed and its details from Tertullian:

> Atquin et in ipso adhuc utero infans trucidatur necessaria crudelitate, cum in exitu obliquatus denegat partum, matricida, ni moriturus.

> But sometimes by a cruel necessity, whilst yet in the womb, an infant is put to death, when lying awry in the orifice of the womb he impedes parturition, and kills his mother, if he is not to die himself.[84]

Thus Tertullian allows such a course of action when it is absolutely necessary, but the only situation when he considers it justified is when birth becomes impossible and so a direct threat to the mother's life. He also lists the instruments used by physicians in his time to perform embryotomy:[85]

> Itaque est inter arma medicorum et cum organo, ex quo prius patescere secreta coguntur tortili temperamento, cum anulocultro, quo intus membra caeduntur anxio arbitrio, cum hebete unco, quo totum facinus extrahitur uiolento puerperio. Est etiam aeneum spiculum, quo iugulatio ipsa dirigitur caeco latrocinio; ἐμβρυοσφάκτην appellant de infanticidii officio, utique uiuentis infantis peremptorium. Hoc et Hippocrates habuit et Asclepiades et Erasistratus et maiorum quoque prosector Herophilus et mitior ipse Soranus, certi animal esse conceptum atque ita miserti infelicissimae huiusmodi infantiae, ut prius occidatur, ne viva lanietur. De qua sceleris necessitate nec dubitabat, credo, Hicesius, iam natis animam superducens ex aeris frigidi pulsu, quia et ipsum vocabulum animae penes Graecos de refrigeratione respondens.

> Accordingly, among surgeons' tools there is a certain instrument, which is formed with a nicely-adjusted flexible frame for opening the uterus first of all, and keeping it open; it is further furnished with an annular blade, by means of which the limbs within the womb are dissected with anxious but unfaltering care; its last appendage being a blunted or covered hook, wherewith the entire foetus is extracted by a violent delivery. There is also (another instrument in the shape of) a copper needle or spike, by which the actual death is managed in this furtive robbery of life: they give it, from its infanticide function, the name of ἐμβρυοσφάκτης, the slayer of the infant, which was of course alive.[86] Such apparatus was possessed both by Hippocrates, and Asclepiades, and Erasistratus, and Herophilus, that dissector of even adults, and the milder Soranus himself, who all knew well enough that a living being had been conceived, and pitied this most luckless infant state, which had first to be put to death, to escape being tortured alive.[87]

The woman first needed to be made ready for the drastic procedure. Soranus advised to lay her down on a hard, slightly tilted bed, with 'thighs spread apart, positioned close to the abdomen, and feet supported'. Her body should also be supported on either side by strong women, and there was the option of tying her down so she would not struggle during the procedure. The doctor sat facing the parturient, and one of the women assisted him to make it easier for him to insert a hand and control his instruments:

> ἔπειτα πειρᾶσθαι τὸ παρεγκεκλικός, εἰ δυνατόν, ἀπευθύνειν καὶ ζητεῖν τόπον εἰς κατάπαρσιν ἐμβρυουλκοῦ πρὸς τὸ μὴ ἐκπεσεῖν ῥᾳδίως.

> Then one should try if possible to make straight what is deviated and should seek a place for the insertion of the hook so that it may not easily fall out.[88]

Further on, Soranus describes the procedure itself, pointing out that if it is to be successful – that is, if the mother is to survive – it must be performed so as to avoid any serious complications.

> ἐπιτήδειοι δὲ πρὸς καταπαρμὸν τόποι τῶν μὲν ἐπὶ κεφαλὴν ὀφθαλμοὶ καὶ ἰνίον καὶ στόμα πρὸς οὐρανίσκον καὶ κλεῖδες καὶ οἱ ὑπὸ πλευρὰν τόποι, μασχάλαι δὲ οὐδαμῶς (ἐν γὰρ ταῖς διολκαῖς ἐπιδιισταμένων τῶν βραχιόνων εἰς σφήνωσιν ἡ τοῦ ἐμβρύου πλατύνεται περιοχή), ἀλλ᾽ οὐδὲ οἱ ἀκουστικοὶ πόροι (δυσπαράδεκτοι διὰ σκολιότητα καὶ στενοὶ λίαν)· τῶν δὲ ἐπὶ πόδας τὰ ὑπὲρ τῆς ἥβης ὀστέα καὶ μεσοπλεύρια καὶ κατακλεῖδες. ὅταν δὲ τῶν εἰρημένων μηδεὶς εὑρίσκηται τόπος, εἰς κατάπαρσιν ἑτοιμάζεται σπάθῃ διαίρεσις. θερμῷ δὲ ἐλαίῳ προκεχλιασμένον τὸν ἐμβρυουλκὸν τῇ δεξιᾷ χειρὶ κατέχειν, τὴν καμπὴν δὲ αὐτοῦ τοῖς δακτύλοις κρύψαντα τῇ εὐωνύμῳ χειρί. πράως συνεισφέρειν καὶ καταπείρειν εἴς τινα τόπον ἄχρι κενεμβατήσεως [ὧν] εἰρήκαμεν.

> places suitable for inserting it are the eyes, the back of the head, the roof of the mouth, the collarbones and the area below the ribs. The armpits, however, are in no wise suitable (for if during extraction the arms are further abducted, the circumference of the fetus is increased so as to lead to impaction); nor are the auditory canals suitable (since they hardly admit the hook, because of their crookedness, and are too narrow). In foot presentation, the bones above the pudenda, the spaces between the ribs and the clavicular region are suitable. But in case none of the said places is found, an incision with a knife is to be made for the insertion. One should hold the hook, previously warmed in olive oil, with the right hand. Covering its curvature with the fingers, one should gently introduce it with the help of the left hand and insert it into any of the said places until it has penetrated deeply. One should also insert a second hook, opposite the first, so that traction may be evenly balanced and not onesided, causing a part to deviate and consequently impaction of the fetus. Next one should give an experienced person the hooks to hold with the admonition that he pull the fetus gently with them, without tearing it to pieces by pulling, nor on the other hand, letting it go

(for if relaxed, the part that has emerged slips back). Rather, when it is necessary to pause in the traction, he should keep the hooks at the previous tension.[89]

The point was to stop the child's body from falling to pieces inside, and its bones from damaging the uterus. Afterwards the physician handed the instruments to a skilled person, so perhaps the midwife, asking them to extract the child slowly and carefully.[90] The author also said to apply warm olive oil or some 'mucous' decoction to the genitals, which should make the process easier.[91]

Soranus recounts the procedure of extracting the foetus should an arm or a leg slip out:

προβεβλημένου δὲ χερίου [ὡς] καὶ ἀνατρέπεσθαι μὴ δυναμένου διὰ τὴν ὑπερβάλλουσαν σφήνωσιν ἢ καὶ ἀποτεθνηκότος ἤδη τοῦ ἐμβρύου (καθὼς συμβάλλομεν ἐκ τοῦ μήτε ἐνερευθὲς εἶναι τὸ μέρος μήτε θερμὸν μήτε σφύζον, πελιὸν δὲ καὶ ψυχρὸν καὶ ἄσφυκτον) περιβάλλοντα δεῖ ῥάκη εἰς τὸ μὴ ὀλισθαίνειν ποσῶς ἐπισπᾶσθαι, κατασχόντα δὲ πρὸς τὸ ἐμφανέστερα γενέσθαι τὰ ὑπερκείμενα ἀποκόπτειν ἀπὸ τοῦ κατὰ τὸν ὦμον ἄρθρου. τὸ δὲ αὐτὸ ποιεῖν καὶ σκέλους προπεσόντος. εἶτα τοῖς δακτύλοις ἀναστρέψαντα τὸ ἄλλο σῶμα διὰ τῆς καταπάρσεως τῶν ἐμβρυουλκῶν κομίζεσθαι. τῶν δυοῖν δὲ χειρῶν προβεβλημένων καὶ μήτε ἀνατρέπεσθαι δυναμένων μήτε παρακρούεσθαι τοῖς σπασμοῖς, ὡς τὴν μίαν καὶ τὰς δύο διὰ τῆς παρὰ τοῖς ἀκρωμίοις περικοπῆς ἀναιρεῖν. εἰ δὲ μείζονος τοῦ κεφαλίου ὑπάρχοντος ἡ σφήνωσις ἀποτελοῖτο, διὰ τοῦ ἐμβρυοτόμου ἢ τοῦ πολυπικοῦ σπαθίου κρυπτομένου μεταξὺ λιχανοῦ καὶ τοῦ μικροῦ δακτύλου κατὰ τὴν ἔνθεσιν, εἰ μὲν ὑγροκέφαλον εἴη τὸ βρέφος, διαιρεῖν, ἵνα τοῦ ὑγροῦ κενωθέντος ἡ περιοχὴ συμπέσῃ τῆς κεφαλῆς, εἰ δὲ φυσικῶς ἁδροκέφαλον, τῇ χειρὶ συνθλαστέον τὴν κεφαλήν, συνείκει [γὰρ] εὐμαρῶς ἁπαλῶν ἔτι τῶν σωμάτων ὄντων. εἰ δὲ μή, τῷ σπαθίῳ καὶ τὸ κρανίον διαιρεῖν καλὸν ἢ κατὰ τὸν τοῦ βρέγματος τόπον, εἰ δὲ μή, καθ' οἱονδήποτε τρόπον· προεκκριθέντος γὰρ τοῦ ἐγκεφάλου συμπίπτει τὸ κεφάλιον. τὰ χείλη δὲ τῆς διαιρέσεως ἀποστρέφειν καὶ συνθραύειν τὰ ὀστάρια δι' ὀδοντάγρας ἢ ὀστάγρας. εἰ δὲ διὰ μέγεθος τοῦ ὅλου σώματος μηδὲ οὕτως ἑλκόμενον ὑπακούοι, τῶν δύο ὤμων ἐνερειδομένων τοῖς πλαγίοις μέρεσιν τῆς μήτρας, καὶ εἰς τὰς σφαγὰς βαπτίζειν τὸ σπαθίον μέχρι κενεμβατήσεως εἰς τὸ ἔμβρυον· ἀποκριθέντος γὰρ τοῦ αἵματος ἰσχνὸν γίνεται τὸ σῶμα. μετὰ δὲ ταῦτα ὅλον τὸ κεφάλιον διαιρεῖν καὶ τὰ μεσοπλεύρια διακόπτοντα καὶ [τὸν] πνεύμονα· πληρωθεὶς γὰρ πολλάκις ὑγρῶν καὶ αὐτὸς ἐπλάτυνε τὸν θώρακα. λύειν δὲ καὶ [τὰ] συνδεδεμένα μέρη τοῦ στήθους διὰ τῶν δακτύλων ἀποσπῶντα τὰς κατακλεῖδας ἀπὸ τῶν ἀντιστέρνων [ἢ μὴ] εἰκόντων ἀπορρηγνύναι· συμπίπτει γὰρ τὰ περὶ τὸ στῆθος μηκέτι διερειδόμενα ταῖς λεγομέναις κλεισίν. εἰ δὲ μηδ' οὕτως ὑπακούοι, τὸ ἐπιγάστριον διαρρινᾶν, ὡσαύτως κἂν ὑδρωπικὸν ᾖ τὸ ἔμβρυον· κενωθέντος γὰρ τοῦ ὑγροῦ συμπίπτει πρὸς ἴσχνωσιν ἡ περιοχὴ τοῦ σώματος. εἰ δὲ καὶ τὰ ἔντερα παρέχει τῷ ἐπιγαστρίῳ τινὰ διόγκωσιν, καὶ ταῦτα πρότερον ἕλκειν καὶ τὰ λοιπὰ τῶν παρακειμένων σπλάγχνων οὕτως τε τὴν ὅλην ἐξενεγκεῖν σύγκρισιν.

If, however, a hand has prolapsed and cannot be turned back because of the severe impaction, or if the fetus is already dead (as we conjecture from the fact that the part is neither flushed nor warm nor pulsating but livid, cold and without pulsation), one should throw a piece of cloth over it to prevent slipping and draw it forward slightly. Then depressing it in order that the parts lying above may become more visible, one should amputate at the shoulder joint. The same should be done if a leg has prolapsed. Then one should turn the rest of the body with the fingers and deliver by inserting the hooks. If both hands have fallen forward and cannot be turned back nor disengaged by pulling, one must remove them both by cutting them off at the shoulders, as has been done with one hand. If, however, the impaction is caused by too big a head, and if the fetus suffers from hydrocephalus, one should split it with an embryotome or a knife for removing polypi, covered during its introduction between the forefinger and the little finger, so that the fluid may be emptied and the circumference of the head collapse. If, however, the fetus naturally has a large head, one should crush the head with the hand, [for] it yields easily when the body is still soft. Otherwise, it is well to lay open the skull with the knife either at the bregma or, if this is not possible, at any other place. For after the brain has been cleared out, the head collapses. The edges of the incision must be turned aside and the little bones fragmented by means of a forceps for drawing teeth, or a forceps for extracting splinters of bone. If, however, because of the large size of the whole body, the fetus does not respond even if so pulled, the shoulders arrested by he lateral parts of the uterus, one must plunge the knife into the jugular region until it has penetrated deeply into the fetus. For when the blood is drained off, the body becomes thin. Afterwards one should lay open the whole head and also cut through the intercostal spaces and [the] lungs. For the latter are often full of fluid and have distended the thorax. One should also free [the] parts of the chest which are bound to one another by tearing away with the fingers the clavicles from the sternum [or], if they [do not] yield, one should break them off. For the chest collapses when its parts are no longer held apart by the so-called collarbones. But if even so the fetus does not respond one should perforate the abdomen; and should do likewise if the fetus is dropsical. For when the fluid is emptied, the circumference of the body collapses and is reduced. In case the intestines too have contributed to the swelling of the abdomen, one must first draw them out together with the other adjacent viscera and thus deliver the whole body."[92]

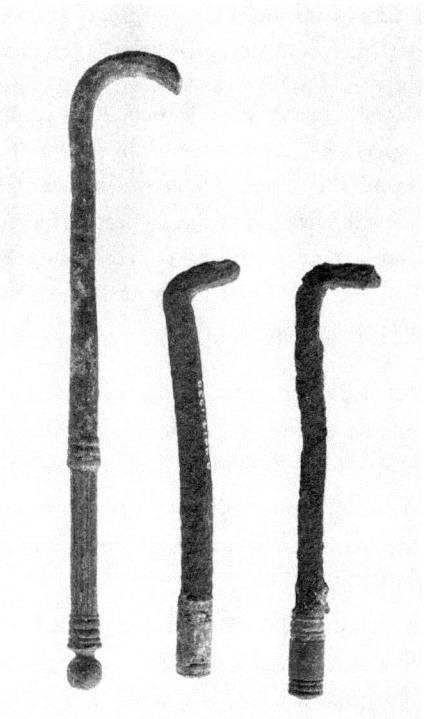

Figure 9 Roman surgical instruments – different hooks © Wellcome Collection (CC BY 4.0).
Source: https://wellcomecollection.org/works/mqy6rxzz

Soranus then writes of the dangers of manipulating the instruments incompetently.[93] To conclude the terrifying description, he adds that all the parts extracted must be put together so that it can be seen if anything remains in the uterus. He remarks that if after the procedure the woman suffers from a genital inflammation caused by injury, it should be alleviated by douching, whereas after a haemorrhage 'appropriate agents' ought to be used, which he unfortunately does not name.

We do not know the mortality rate of women after that kind of surgery, although high mortality is to be expected. It is possible such a procedure killed the mother mentioned in this inscription:

[multa tulit nimis adversi]s incommoda rebus / [infelix misero e]st fine perempta quoq(ue) / [quadraginta a]nnos postquam trans/[egit in aevo] / [fu]nesto grauis heu triste puerperio / nequiuit miserum partu depromere fetu(m) / hausta qui nondum luce peremptus abiit / adque ita tum geminas g[e]mino cum corpore /

praeceps / laetum(!) ferali [transtu]lit hora an[imas] / at nos maerentes coniux natique / generque / carmen cum lacrim[is] hoc tibi [condidimus]

> This unfortunate woman met a pitiable end after completing forty years. Pregnant, alas, she experienced a grievously difficult labour and was not able to drive out from her womb the wretched fetus which, destroyed, passed away not yet in the light. And in this way then she, at peace, suddenly transferred in a funereal hour two souls along with one twinned body. But those of us left grieving, your husband, your children, and your son-in-law, through our tears we composed these verses for you.[94]

As can be seen, Soranus offers a detailed discussion of the causes of difficult birth and exhaustive advice, taking into account a number of potential scenarios, on how to save the child, or, if that is impossible, the mother. I have quoted this excerpt word for word more than once, because it may indicate that such surgery had to be performed quite often, and its description is based on the experiences of physicians who carried it out.

The advanced and detailed nature of those procedures demonstrates how valuable a woman's life was, and that it would be saved at all cost, especially if the child was unfortunately already doomed. Clearly it was believed possible for the woman to survive such surgery;[95] perhaps it was even thought she could still become a mother in the future.

Archaeological finds do confirm that embryotomy was practised in cases when the foetus was dead. For instance, the two child corpses discovered at the Roman cemetery in Poundbury[96] and Hambleden, England,[97] indicate the procedure was performed in the way described by Soranus.

The myth of caesarean section

It is common opinion that the term *caesarean section* comes from the way Julius Caesar was born. The historical misunderstanding regarding his birth is deeply rooted in our culture, even though no ancient historian, not even the curiosity collector Pliny, mentions the most famous Roman being born in that way. The myth is well illustrated by a mediaeval woodcut from an edition of Suetonius' *Lives of the Twelve Caesars*: in it, Caesar's mother lies on an operating table, her abdominal cavity cut open, while he is being taken out by a midwife and a surgeon, who holds a knife.[98]

However, it is widely considered indisputable that Caesar's mother, Aurelia Cotta, died at sixty-six, only ten years before he did, which strongly indicates he

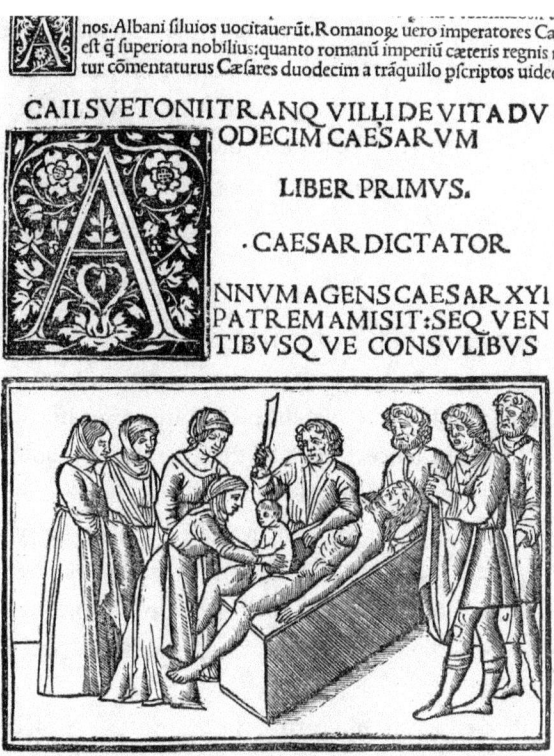

Figure 10 *The Birth of Caesar*. A woodcut from Suetonius' *Lives of the Twelve Caesars*, published in 1506 © Wellcome Collection.

Source: https://wellcomecollection.org/works/uzmukqh2

could not have in fact been born through caesarean section, as doctors were not able to perform it at the time, and even if they had been, it would not have been possible to keep the woman operated on alive. Indeed, most researchers agree the name of the surgical procedure comes from a law laid down by Numa Pompilius which forbade the burial of a pregnant woman's body before taking the child out of her womb.[99]

How should one interpret the silence on caesarean section in medical sources? A few explanations have been considered. Either (1) the procedure was so common that there was no need to mention it; or (2) caesarean section was only practised on dead women, and so it was not a medical procedure as such; or (3) it was a religious rather than a medical operation.[100] Those explanations, particularly the one suggesting the procedure was quite common, do not seem justified in the light of the sources. It would be unlikely for Soranus, who was very systematic, went into a lot of detail, and even wrote about preparing the most basic things useful for a normal delivery, and who describes abnormal births and the process of saving the mother and the child if they were in danger, to have decided caesarean section was too trivial an intervention to mention.

Death in childbirth and the postpartum period[101]

It is under a lucky star, Pliny wrote, that the people are born whose mothers die after they gave birth to them: 'Instances are the birth of the elder Scipio Africanus ... Also Manilius who entered Carthage with his army was born in the same manner.'[102] The increased number of deaths of women in their childbearing years most likely indicates high perinatal mortality rate, caused by a number of factors, including early marriages, numerous births, lack of hygiene and abortion practices.[103] The reproductive period was then a time of excess mortality of women relative to men in the same age group.[104]

Women often died either in childbirth or because of perinatal complications.[105] Some died unable to give birth; others lived through the delivery, but then died from complications, haemorrhages, or inflammations. The tragedy of one such death is recounted by Pliny the Younger in a letter to Velius Cerealis.[106] Pliny refers to the two daughters of his friend Helvidius as 'victims of their own motherhood', since they died in childbirth (the children were girls). He had a lot of compassion for the two young women who had died, but also commiserated with the children, who would be brought up motherless, and the widowed husbands.

Another, maybe even better-known 'victim of motherhood' was Cicero's daughter Tullia, who died at the beginning of 45 BCE after bearing a son. The child, Lentulus, probably died soon after, as his grandfather mentioned him for the last time in a letter to Atticus in March of that year.[107]

It was not a rare occurrence. Thanks to epigraphic texts we get a closer look at the presumable tragedy of losing a wife, daughter, or granddaughter who died while trying to give birth or a little later, in puerperium. Still, we cannot always say for sure in those cases that the death was directly caused by childbirth.[108] One family remembered a young mother who died in her first childbirth; the text of the inscription conveys genuine sadness and grief over the loss of a loved one.[109] Veturia of Aquincum married at sixteen and died at twenty-seven, after six deliveries, the last of which ended tragically.[110] The tombstone of the slave Gemina was set up by the freedman Gaius Aerarius. The inscription said she died at twenty-five, and the cause was giving birth.[111]

Another moving sepulchral inscription also confirms a woman's death in childbirth:

> [Dis in]fernis memoriaeq(ue) semper habendae / Hi[ppoda]miae suae constituit pignora post gemina / nat[a at a m]atre relicta dilectae nimium gratus uir Apolaustus / co[mes tu] qui pergis iter mane quaeso parumper / [siste g]ressum dunc perlegens an{c}xia fata / [- - -]pus quondam dunc uita manebat / [- - -fl] orente iuuenta / [- - - co]ntraria uoti[s/- - -] maero[re- - -] parent[- - -] / [- - - d] ilecto c[- - -]ro / [- - -] semperq(ue) [... m]arito / [- - -]ro forma [- - -]te beata / [- - -e]t transeg[it o]rbes / [- - -f]ugiens m[- - - r]eliquit / [- - -]o mar[- - -]rgine et una / [- - -] per[...] aq. litora uisa / quo na[sc]or mo[r]io[r m]orte[m m]ihi uita parauit / nam partu genitam partu[s me] tradidit umbris / [H]ippodamia fuit n[o]men d[unc] uita manebat / haec tamen ex[t]remi te [- - -] / quod quae me genuit pat[ria- - -] / adque ubi uita data est i[- - -] / apte nam genitam t[r] ist[- - -] / hoc mihi dilecte con[iu]x p[- - -]

(Lines 1 to 5) To the gods below and for the memory always to be preserved of his very own Hippodamia, her grateful husband, Apolaustus, erected this after the birth of their twin pledges, but the children were left behind by their mother. I implore you, companion, rest here for a little while (and continue your journey later). Halt your step, while reading all the way through the distressing fate (of my wife) . . .
(Line 17) Because I gave birth, I died. My life set up my death: for I was born through labour, and my own labour delivered me to the underworld. Hippodamia was my name while life remained to me. Nevertheless these things at the end you . . . Because this country bore me . . . and where life was given . . . for born fittingly . . . My husband lovingly for me (set up this monument?) . . .[112]

In the epitaph of Rusticea, a young woman from Mauretania, we read, 'The cause of my death was childbirth and malicious fate'.[113] Unfortunately, we do not know what happened during the delivery, but Rusticea tries to comfort her husband and asks him not to waste tears on her, but instead to take care of their son. Unfortunately another thing we do not know is whether the son she means is the child she died giving birth to or another one, born earlier. There is also an inscription from Alba Fucens which indicates the child lived (it was a daughter), but the mother, Aedia, died in childbirth.[114] Meanwhile, Cornelia Calliste, a fifteen-year-old girl, survived the delivery itself, but died seven days later.[115]

Another woman who died in her postpartum period was Daphnis from Carthage. The evidence is the phrase 'I have recently given birth'.[116] Rubria Festa was probably another victim of perinatal complications. The inscription in her honour was set up by her husband, Iulius Secundus:

> [h]anc struem perennis arae posuit his in sedibus / Iulius Festae Secundus coniugi karissimae / uixit annos sextriginta bisque uiginti dies / pondus uteri enisa decimum luce rapta est tertia / nata claro Rubriorum genere de primoribus / sancta mores pulchra uisu praecluens prudentia / exornata summo honore magno iudicio patrum / aurea uitta et corona Mauricae prouinciae / haec et diuum consecuta est summa pro meritis bona / quinque natos lacte mater ipsa quos aluit suo / sospites superstitesque liquit uotorum potens.

> Iulius Secundus [made] in this place, an altar, destined to endure, for Festa, his most beloved wife. She lived thirty-six years and twice twenty days. It was her tenth delivery. On the third day she died. Born into the gens Rubria, celebrated among the leading families, flawless in her character, beautiful to behold, outstanding in her wisdom, she received – the highest honour which can be given by the judgment of the senators – the golden ribbon and the crown of the province of Mauretania. For her merits, she received the greatest blessings from the gods. As a mother, she left behind five children safe and sound whom she herself nursed with her own milk, and thus saw her vows fulfilled.[117]

Aeturnia Zotica, who 'lived fifteen years, five months and eighteen days' and 'died sixteen days after giving birth' was probably another of the many women and girls who died in childbirth.[118]

M. Carroll thinks that in the case of women who died in childbirth, highlighting their age at death is meant not just to express the depth of their husbands' grief, but also, especially if the women were quite young, to point to the accompanying loss of potential future descendants. One possible reason why that intention is poorly documented is the cost of inscriptions.[119] Every inscription intended to commemorate a dead person was a result of the conscious choice of people who decided to include or omit certain facts. Every extra letter, every cut meant additional costs.

Is there any other way to show a woman most likely died in childbirth, even if the epitaph does not say so explicitly? Carroll supposes that mourning steles depicting women holding swaddled children are images of women who died under exactly such circumstances, but considering the importance of female fertility in the Roman world, sepulchral images of women holding infants in their arms may simply show them as mothers and be evidence of their fertility, regardless of whether those specific women died in childbirth. It could simply be a model way of indicating or symbolizing motherhood, used regardless of a mother's cause of death or the number or age of the children, whether she survived giving birth or died because of it. It might also, perhaps even primarily, stand for lost hopes for grandchildren who would extend the lineage.[120]

Funeral portraits, too, include many depictions of women holding a baby. Carroll thinks they can be understood as images of mothers with children who died soon after them.[121]

Divine protection during childbirth[122]

Requests for divine protection

The Romans believed that the time of pregnancy, childbirth and infancy was, like all other stages of human life, under divine protection. Some deities had specific roles, while others, known only from their names, were invoked in order to promote or prevent a specific result. Many of those minor 'deities of the moment' (*dii indigenes*) have only been preserved in Christian polemic works, whereas deities as important as Juno Lucina are known from many and diverse sources.[123] In fact, her popularity and significance were such that for many Romans she became a counterpart of the Greek Eileithyia,[124] called upon by women during childbirth.[125] Future parents worshipped her more than any other gods, and information regarding her and her protection of women appear quite often in numismatic, epigraphic and literary sources alike.[126]

Each year on 1 March was held the festival of Matronalia,[127] during which married women, mothers and pregnant women went to the temple of Juno Lucina.[128] Literary sources also confirm that there was an old sacred grove of the goddess near the Esquiline Hill, where a temple would be erected to her in historical times.[129] The time, place and course of the festival are recounted by Ovid in the *Fasti* as follows:

> tempora iure colunt Latiae fecunda parentes, / quarum militiam votaque partus habet. / adde quod, excubias ubi rex Romanus agebat, / qui nunc Esquilias nomina collis habet, / illic a nuribus Iunoni templa Latinis / hac sunt, si memini, publica facta die. / quid moror et variis onero tua pectora causis? / eminet ante oculos, quod petis, ecce tuos. / mater amat nuptas: matris me turba frequentat: / haec nos praecipue tam pia causa decet.' / ferte deae flores: gaudet florentibus herbis / haec dea: de tenero cingite flore caput: / dicite 'tu nobis lucem, Lucina, dedisti': / dicite 'tu voto parturientis ades.' / si qua tamen gravida est, resoluto crine precetur, / ut solvat partus molliter illa suos.

> 'tis right that Latin mothers should observe the fruitful season, for in their travail they both fight and pray. Add to this that where the Roman king kept watch, on the hill which now bears the name of Esquiline, a temple was founded, if I remember aright, on this very day by the Latin matrons in honour of Juno. But why should I spin out the time and burden your memory with various reasons? The answer that you seek stands out plainly before your eyes. My mother loves brides; a crowd of mothers throngs my temple; so pious a reason is above all becoming to her and me.' Bring ye flowers to the goddess; this goddess delights in flowering plants; with fresh flowers wreathe your heads. Say ye, 'Thou, Lucina, hast bestowed on us the light (lucem) of life'; say ye, 'Thou dost hear the prayer of women in travail.' But let her who is with child unbind her hair before she prays, in order that the goddess may gently unbind her teeming womb.[130]

Roman women wanted to believe the goddess would ensure they gave birth safely. Her help was especially counted on in cases as hard as this one, recounted in Statius' Silvae:

> quippe bis ad partus venit Lucina manuque / ipsa levi gravidos tetigit fecunda labores. / felix a! si longa dies, si cernere vultus / natorum viridesque genas tibi iusta dedissent / stamina.
>
> for fruitful Lucina came twice for a delivery and herself lightly touched the pangs of labor. Happy, ah, if length of days and just threads had vouchsafed you to see your children's faces, their youthful cheeks![131]

Like the heroines of Terence, Plautus and Catullus, women called upon her during childbirth not only hoping for a sense of security, but also believing that she would soothe actual, physical pain:

> tu Lucina dolentibus / Iuno dicta puerperis, / tu potens Trivia et notho es / dicta lumine Luna. / tu cursu, dea, menstruo / metiens iter annuum.
>
> thou art called Juno Lucina by mothers in pains of travail, thou art called mighty Trivia and Moon with counterfeit light.[132]
>
> Miseram me, differor doloribus. / Iuno Lucina, fer opem. serva me, obsecro.
>
> Pamphila [cries from inside] Oh! oh! I'm wracked with pain. Juno Lucina,[24] help me, save me, I beg you.[133]

Or:

> Perii, mea nutrix. obsecro te, uterum dolet. / Iuno Lucina, tuam fidem! / Em, mater mea / tibi mea, / tibi rem potiorem verbo: clamat, parturit.

I'm done for, my nurse. I entreat you, my womb hurts. Juno, goddess of childbirth, help me! There, mother! There's better proof for you than mere words: she's screaming, she's giving birth.[134]

Finally, Juno received offerings and thanks for safe and quick delivery. Usually, they are typical expressions of gratitude and declarations of having fulfilled one's promise to the goddess, as in this inscription from Lusitania, set up, perhaps, by a happy father:

Abru[n]us / Luci[nae] Div/inae v(otum) s(olvit) / a(nimo) l(ibens)

Aburnus gladly gave the divine Lucina the promised offering.[135]

Juno supported not just commoners, but also the women of the reigning family.[136] She is also depicted on coins. Holding an infant in her arms, she can be seen on the coinage of Faustina, Marcus Aurelius' wife, as well as of Lucilla and Julia Mamaea. On the reverse of a silver *denarius* of Julia Mamaea, the seated Juno holds a flower in her right hand and a swaddled child on her left shoulder. The *denarius* with Lucilla, Marcus Aurelius' daughter and Lucius Verus' wife, bears an identical image.[137]

Magical practices assisting childbirth

Regardless of their social standing, pregnant women feared childbirth and looked for help not only to humans and gods, but also magic. That is why delivery scenes can be seen on engraved gems, although due to their size, the images are very schematic. One relief sculpture on an engraved gem shows a naked pregnant woman sitting in a birthing chair. Three ring-shaped grooves highlight the convex belly. The woman's hair is loose. The object is so small that it comes as no surprise that the face is barely sketched. Although pregnant women's hair is often tied, they were advised to loosen it for childbirth, as here. One piece of folk advice is that loose hair 'makes birth easier', and strengthens the head.[138] That will probably be why the woman on the engraved gem holds her hands clasped together above her head.[139] The birthing chair is only indicated with a few lines, two vertical ones for legs and one horizontal one for the back, while the armrests end in decorative heads, perhaps a ram's. On another engraved gem, there is clearly visible the round belly of the woman giving birth, indicated with curved lines.[140] She faces left, and the image underlines her sharp nose, prominent lips and large eyes. She is shown nude as well, her long, loose hair falling onto her shoulders. Her hands grasp the armrests. In this case the birthing chair is very schematic too.

In 2007 near Oxford, UK, a small gold amulet was discovered bearing a magical text in Greek, requesting health for the mother and a safe birth for her child. While of course we know such amulets had no real influence on how the birth went, they certainly could have acted as a placebo of sorts, improving the would-be mother's mood, and, as Soranus wrote, her good mood and faith in the birth going smoothly were two factors increasing the chance that it would in fact be safe.[141]

6

Dies lustricus: The Birth of ... a Mother?

If one were to ask why birth was mostly the subject of medical texts, and rarely of narrative and visual sources, then the answer could be that the time of giving birth was regarded as part of the 'space reserved for women', and it was in that space that birth as a biological phenomenon occurred.[1] Nonetheless, in Rome, the act of bearing a child was never only understood in its biological sense. The legal-and-custom-related aspect was just as important. For a long time, it was assumed in scholarship that a newborn baby laid on the ground by the midwife would be symbolically picked up by the father,[2] who thus demonstrated he acknowledged the child as his.

The meaning of the gesture, known as *infantem tollere*, was long accepted at face value, and it was only T. Köves-Zulauf who first questioned its very existence. Other researchers also believed it should only be taken figuratively. V. Dasen writes that no legal text mentions the gesture because no special act was needed for a child to be legitimate. From the legal standpoint, the child only had to be born in a legal marriage to automatically come under the power (*patria potestas*) of the mother's husband. Dasen proposes this interpretation of the event in question based on the theory put forward by Arnold van Gennep, whose research centred on tribal rituals understood as a way to maintain the continuity of communal experience. Among those, rites of passage were important, accompanying transitions from one state or world to another in all those areas of human life where change took place. Gennep distinguished and described three stages of passage: pre-liminal (exclusion), liminal (transition) and post-liminal (inclusion). For an individual's social role or position to change, they first had to be excluded from their 'old world'. For a while, their status was suspended between the old role and identity and the new. Finally, there was inclusion in a 'new world'. Following T. Köves-Zulauf's study, historians concluded that if the ritual of the father lifting the baby off the ground did not exist in the Roman world then, until the *dies lustricus*, the child likewise did not *exist*, being instead a liminal entity without an identity.[3]

The act of placing the child on the floor does feature in medical texts but, as Dasen emphasizes, it was done not by a man, but rather by a woman: the midwife who had delivered the infant.[4] Soranus is one of the sources that indicate this:

> Ἡ τοίνυν μαῖα τὸ βρέφος ἀποδεξαμένη πρῶτον εἰς τὴν γῆν ἀποτιθέσθω προεπιθεωρήσασα, πότερον ἄρρεν τὸ ἀποκεκυημένον ἐστὶν ἢ θῆλυ, καί, καθὼς γυναιξὶν ἔθος, ἀποσημαινέτω·· κατανοείτω δὲ καί, πότερον πρὸς ἀνατροφὴν ἐστιν ἐπιτήδειον ἢ οὐδαμῶς.
>
> Now, the midwife having received the newborn. Should first put it upon the earth, having examined beforehand whether the infant is male or female, and should make an announcement by signs as is the custom of women. She should also consider whether it is worth rearing or not.[5]

What did that mean for the woman? If she did not become a mother either as she gave birth or at the moment of *tollere liberos*, then when did that occur? According to the content of the *lex Malacitana*, candidates for officials underwent evaluations which included the number of children they had, and dead children were counted provided they had been given names.[6] That would point to the naming, rather than the 'lifting', as the crucial moment. It was naming that included the newborn among the living.

Another piece of evidence is a story quoted by Aulus Gellius, where the goal was to acquire the *ius trium liberorum*.[7] There was some discussion as to whether a child born in the eighth month of pregnancy who died straight after birth could be taken into account when granting the parents the right of three children. Gellius' account suggests there was in fact no such possibility, because according to lawyers, an eighth-month birth should be treated as a miscarriage, but the question remains if in this case the birth could not be counted because it occurred in the eighth month, or because the child died immediately. Perhaps, as I have written above, Aulus Gellius thought that only miscarriages and not births were possible in the eighth month, as he could hardly not have known that for the *ius trium liberorum* to apply, the child, even one born in the ninth or tenth month, had to live until the *dies nominum / lustricus*.[8] It is usually assumed that in antiquity, almost 30 per cent of children did not live to reach one year. It is impossible to determine the percentage of deaths in the first few days of life. It seems people in antiquity did know how important those days immediately after childbirth were, for both the mother and the child. Dasen suggests we redefine the days preceding the *dies lustricus*, believing that the time of transition was not just about waiting to see if the child would live; on the contrary, it was a period of an intense humanization of the newborn, of preparing it for independent existence as a separate entity.⁹ The stage of accepting the child into the society began with bathing, and went through massage to fashioning with swaddling bandages, which were supposed to give the child's body the right shape.¹⁰

Caring for a woman in puerperium

Many women who survived the birth safely did die in their postpartum period. Julius Caesar, for instance, during whose dictatorship Cicero wrote his treatise on old age, lost in such circumstances both his first wife Cornelia and his daughter with her, Julia, who had married Pompey the Great. In 46 BCE, in turn, Cicero himself mourned his beloved daughter Tullia, who also died in puerperium. However, with other sources that supply information of similar cases – that is, inscriptions which mention young mothers dying – it is usually hard to tell which apply to women who actually died during childbirth, and which mean mothers who died a few days later. Our knowledge regarding the care women in confinement received is unfortunately rather scant, but

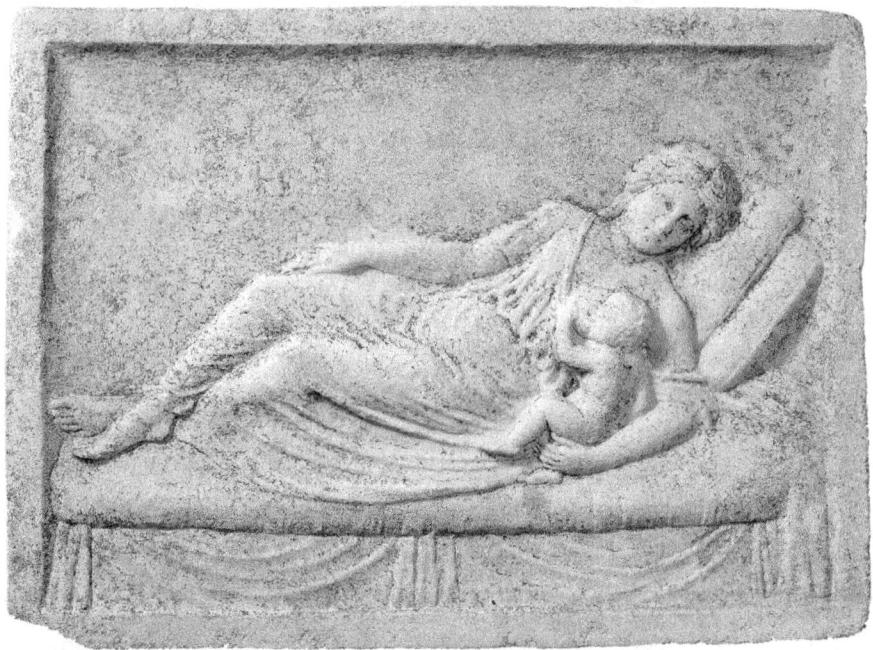

Figure 11 Plaque in tomb relief showing mother and child © Wellcome Collection
Source: https://wellcomecollection.org/works/mm7hrruc

occasionally, wording does come up which indicates a woman died because of post-natal complications. Such was the case of the Cornelia Calliste[11] mentioned above and of Festa, Iulius Secundus' 'beloved wife'.[12]

Daphnis, from Carthage, suffered a similar fate. We do not know how many days after giving birth she died, there is only the information she had given birth 'recently' (*dedi proxime nato*).[13] Sometimes such inscriptions also feature the mother's fear for the baby's future, perhaps as a trope of a sort: who will feed and take care of the child during their long life? (*quis alet natum quis vitam longa(m) ministrat?*)

Unfortunately, rather few medical texts remain containing advice on how to take care of a woman in her postpartum period. In Caelius Aurelianus' opinion, a woman who has recently given birth ought to lie down in a dark room. If the delivery was smooth, her genitals should be rinsed with olive oil mixed with wine; if it was hard, warm olive oil should be used, and she should fast for two days, after which her diet should be light. Doctors also paid attention to the stool excreted during puerperium. Caelius Aurelianus wrote that during that time,

> Oportet spongiis aqua tepida expressis ea loca tergere; tunc ne frigore concepto vexetur, de cathedra vel duro lecto surgere parientem et collocari in cubiculo molli calido mediocriter et obscuro; neque iunctis femoribus, ne materia labens in exitum arceatur, neque nimis distantibus, ne facile frigore partes penetrentur, set modice separatis, ut quicquid ex ea foris exire ceperit non impediatur. tunc ad fluorem lapsum excipiendum spongia mollis sive lana vel latus pannus fibris imponantur, et frequentius commutentur. tunc clunes et pubes usque ad umbilicum munda lana contegantur. et si sine quassatione partus effectus est, oleo spano, id est viridi, admixto modico vino ipse partes irrigentur, quo matricem velud recenti vulnere affectam medela denssemus. si vero laboriosus processit partus, oleo dulci et calido ipsa loca calefiant. tunc requies et abstinentia cibi, ut in ceteris causis, usque ad tertium diem adhibeatur, nisi vires coegerint resumptionem. Tertio vero die sessiones adhibende ex aqua calida aut oleo et tepida, et totum corpus oleo perunguendum, atque ita cibus dandus parvus et digestibilis, ut panis et aqua calida aut pultes et ova apala, et aqua bibenda. est enim numquam tutum, etiam si plerisque consuetum vinum, sumere cibum vini potione coniuncta. tunc post secundam diatriton lavationem convenit adhibere et vinum dari adiuncta cibatione. set tunc quoque vinum parvum dabitur et aquatum, et usum omnium sensim permittimus rerum. set quoniam de conatu et tensione frequentius in partu ruptiones occurrunt, post aliquos dies partus cerotaria imponimus que conficientur cera et oleo roseo, spuma argenti, et cerusa, et alumine rotundo.[14]

Those places should be rubbed with sponges wet with lukewarm water and squeezed partly dry. Also, lest the parturient break out in shivers from cold, she should be lifted off the chair or hard bed and laid in a comfortable, moderately warm and dark sleeping chamber. Her thighs ought ne to be pressed togrther, so that the secretions may flow freely from the exit of the uterus, or spread too wide lest cold reach those parts easily, but rather slightly open, so as to provide no obstruction to anything that might be secreted. Moreover to remove the fluid secreted one should apply a soft sponge or wool or a wide piece of fabric, to b changed frequently. In addition, the woman's buttocks and genital area as far as the navel must be bound in clean wool, and if the birth was smooth, those same parts must be sprinkled with Spanish olive oil with a small admixture of wine. In that way the medicinal drug will fortify the uterus, which has just suffered a wound, so to speak. If the birth was very difficult, those parts should be warmed with sweet, warm olive oil; moreover, let the woman rest and abstain from food (as in other cases) until the third day when her strength will begin to return. However, on the third day apply sitz baths in warm and lukewarm water or oil, anoint the whole body with oil as well, and offer a modest, light meal, such as bread soaked in warm water, or flour-and-vegetable congee with soft-boiled eggs; and water must be drunk too, for it is never safe to ingest food and chase it down with wine, even though most people find it ordinary. Further more, after three more days it is proper to wash the woman's body and serve wine with her food, but only a little wine, and mixed with water. Gradually one should allow her the use of all other things, but since frequent pushing during parturition causes ruptures, after a few days apply poultices composed of wax, rose oil, *spuma argenti* (possibly lead oxide?), the cherry, and alum.

According to Galen, another authority on the subject, after giving birth, a woman should act calmly, sweat, and observe a strict diet. Defecation should be regular, and the faeces the right colour. The woman ought to breathe steadily, have warm feet and a moist tongue, and sleep well. Her urine, Galen believes, should be ample and pale yellow, neither too thin nor too thick. During puerperium, a healthy woman's stool is yellow or pale yellow; red, black or green stool may indicate a pathology. The stool should also be ample and dark in colour. Soranus, meanwhile, thought that puerperium pathologies could already be predicted during labour: difficult labour with fever could be a sign of trouble later. Convulsions, fever, delirium, insomnia, thirst, pain in the heart, pain in the abdomen, cold feet and cloudy urine were all listed as alarming symptoms, but when coma and foul-smelling vomit joined them, one should expect the patient to die soon.

Men believed Roman women spent a long time – too much time, in fact – in confinement after giving birth. Varro notes that in Illyria, women give birth quickly and return to work virtually straight away, as if they had not so much borne a child as found one.[15] Ligurian women were also said to go back to their household duties immediately after delivery.[16]

Caring for a newborn: Fashioning a human being

Unfortunately, no handbook survives of paediatrics, even though the subject matter does of course come up in works dealing with general medicine,[17] and so we can see how taking care of a newborn child was envisioned.[18] One would draw on family tradition and stories told and advice given by experienced mothers, female neighbours and specialized midwives.

To fully understand Soranus on this, we must also take into account one fundamental difference in how young children, and newborn infants in particular, are seen: unlike to us, to the Romans a newborn baby was closer to an animal than a human being, and it was believed that only proper care could make them actually human.[19] This could be achieved thanks to three main factors: baths, massage and swaddling bandages, which were supposed to shape, literally and figuratively, a future Roman citizen.[20] First, though, another crucially important thing happened (or at least, it was important to the father): the baby's gender was officially announced. This was done by the midwife, who then evaluated the child. A test was used to that purpose resembling our present-day Apgar score.[21] On that important matter, Soranus advised one to pay close attention to whether the child's body

> τοὺς πόρους ἔχειν ἀπαρεμποδίστους, οἷον ὤτων, ῥινῶν, φάρυγγος, οὐρήθρας, δακτυλίου, καὶ τὰς ἑκάστου [μορίου] φυσικὰς κινήσεις μὴ νωθρὰς [καὶ] μηδὲ ἐκλύτους καὶ τὰς τῶν ἄρθρων κάμψεις τε καὶ ἐκτάσεις μεγέθη τε καὶ σχήματα καὶ τὴν πᾶσαν ἐπιβάλλουσαν εὐαισθησίαν, ἣν γνωρίζομεν κἀκ τῆς ἐπιφανείας ἐπερείδοντες τοὺς δακτύλους· κατὰ φύσιν γάρ ἐστι τὸ πρὸς ἕκαστον ἀλγεῖν τῶν νυσσόντων ἢ θλιβόντων. ἐκ δὲ τῶν ἐναντίων τοῖς εἰρημένοις τὸ πρὸς ἀνατροφὴν [ἀν]επιτήδειον.

is perfect in all its parts, members and senses; that its ducts, namely of the ears, nose, pharynx, urethra, anus are free from obstruction; that the natural functions of every [member] are neither sluggish nor weak; that the joints bend and stretch; that it has due size and shape and is properly sensitive in every respect. This we may recognize from pressing the fingers against the surface of the body, for it is natural to suffer pain from everything that pricks or squeezes.[22]

It was probably the midwife who, based on this kind of inspection and her own expertise, estimated the baby's overall chances of survival.

Cutting the umbilical cord: The child as a separate entity

Divine (and of course, human) care for the mother and child did not end with a safe birth at all. With the help of the goddess Levana, the midwife presented the newborn, carefully inspected and with the umbilical cord cut off, to the mother.[23] In Soranus' opinion, the umbilical cord was best cut with an instrument made of gold or iron, but both Soranus and Oribasius (who drew on him in his work) wrote that most of the women who delivered children regrettably used a shard of glass instead, a reed, or even bread crust, or linen thread wound tightly around the cord. Their unwillingness to use metal objects for the purpose stemmed from a folk superstition which made it a bad sign to use iron during delivery.[24] Actually, this all-important moment of cutting and tying up the umbilical cord does not feature in images at all. However, one engraved gem, on which one can see the Parcae, or the deities who decided a person's fate, does seem to refer to it figuratively, since centrally in the image we see a length of thread unspooled directly above the head of a baby lying on the ground, naked. As Catullus emphasizes more than once in a poem, the yarn spun by the Parcae was woollen.[25] Dasen thinks we can interpret that as a metaphor: the thread the Parcae will spin in the future is the same as the thread that lets a person begin their independent life on earth, out of the mother's womb,[26] and it will only be able to do so once the midwife ties the thread of life to the child's body.

The aforementioned woollen yarn or thread also appears in medical texts. Soranus advises that just this kind of thread should be used to tie up the umbilical cord stump, since linen thread causes pain by cutting into the body. Tying the umbilical cord correctly was also necessary to prevent a haemorrhage.[27]

According to Soranus, the umbilical cord should dry up and, after three or four days, wither away, leaving at the base a wound, which should be treated.[28] To speed up the process, many women applied to the stump ground pig trotters, snails, onions, and even lead, 'burnt and rinsed', as applying lead to the umbilical cord was believed to be the most efficient way of causing the wound to heal quickly:

ἄμεινον δὲ τοῦτον καὶ σφονδύλῳ τῷ ἐριουργικῷ παραπλησίως σχηματίσασαι κατὰ τῆς τοῦ ὀμφαλοῦ χώρας ἐρείδουσιν, διὰ τὸ ἐμψυκτικὴν [μὲν] εἶναι τὴν ὕλην ἐπουλωθησομένης τῆς ἑλκώσεως, διὰ δὲ τὸ βαρεῖαν εὐπρεπῶς εἰς κοιλότητα τυπωθησομένου τοῦ ὀμφαλοῦ.

It is still better if they mould the lead in the shape of a spinning whorl and press it upon the region of the umbilicus. Since the material is cooling, the wound will cicatrize and since it is heavy, the umbilicus will be properly moulded into a cavity.[29]

Washing the newborn child

After the wound at the navel was treated, the baby's first bath was prepared. Soranus says that because of the mother's weariness after labour, the task ought to be left to the midwives.[30] The symbolic and religious import of the first bath is emphasized on a whole series of empire-era sarcophagi. One can see the infants with midwives, wet-nurses, or nannies, as whole groups of women tend to be pictured, one of them holding the baby and kneeling next to the tub (*alveus*), while the others hold a long stretch of fabric, presumably a towel of sorts.[31] In the background, the images often show the Parcae, deciding the child's future.[32]

Of course, the significance of bathing went beyond ritual. It was primarily meant to clean the child's body of the sticky layer of *vernix caseosa* and blood, as well as strengthening the skin and giving it resistance to ailments such as rashes. To that purpose, Soranus also recommended a form of salt therapy. Before bathing, the newborn was gently sprinkled with ground salt, natron, or even lye, naturally while carefully protecting the child's eyes and mouth, since the agents in question could lead to sores, burning pain and shortness of breath, and using too much salt could irritate the baby's skin. On the other hand, if too little was used, it would not work and the skin would not gain the resistance expected.[33] In the case of weak and small children with very delicate skin, the physician advised the reader to add the salt to honey, olive oil, or 'juice from barley, fenugreek, or mallows' so as to protect the skin of the most vulnerable babies from irritation. After these were applied to the skin, the baby was bathed in lukewarm water. All of the salt paste needed to be washed off very carefully. The action was then repeated, but this time, slightly warmer water was used. The recommendation was to use fingers to remove mucus from the nose, mouth and ears during this second ablution. Soranus thought the eyes should be cleaned with olive oil,

> σμῆξαι γὰρ ἀγαθὸν τούτῳ τὸ παχύτατον ἐν αὐτοῖς ὑγρόν, οὗ μὴ γενομένου κατὰ τὸ πλεῖστον ἀμβλυωπεῖν συμβαίνει τὰ τρεφόμενα.
>
> for it is good thus to wash off the thickest moisture in them; if this is not done, in most cases the nurslings become dim-sighted.[34]

The first bath ended with a check-up of the anal opening, which one was to delicately open up with one's little finger so as to break the thin membranous tissue often found there and enable the child to pass stool freely. After that procedure, the child would often excrete meconium. Having bathed the baby, one ought to dress the umbilical stump again with some folded cloth or wool soaked in olive oil.[35]

Newborn babies were to be washed every day, with special attention paid to the conditions in which all hygienic procedures were carried out, so the child would not catch a cold.

Massage: 'Fashioning' a human being

After the bath, treatments were recommended aimed at shaping the little human being (physically). The child was to be held head down by the ankles. This was supposed to widen the vertebrae and make the spine more flexible. Next, a massage was called for to soften the tendons. One gave the buttocks their proper shape by kneading them with one's index and middle fingers, while the parts above the last vertebra were kneaded with the fist so they would not protrude. The back was given similar treatment; the whole procedure was meant to prevent the formation of a hunched back in the future. If needed, Soranus also recommended massage that would mould the head into the perfect shape,[36] and in boys, careful attention was paid to the form of the foreskin. If the foreskin was not fully developed, the author advised his readers to stretch it gently so as to extend it, or to wrap it in a scrap of wool for protection. Wool was also to be placed under the scrotum to keep it separate from the thighs and prevent unnecessary pressure on it.[37]

Soranus pointed out it was necessary to clean the baby's eyes, although it should not be done too often, or else it could result in 'an irritation of the membranes'.[38] 'The eyes should be wiped with two thick fingers, and the nose, moulded, that is, raised where it is concave and pressed in where its is aquiline; however, in the latter (that is, aquiline), one must not knead at the spot where it is raised, but rather extend the wings of the nose away from its curve and pull them up.'[39]

Only after all those ministrations could the infant be swaddled. As primitive diapers, swaddling clothes and bandages 'humanized' the newborn and were widely believed to help the child shift from the foetal position to an upright one. They were meant to help shape the 'little wrinkled animal' into a human being and help it grow properly. This brand of diapering was on the one hand to protect the child's sensitive skin from external factors, and on the other, just like the massage described above, to 'shape' their body, correct any deformities, and even keep them warm.[40] Soranus emphasized that owing to correct swaddling, boys would later feel no shame of their appearance and would train eagerly, whereas girls would develop bodies suited to their reproductive functions. The significance of the act, the ritual even, is indicated by the level of detail in its descriptions. The mother (or the midwife, or the nanny) would gently lay the baby in her lap, her thighs covered with a piece of warm soft fabric, and begin to swaddle the child. The swaddling bandages were strips of soft, clean wool three to four fingers wide. Linen diapers were avoided, since linen cloth shrinks when wet (for example, with sweat), which might irritate the child's delicate skin or make the swaddling strips cut into the flesh, whereas wool is soft:

> λαβοῦσα τοίνυν τὴν ἀρχὴν τοῦ τελαμῶνος κατὰ τοῦ ἀκροχειρίου τιθέτω καὶ τὴν ἐπείλησιν ἐγκύκλιον ἀγέτω κατὰ τῶν δακτύλων ἐκτεταμένων, εἶτα κατὰ τοῦ ἐπικαρπίου, πήχεώς τε καὶ βραχίονος, πιέζουσα μὲν τὰ κατὰ τοὺς καρποὺς ἡσυχῇ, τὰ δὲ ἄλλα μέχρι μασχάλης ἀνιεῖσα. τῷ δὲ αὐτῷ τρόπῳ καὶ τὴν ἑτέραν σπαργανώσασα τῷ θώρακι λοιπὸν κυκλοτερῶς περιειλείτω τελαμῶνα τῶν πλατυτέρων, ὁμαλῶς μὲν ἐπὶ τῶν ἀρρένων πιέζουσα τὴν ἔνδεσιν, μᾶλλον δὲ τὰ κατὰ τοὺς μαστοὺς σφίγγουσα τῶν θηλειῶν, ἀνιεῖσα δὲ τὸ περὶ τὴν ὀσφύν, εὐπρεπέστερον γάρ ἐστιν ἐπὶ γυναικῶν τοῦτο τὸ σχῆμα. μετὰ δὲ ταῦτα σπαργανοῦν κατ' ἰδίαν ἑκάτερον τῶν σκελῶν, τὸ γὰρ ζυγώσασαν αὐτὰ γυμνὰ συνεπιδεσμεῖν ὁμοῦ ποιητικόν ἐστιν ἑλκώσεως· αἱ γὰρ τρυφερῶν ἀκμὴν ἔτι τῶν σωμάτων παραθέσεις τῇ πυρώσει ταχέως ἐπικαίουσιν. τὰς δὲ περιειλήσεις τῶν τελαμώνων ἕως ἄκρων ποιείσθω δακτύλων, ἀνιεῖσα μὲν τὰ κατὰ τοὺς μηροὺς καὶ τὰς γαστροκνημίας, σφίγγουσα δὲ τὰ πρὸς τοῖς γόνασι καὶ ταῖς ἰγνύαις τά τε κατὰ τοὺς ταρσούς τε καὶ τὰ σφυρά, ἵνα τὰ μὲν ἄκρα πλατύνηται τῶν ποδῶν, τὰ δὲ μέσα συνάγηται. μετὰ δὲ ταῦτα παραβάλλουσα τοὺς μὲν βραχίονας τοῖς πλευροῖς, τοὺς δὲ πόδας ἀλλήλοις, πλατεῖ τελαμῶνι κυκλοτερῶς ὅλον τὸ βρέφος ἀπὸ θώρακος ἄχρι ποδῶν κατειλείτω· παραβεβλημέναι γὰρ αἱ χεῖρες ἔνδοθεν τῆς περιειλήσεως εἰς ἔκτασιν ἐθίζονται. παχυντικαὶ γὰρ τῶν νεύρων αἱ μέχρι πλείονος τῶν ἄρθρων εἰσὶ συζεύξεις (ὥστε καὶ ἀγκύλας ἐπιφέρειν), τῷ μέντοι πρῶτον κατειλῆσθαι τὰ χέρια κωλύεται [τὸ] διὰ τῆς ἀτάκτου παραφορᾶς διαστρέφεσθαι, πολλάκις δὲ καὶ διὰ τοῦ κατὰ τῶν ὀφθαλμῶν τοὺς δακτύλους ἐπιφέρειν κακῶς διατίθεται τὰς ὄψεις. μεταξὺ μέντοι τῶν ἀστραγάλων καὶ τῶν γονάτων, ἔτι δὲ καὶ τῶν ἀγκώνων ἔριον παρεντιθέσθω πρὸς τὸ μὴ ἑλκοῦσθαι τὰς ἐξοχὰς τῇ βιαιοτέρᾳ θλίψει καὶ παραθέσει τῶν μερῶν. τὸ δὲ κεφάλιον σκεπαζέσθω κυκλοτερεῖ περιειλήσει ῥάκους ἢ ἐρίου τρυφεροῦ τε καὶ καθαροῦ. ἐνδέχεται δὲ καὶ ὑπὸ τὸ μετάφρενον ἐπίμηκες καὶ πλατὺ ῥάκος ἢ ἔριον προϋποβάλλειν· εἶτα μετὰ τὴν ἔμπροσθεν εἰρημένην σπαργάνωσιν (δίχα τοῦ ἔξωθεν ἑνὸς καὶ κοινοῦ κατὰ πάντων τελαμῶνος)

ἀναδιπλοῦν τὸ ὑποκείμενον ῥάκος ἢ τὸ ἔριον πρῶτον μὲν κατὰ τὰ ἄνω μέρη ὑπὸ τὸν τράχηλον, εἶτα καθ' ὅλου τοῦ νηπίου δίχα τῆς κεφαλῆς· ὕστερον δὲ πλατυτέρῳ τελαμῶνι καὶ ὡσανεὶ πέντε δακτύλων τὸ πλάτος ὅλον περιτυλίττειν τὸ βρέφος, τὴν δὲ κεφαλὴν ὡς ὑπεδείξαμεν σκέπειν. ἐνδέχεται δὲ καὶ δύο μὲν ὑποστρωννύναι ῥάκη, ἵν' ᾖ τὸ μὲν εὐμέγεθες καὶ τὸ ὅλον περιλαβεῖν σῶμα δυνάμενον, τὸ δὲ χάριν τοῦ μόνην τὴν ὀσφὺν περιελθεῖν αὔταρκες εἰς ὑποδοχὴν τῶν σκυβάλων. οὐ δεῖ γάρ, ὡς ἐπαχθέστερον, ἐρίῳ μὲν καθαρῷ τὸν θώρακα μετὰ τοῦ ἐπιγαστρίου περιλαβεῖν, τὰ δὲ λοιπὰ [μὴ] περιλαβεῖν, ὡς ἔμπροσθεν εἰρήκαμεν.

The midwife then should take the end of the bandage, put it over its hand and, winding it round, carry it over the extended fingers; then over the middle of the hand, the forearm and the upper arm, slightly compressing the parts at the wrist but keeping the rest up to the armpit loose. Having also swaddled the other arm in the same manner, she should then wrap one of the broader bandages circularly around the thorax, exerting an even pressure when swaddling males, but in females binding the parts at the breasts more tightly, yet keeping the region of the loins loose, for in women this form is more becoming. After this one must swaddle each leg separately, for to join them naked and bind them up together is apt to produce ulceration; for the juxtaposition of bodies which are as yet soft makes them quickly burn with inflammation. The midwife must wind the bandage to the very tips of the toes, keep the region of the thighs and the calves loose, but tighten the parts at the knees and their hollows as well as the instep and the ankles, so that the ends of the feet be broadened but their middle be contracted. Afterwards she should lay the arms along the sides and the feet one against the other, and with a broad bandage she should wrap up the whole infant circularly from the thorax to the feet; since if the hands are put inside the wrapping, they become accustomed to extension. For the confinement of the joints for any length of time is apt to thicken the sinews (so as even to bring about ankylosis); however, by wrapping up the little hands just at first, they are prevented from becoming twisted by inordinate movements. Also, putting the fingers to the eyes, often causes impaired vision. Now between the ankles, the knees, and the elbows too, a piece of wool should be inserted so that the prominences may not be ulcerated by the relatively forcible pressure and juxtaposition of the parts. The little head should be covered by bandaging it circularly with a soft clean cloth or piece of wool. It is also possible first to put a long broad cloth or piece of wool beneath the back; then after the swaddling mentioned before (omitting the one external bandage which all parts have in common) one must first fold the underlying cloth or piece of wool over the upper parts below the neck, then over the whole child except the head; afterwards one must wrap the whole newborn around with a broader bandage about five

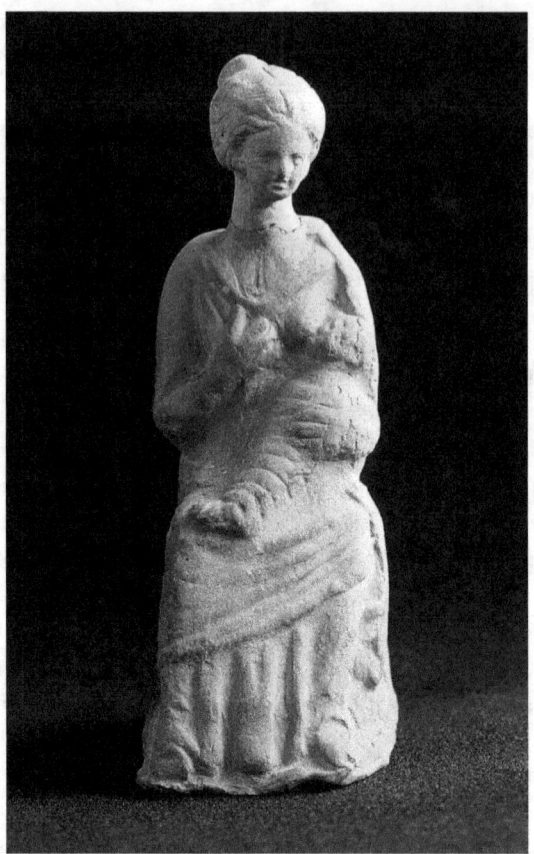

Figure 12 A mother feeding a swaddled infant © Wellcome Collection (CC BY 4.0). Source: https://wellcomecollection.org/works/mj8kvw57

fingers in breadth, covering the head, however, as we have shown. Another possibility is to put two pieces of cloth underneath, so that one is of good size and capable of embracing the whole body, the other one large enough for the reception of the faeces, to go around the loins only. For, as we have said before, one should not, because it is too burdensome, cover the thorax together with the abdomen with clean wool yet leave the other parts [un]covered.[41]

For convenience, Soranus allows the use of an external cloth layer made of two parts when changing the swaddling bandages. One part should be long enough to wrap the child's whole body in it, and the other should reach the hips and catch the stool.[42]

The social birth of the child – and the mother

Being born was often a well-documented event among the Romans.[43] Epigraphic material survives indicating that the family friends, and neighbours were all notified of the joyous occasion.[44] Inscriptions were discovered in Pompeii informing the reader that a child had been born.[45] A laurel wreath was hung on the door of a house where a baby had just been born.[46] Remembering his disappointment when he was not informed that a friend of his now had another son, and scolding him for that, Statius wrote:

> cumque tibi vagiret tertius infans, / protinus ingenti non venit nuntia cursu / littera, quae festos cumulare altaribus ignes / et redimire chelyn postesque ornare iuberet / Albanoque cadum sordentem promere fumo / et cantu signare diem?

> When your third child was wailing, did no letter come straightway posthaste to bring me word, telling me to heap my altar with festal fire and wreathe my lyre and decorate my doorway and bring out a jar begrimed with Alban smoke and mark the day with chalk?[47]

Juvenal also advised his audience to prepare house decorations for the occasion of a child's birth:

> ornentur postes et grandi ianua lauro.

> Let's decorate the doorposts and the doors with abundant laurels.[48]

while in another satire, one character admonishes another:

> foribus suspende coronas: iam pater es.

> Hang the garlands over your doors: now you're a daddy.[49]

Meanwhile, the child was under the protection of deities, for whom special altars and places of honour were made ready in the atrium, such as *lectisternia* for Picumnus and Pilumnus or Juno and Hercules. Politeness dictated that friends and neighbours come over and congratulate the father. Aulus Gellius recounts the visit the philosopher Favorinus paid to a disciple of his whose wife had just given birth to a son:

> Nuntiatum quondam est Favorino philosopho, nobis praesentibus, uxorem auditoris sectatorisque sui paululum ante enixam auctumque eum esse nato filio. 'Eamus' inquit 'et puerperam visum et patri gratulatum.'

Word was once brought in my presence to the philosopher Favorinus that the wife of an auditor and disciple of his had been brought to bed a short time before, and that his pupil's family had been increased by the birth of a son. 'Let us go,' said he, 'both to see the child and to congratulate the father.'[50]

Besides receiving guests, the father's duties included following legal regulations. The available sources clearly indicate one general rule which applied in the empire: newborn children had to be registered within thirty days from birth (or from the day they were named).

> Inter haec liberales causas ita munivit, ut primus iuberet apud praefectos aerarii Saturni unumquemque civium natos liberos profiteri intra tricensimum diem nomine imposito. Per provincias tabulariorum publicorum usum instituit, apud quos idem de originibus fieret, quod Romae apud praefectos aerarii.

> In the meantime, he put such safeguards about suits for personal freedom—and he was the first to do so—as to order that every citizen should bestow names upon his free-born children within thirty days after birth and declare them to the prefects of the treasury of Saturn. In the provinces, too, he established the use of public records, in which entries concerning births were to be made in the same manner as at Rome in the office of the prefects of the treasury.[51]

While introducing the custom is attributed to Marcus Aurelius, it had already been practised before, as children needed to be registered within thirty days of birth from Augustus' times. Registration of births is mentioned in two well-known legal acts from Augustus' reign, the *lex Aelia Sentia* of 4 CE and the *lex Papia Poppaea* of 9 CE.[52]

The documents pertaining to the registration were kept in archives, but perhaps the people who submitted their declarations about children just born received some manner of an official receipt to verify the fact, as apparently indicated by a passage in Apuleius' *Apologia*, where the author defends the honour of his wife Pudentilla. Addressing his accusers, he wishes to submit at the trial the proper documents to verify his wife's age. He writes:

> De aetate vero Pudentillae, de qua post ista satis confidenter mentitus es, ut etiam sexaginta annos natam diceres nupsisse, de ea tibi paucis respondebo: nam [non] necesse est in re tam perspicua pluribus disputare. Pater eius natam sibi filiam more ceterorum professus est. Tabulae eius partim tabulario publico, partim domo adservantur, quae iam tibi ob os obiciuntur. Porrige tu Aemiliano tabulas istas: linum consideret, signa quae impressa sunt recognoscat, consules legat, annos computet, quos sexaginta mulieri adsignabat.

Now about Pudentilla's age you went on to tell such a barefaced lie as to say that she married at sixty. On this matter my answer will be brief, since there is no call for lengthy argument when the facts are so clear. Like other fathers, her father registered his daughter's birth. The records are kept both in the public record office and at home, and they are now being brought for you to see You, hand those records to Aemilianus; let him examine the thread, acknowledge the stamped seals, read the names of the consuls, calculate the years, of which he bestowed sixty on the lady.[53]

The custom of offering a coin in the temple of Juno Lucina was another indication that a newborn child (in this case, a son) was accepted into the family. Dionysius of Halicarnassus reports:

ὡς δὲ Πείσων Λεύκιος ἐν τῇ πρώτῃ τῶν ἐνιαυσίων ἀναγραφῶν ἱστορεῖ, βουλόμενος καὶ τῶν ἐν ἄστει διατριβόντων τὸ πλῆθος εἰδέναι, τῶν τε γεννωμένων καὶ τῶν ἀπογινομένων καὶ τῶν εἰς ἄνδρας ἐγγραφομένων, ἔταξεν ὅσον ἔδει νόμισμα καταφέρειν ὑπὲρ ἑκάστου τοὺς προσήκοντας, εἰς μὲν τὸν τῆς Εἰλειθυίας θησαυρόν, ἣν Ῥωμαῖοι καλοῦσιν **Ἥραν φωσφόρον**, ὑπὲρ τῶν γεννωμένων· εἰς δὲ τὸν τῆς Ἀφροδίτης τῆς ἐν ἄλσει καθιδρυμένης, ἣν προσαγορεύουσι Λιβιτίνην, ὑπὲρ τῶν ἀπογινομένων· εἰς δὲ τὸν τῆς Νεότητος, ὑπὲρ τῶν εἰς ἄνδρας ἀρχομένων συντελεῖν· ἐξ ὧν ἤμελλε διαγνώσεσθαι καθ᾽ ἕκαστον ἐνιαυτόν, ὅσοι τε οἱ σύμπαντες ἦσαν καὶ τίνες ἐξ αὐτῶν τὴν στρατεύσιμον ἡλικίαν εἶχον.

And wishing also, as Lucius Piso writes in the first book of his Annals, to know the number of the inhabitants of the city, and of all who were born and died and arrived at the age of manhood, he prescribed the piece of money which their relations were to pay for each—into the treasury of Ilithyia (called by the Romans Juno Lucina) for those who were born.[54]

However, the most significant event was probably the *dies lustricus*, when the child was named.[55] It was usually held on the eighth day following birth (for girls), or on the ninth (for boys).[56] Plutarch explains that was because women reached maturity earlier than men. Until the umbilical stump fell off, the infant was considered more a vegetable than a living being, so the *dies lustricus* was only celebrated once the last thing to connect the child with the mother's body 'withered away'. It was then that the child commenced independent existence, which justified it receiving a name of its own.

We do not know how the celebration went, but Dasen believes it was that day's rituals that Persius had in mind when he wrote:

> Ecce avia aut metuens divum matertera cunis / exemit puerum frontemque atque uda labella / infami digito et lustralibus ante salivis / expiat, urentis oculos inhibere perita;

> Look—a grandma or superstitious aunt has lifted the boy from his cradle and first protects his forehead and wet lips with her wicked finger and magical saliva, an expert at warding off the withering evil eye.[57]

From the legal standpoint, the naming was more important than the day of actual, physical birth, because it meant 'the birth of a Roman'.[58] Tertullian compared the day to events as important in a Roman man's life as donning the *toga virilis* or marriage.[59] According to the text of the *lex Malacitana*, candidates for offices were evaluated, in part, based on how many children they had, and dead children were counted provided they had been named before their deaths.[60]

Certainly the celebration was very significant from the perspective of a Roman family, possibly especially from a woman's perspective. A woman who had been through the whole pregnancy had already moved beyond her old status but had not arrived at the new one, since officially she was not yet a mother.[61] If we assume that until the *dies lustricus* a child was not so much a separate entity as part of the woman, she was at that point still at the transitional stage, and only after the *dies lustricus* could she enjoy motherhood.

Conclusion

'I have fulfilled my votive pledge; much offspring of mine remains. As I wished, I got a splendid funeral from my husband'[1]

The goal of this book has been to depict *mater in statu nascendi*, a woman as she became a mother, in the context of the interest in reproductive health in Rome. I have tried to distinguish and describe several moments in the life of a Roman woman which made the successive stages of that process, and were a part of a woman's life. The term I use to refer to it, *cursus laborum feminae Romanae*, has been coined especially for this book. Those moments include the birth of a girl, her wedding, then childbirth which, although biologically speaking means a child's birth, is also a mother's psychologically, and finally the *dies lustricus*, which can be considered the legally sanctioned social birth of both the child and the mother.

Taking into account the specific character of my source material, I have tried to make use of narrative and epigraphic texts, visual sources and medical literature alike to discuss aspects of women's reproductive health which aroused the interest of historians, poets, prose authors, lawyers, physicians and ordinary Roman people. Most of those sources are dated to the period from the first century BCE to the third century CE, but of course I have occasionally used earlier and slightly later materials, although they comprise a small fraction of the whole. I decided not to use Christian sources and, as I have already indicated in the Introduction, that was deliberate.

I wrote the book with the conviction that we owe everything we know of those aspects of women's life in the era to sources created by men, which limits certain research perspectives without ruling them out altogether.

***

Marriages of Roman citizens were made so that children would be born in them. Dionysius of Halicarnassus reports that already Romulus' legislation contained regulations which obligated citizens to marry and have children. Because of how

Romans understood fertility and pregnancy, any Roman women who wished to use a natural method of fertility control would have encountered serious problems, since at the time it was believed conception was most likely to occur at the beginning and end of a woman's menstrual cycle. The effects of that belief were twofold: on the one hand, couples who wanted a child could easily miss the best time for impregnation; on the other, couples trying to avoid pregnancy or simply not trying for it inadvertently increased their chances of conception by having intercourse at other times.

A married couple's fertility, proven by the birth of a child, offered a sense of contentment and respect, but also tangible benefits granted by the state. Interestingly, both spouses benefited. The *ius trium liberorum* referred to here was also applied to people with no offspring if their merits with the emperor were deemed of equal worth with parenthood, but it was a privilege of the very few. However, it must be remembered that while that imperial-era privilege could solve a number of legal issues, it did nothing to satisfy a person's need for an heir or their emotional desire to have children.

Infertility was unambiguously seen as a gender-related issue in Rome, blamed almost exclusively on women. In the social dimension, at least, it seldom applied to men. It was widely believed in the Roman society that if a man suspected his spouse was infertile and was determined to sire children, he could divorce her, marry another woman and try again for children with her. The wife had no such options, even if she suspected it was actually her husband who was infertile. The label of infertility must have led to a sense of failure in women, particularly those of the Roman elite. According to the society's concept of motherhood, a woman who could not give birth was simply not needed.

Still, not everyone wanted to have children, so all of the medical knowledge of the time was harnessed when people attempted to regulate their fertility. Even so, S. Dixon emphasizes that our present-day interest in ancient fertility control, and especially in contraception and abortion, has completely eclipsed the much stronger concerns then felt to *ensure* fertility. For Roman families, having too few children (who survived their childhood) was much more of a problem than having too many unwanted pregnancies. Neither is it a surprise that, with life expectancy fairly low, people married young to preserve generational continuity and provide the state with enough citizens, thus the high number of very young mothers.

Virtues such as fertility, chastity and modesty played an important part in arranging marriages, but so did the dowry brought into the family and political alliances. Roman jurists decided that girls could legally marry as early as at twelve, an age corresponding to natural puberty and menarche. The Romans did not doubt that menstruation had a connection to fertility – in fact, guaranteed fertility – and that a woman who did not menstruate could not become pregnant, but the arrival of monthly periods and marriage did not automatically mean the girl was ready to become a mother. Ancient physicians did stress that such a young age was not suitable for giving birth to one's first child, since the reproductive organs might well not be ready for the girl to carry to term and give birth safely. However, from the extant sources we know their opinion was not necessarily respected by the society (or, actually, by its elite).

As there are no sources on the matter, we do not know whether a girl just about to marry had had any sexual experiences; most likely she was expected not to have had any. Suddenly confronting sexuality on their wedding night probably marked a drastic change in the life of teenage girls who had commemorated their childhoods only the day before. We can, however, suspect that girls were prepared for the transition in some way, perhaps through conversations with their mothers, nurses or midwives. Some researchers think dolls could have been helpful, since, as educational toys, they played an important role in girls' socialization and sexual education. Perhaps they also helped girls familiarize themselves with their future role of a wife and mother.

Not all the girls thus prepared to take on the role of a matron lived long enough to become one, but the way they were commemorated after death is priceless evidence for the importance that transition into a wife and mother had for Roman families, and for the scale of the pain they felt at their lost expectations that their daughters would become mothers themselves. Young girls' graves often held objects connected with the transition from childhood to wifehood (and motherhood), a transition brutally interrupted by death. This wealth of feminine items in their tombs not only constituted a kind of compensation for unfulfilled motherhood, but also had an important psychological function in the family's life, by allowing the mourners to see the young woman at the moment they had all been looking forward to. The tombs were often meant to reflect both childhood and unachieved maturity, thus on the one hand acknowledging the past, and on the other, expressing longing for a future that would never come. Such burials were in a sense compensational.

The same principle applied when hopes were lost for a descendant, that is, when a woman died during or as a result of childbirth. Tombstones set up by women's parents, depicting them holding swaddled infants, display a pattern which symbolized motherhood and was employed regardless of why the mother died, how many children she had, how old those children were, and whether she survived childbirth or died because of it. It might have also symbolically expressed (indeed, that may have been its primary purpose) the belief that to a woman's family, her death meant the loss of hopes for grandchildren who would extend the lineage.

Relief sculptures and inscriptions mentioning dead women are a sad, but also a magnificent testimony to the Roman way of life. The high mortality rate among women – and it was not just high in the perinatal period – was caused by ignorance, not so much of medicine in general as of antiseptic principles and procedures. Women were taken care of by midwives and doctors. In the preface to his Latin translation of Soranus' Greek *Gynaecology*, Caelius Aurelianus wrote that the ancients eventually decided to establish women doctors so that female patients in need of examination or help did not have to face the discomfort of being seen by men. Thus it was shame that lay behind the admittance of women into the profession and shame that motivated authors to write down their practical knowledge of obstetrics. Of course we know little about the women deprived of that kind of care (for instance, because their finances did not permit it).

Midwives and female physicians made a small group in ancient Rome, but one important to the society of the time. Although our sources are rather few, they not only prove that professional group did in fact exist, but also indicate that male doctors, teachers, husbands and parents of the women known as *medicae* and *obstetrices* treated them with enormous respect and appreciated their professional skills. In addition, their very presence may have led to an increase in Roman women's trust in medicine, thereby also raising the level of prevention and care extended to the reproductive health and life of Roman women.

The scarcity of visual sources depicting pregnancy *in extenso* goes hand in hand with the surprising, even 'amazing' absence of any discussion of pregnant women – their appearance, moods and states of mind. Of course, that is largely because those sources were written and otherwise created by men, for whom the end result (that is, children) was much more interesting than the process (that is, pregnancy).

Like N. Kampen, I perceive a dissonance in the source material here. On the one hand, children born alive, miscarriages, stillborn children, children who died in their infancy, and the fear of childlessness, which comes up in so many sources, are all symptoms of the patriarchal concerns of men from the elite, for whom heirs were of importance. However, that is accompanied by a lack of discussion of pregnancy and a lack of depictions of it. This could stem from a fear of investing emotions and attention into a person who might soon die in childbirth. Unfortunately, we do not know what women themselves thought about their relationship with their bodies, including pregnancy, since their images were made by men too.

The same applies to birth and labour. Why is the act of birth mostly covered by medical works and so rare in narrative and visual sources? It could be because birth was seen as part of 'women-only space', and it is in that space that childbirth occurred as a biological phenomenon. Still, social birth, the *dies lustricus*, the ceremony at which the child was given a name, was probably the most significant event. It was usually held on the eighth or ninth day after birth, for girls and boys respectively. Until the umbilical stump fell off, the child was regarded as a plant more than an animal, so the *dies lustricus* was only celebrated after the last thing was gone which had tied the baby to the mother's body.

From the legal standpoint, naming the child was more important than the day of their birth, as it was on the naming day that a Roman was born. The importance of the celebration was great to the Roman family, but even greater, perhaps counter to what has been written on the subject before, to the Roman woman. After all, it was the woman who, having gone through puberty, became pregnant, and by giving birth left her old status behind (but had not yet gained a new one, as we assume that until the *dies lustricus* the baby was not an independent entity, but rather part of the woman) and remained at a transitional stage. It was only then that she achieved what the Roman society expected of her, only then (from the *dies lustricus* on) could she fully enjoy motherhood. Such was the story of Claudia, who would now appreciate it if we paid attention to her:[2]

> Hospes, quod deico paullum est, asta ac pellege./ Heic est sepulcrum hau plucrum pulcrai feminae./ Nomen parentes nominarunt Claudiam./ Suom mareitom corde deilexit souo. / Gnatos duos creavit, horunc alteriumin / terra linquit, alium sub terra locat. /Sermone lepido, tu, autem incessu commodo./ Domum servavit, lanam fecit. Dixi. Abei.

> Stranger, my message is short. Stand by and read it through. Here is the unlovely[1] tomb of a lovely woman. Her parents called her Claudia by name. She loved her husband with her whole heart. She bore two sons; of these she leaves one on earth; under the earth has she placed the other. She was charming in converse, yet proper in bearing. She kept house, she made wool. That's my last word. Go your way.

Notes

Introduction

1 Considering the meaning of Latin *labor* (toil), I would like to suggest this expression as a mock contrast of sorts with the *cursus honorum*, only relevant to men: Tatarkiewicz 2018.
2 Gourevitch 1994: 200–6.
3 Among the few exceptions are papyri from the Roman Egypt, which include correspondence (some of it by women or addressed to women) with mentions in them of pregnancy, childbirth and miscarriage. See e.g. Bagnall, Cribiore 2006.
4 Gell. 18.6.8.
5 Gromkowska-Melosik 2013: 33; although S. de Beauvoir's famous words bear repeating here: 'one is not born, but rather becomes, a woman.' For a broad discussion of motherhood and women's involvement in caring for infants in the context of the so-called motherly love, see e.g. Badinter 1998, 2013.
6 Interestingly, the Latin word *maternitas* only first appears in texts in the ninth century CE, and comes from the Greek μητρίς (*mother country*). It only came to be used in the context of motherhood in the eleventh–twelfth centuries CE (and then rarely): Tombeur 2005: 139–49.
7 Hänninen 2005: 49.
8 I must emphasize most of the extant material depicts the Roman elites, and women are no exception. Nonetheless, I decided against narrowing down the scope of this study in the title already, since I have attempted to use a variety of sources, including epigraphic and visual ones, which often include non-elite women, even slaves and freedwomen. Even so, due to the sources preserved, the heroines of this study are still higher-class women.
9 Dixon 1988: 7.
10 This work is a modified and supplemented version of my book *Mater in statu nascendi. Społeczne i medyczne aspekty zdrowia reprodukcyjnego kobiet w starożytnym Rzymie* (Poznań 2018).
11 Plut., Amatorius liber 771c: τὰς δ' ὠδῖνας αὐτὴ καθ' ἑαυτὴν διήνεγκεν, ὥσπερ ἐν φωλεῷ λέαινα καταδῦσα πρὸς τὸν ἄνδρα.
12 Chodorow 1978.
13 Nussbaum 1998: 197–8; Nussbaum is considered a pioneer of 'new' research into women in antiquity by S. Pomeroy in *Goddesses, Whores, Wives, and Slaves*; she did

create a model of roles assigned to women in the ancient world and a model for describing them, but mainly she included the history of women in the broadly conceived perspective of social history. See Pomeroy 1975. Other studies deserving of mention are: Rabinowitz, Richlin 1993; Pomeroy 1991; King 1995: 199–216; Foxhall 2013: 165–84; Musiał 2013: 5–22; Gillmeister 2013: 3–16, 2015: 22–32; Olszewski 2002; Kompa 2015: 49–69.

14 The literature is so abundant it cannot possibly be listed in full. What follows is a modest and subjective selection: Budin, MacIntosh Turfa 2016; Hemelrijk, Woolf 2013; James, Dillon 2012; Bauman 1992; Hemelrijk 1999; Wood 2000; Staples 1998; Cantarella 1987.

15 Nifosi 2019 should be mentioned here, as well as the unpublished but fascinating doctoral dissertation by Hug: Hug 2014.

16 Dixon 1988.

17 Dixon 1992.

18 Hackworth Petersen, Salzman-Mitchell 2012.

19 Augoustakis 2010.

20 Morelli 2009. This book does not include that imperial propaganda of fertility (*fecunditas*), featured not merely on coins, but also in inscriptions and visual images.

21 Sharrock, Keith 2020.

22 In the state of being 'born', that is, made.

23 D. N. Stern claims the child's physical birth corresponds to the psychological birth of the mother, expressed in the forming of a new identity, the sense that one is a mother: Stern, Bruschweiler-Stern, Freeland 1999.

24 Gourevitch 1984; Gourevitch was also a member of the team responsible for preparing a critical edition and French translation of Soranus for Les Belles Lettres (P. Burguière, D. Gourevitch, Y. Malinas, *Soranos d'Éphèse, Maladies des femmes*, Tome I–IV, Paris 1988–2000), and the author of hundreds of papers on ancient medicine.

25 Primarily: Dasen, 2015, 2004, 2005; Dasen, Boudon-Millot, Maire 2008; and numerous articles.

26 Flemming 2000.

27 Dierichs 2002.

28 https://www.academia.edu/43671077/WOMEN_IN_ANTIQUITY_A_BIBLIOGRAPHY_A_new_corrected_5th_edition_667_pp_9_935_entries_on_feminity_womanhood_gender_sexuality_prostitution_marriage_family_pregnancy_childbirth_motherhood_nursing_breastfeeding_abortion_gynecology_female_anatomy_and_physiology_by_Yiannis_Panidis (accessed on 20 January 2022).

29 Rudolf 2016: 24.

30 Rudolf 2016: 25–6.

31 Hopwood, Flemming, Kassell 2019.

32 Rudolf 2016: 25–6.
33 Treggiari 1991: 5.
34 Plut., Περὶ παίδων ἀγωγῆς 2.
35 Soranus 1.7.30.
36 Soranus 1.11.42. He does, however, mention that some authors believe women who do not engage in intercourse have health problems and menstrual difficulties. As his example, he cites widows, whose flow is scant, but who face no such problems once they remarry.
37 Flemming 2007: 257–79; Tsoucalas, Kousoulis, Androutsos 2012: 337–8; Tsoucalas, Sgantzos 2016: 1–5 http://www.jusurgery.com/universalsurgery/aspasia-and-cleopatra-metrodora-twomajestic-female-physician-surgeons-in-theearly-byzantine-era.pdf (accessed on 12 September 2016).
38 Περὶ γυναικείων παθῶν τῆς μήτρας (manuscript, Flor. Laur. 75,3); even the name *Metrodora*, occasionally translated as *mother's gift*, may indicate she was fictional, or the name was a pseudonym; see e.g. Touwaide 2002: 132.
39 There is much discrepancy in literature (from the second to the twelfth century CE); Tsoucalas, Sgantzos 2016: 1–5.
40 Although in one of Seneca's letters it is the concerned father who runs to get the midwife when his daughter goes into labour, heedless of his surroundings: 'Who anxiously calls for a midwife to attend to his daughter about to enter confinement, does not read an announcement then or the programme of the games' (Sen. *Ad Luc.* 117).
41 Plin., HN 28.9.
42 Ovid. *Fasti* 3.257–8: Si qua tamen gravida est, resoluto crine precetur / ut solvat partus molliter illa suos.
43 van Gennep 2006: 37–50; Jaskulska 2013: 79–82.
44 Σωρανός ὁ Ἐφέσιος, but I have decided to consistently employ the Latinized variant of his name (*Soranus*) rather than the Greek (*Soranos*), mostly for consistency with other Latinized Greek proper and geographical names.
45 *Sorani Gynaeciorum libri IV,* ed. J. Ilberg, Berlin 1927.
46 *Soranus of Ephesus, Soranus' Gynecology,* ed. and transl. O. Temkin, Baltimore 1991.
47 Green 2008; Green, Hanson, 1994: 968–1076.
48 Caelius Aurelianus, *Gynaecia. Fragments of a Latin Version of Soranus' Gynaecia, from a Thirteenth Century Manuscript,* ed. M. F. Drabkin, I. E. Drabkin, Baltimore 1951; Bendz 1943: 65–76.
49 *Theodori Prisciani Euporiston libri III cum Physicorum fragmento et additamentis pseudo-Theodoreis,* ed. V. Rose, Leipzig 1894, pp. 427–61.
50 *La Gynaecia di Muscione: manuale per le ostetriche et le mamme del VI sec. d.C.,* ed. R. Radicchi, Pisa 1970.
51 A. Prenner, *Mustione 'traduttore' di Sorano di Efeso. L'ostetrica, la donna, la gestazione,* Napoli 2012.

52 Dionysius of Halicarnassus, *Roman Antiquities*, transl. E. Cary, Cambridge 1937.
53 Cornelius Tacitus, *Annales*, Hrsg. E. Koestermann, Leipzig 1960.
54 Suétone, *Vie des douze Césars*, tr. H. Ailloud, Paris 1931–2.
55 Plutarch, *Moralia, Volume VI: On Affection for Offspring*, transl. W. C. Helmbold. Cambridge 1939; Plutarch, *Lives, Volume I: Theseus and Romulus. Lycurgus and Numa. Solon and Publicola*, transl. B. Perrin, Cambridge 1914.
56 Dio Cassius, *Roman History, Volume V*, transl. E. Cary, H. B. Foster, Cambridge 1917; Dio Cassius, *Roman History, Volume VII–VIII*, transl. E. Cary, H. B. Foster, Cambridge 1924.
57 *Scriptores Historiae Augustae*, Hrsg. E. Hohl, Leipzig 1965.
58 Cicero, *On the Republic. On the Laws,* transl. C. W. Keyes, Cambridge 1928; Cicero, *Letters to Atticus,* ed. and transl. D. R. Shackleton Bailey, Cambridge 1999; Cicero, *On Ends,* transl. H. Rackham, Cambridge 1914; Cicero, *Pro lege Manilia. Pro Caecina. Pro Cluentio. Pro Rabirio Perduellionis Reo*, transl. H. Grose Hodge, Cambridge 1927.
59 *Plinius Caecilius Secundus Gaius: Epistularum libri novem. Epistularum ad Traianum liber. Panegyricus*, Hrsg. M. Schuster, R. Hanslik, Lipsiae 1958.
60 Apuleius, *Apologia. Florida. De Deo Socratis,* ed. and transl. Ch. P. Jones, Cambridge 2017; Apuleius, *Metamorphoses (The Golden Ass),* ed. and transl. J. A. Hanson, Cambridge 1996.
61 Pliny, *Natural History, Volume VI: Books 20–32,* transl. W. H. S. Jones, Cambridge 1951–63.
62 Solinus, *Wunder der Welt. Collectanea rerum mirabilium. Lateinisch und Deutsch*, Hrsg. Kai Brodersen, Darmstadt 2014.
63 *A. Gellii Noctium Atticarum libri XX*, Hrsg. M. Herz, C. Hosius, Lipsiae 1903.
64 Quintilian, *The Lesser Declamations,* ed. and transl. D. R. Shackleton Bailey, Cambridge 2006.
65 Seneca the Elder, *Controversiae*, transl. M. Winterbottom, Cambridge 1974.
66 Seneca, *Moral Essays, Volume II: De Consolatione ad Marciam,* transl. J. W. Basore, Cambridge 1932; Seneca, *Moral Essays, Volume II: De Consolatione ad Helviam,* transl. J. W. Basore, Cambridge 1932.
67 Ammianus Marcellinus, *History,* ed. and transl. J. C. Rolfe, Cambridge 1950.
68 *Artemidori Daldiani Onirocriticon libri V*, Hrsg. R. Ambrose, Leipzig 2011.
69 *Livre de Censorinus sur le jour natal*, tr. J. Mangeart, Paris 1843.
70 *Estudios y traduccion Dioscorides. Sobre los remedios medicinales. Manuscrito de Salamanca*, trad. A. López Eire, F. Cortés Gabaudan, Salamanca 2006.
71 *Plinii Secundi, quae fertur una cum Gargilii Martialis, Medicina*, ed. V. Rose, Lipsiae 1875.
72 Lucretius wrote as an Epicurean, and meant to make Epicurus' philosophy accessible to Romans, as well as to popularize the Epicurean lifestyle; see e.g. L. Fratantuono,

A Reading of Lucretius' 'De rerum natura', London 2015; *T. Lucreti Cari De rerum natura libri sex*, Hrsg. J. Martin, Leipzig 1953.

73 Ovid, *L'Art d'aimer*, ed. and transl. H. Bornecque, Paris 2011; Ovid, *Fasti*, transl. J. G. Frazer, Cambridge 1931; Ovid, *Heroides. Amores*, transl. G. Showerman, Cambridge 1914.
74 Horace, *Odes and epodes*, ed. N. Rudd, Cambridge 2004.
75 *Sexti Properti Elegiarum libri IV*, Hrsg. P. Fedeli, Leipzig 2006.
76 Martial, *Epigrams, Volume II–III*, ed. and transl. D. R. Shackleton Bailey, Cambridge 1993.
77 Juvénal, *Satires*, transl. P. De Labriolle, F. Villeneuve, Paris 2004.
78 *Corpus Iuris Civilis, t. 1, Institutiones. Digesta*, Hrsg. P. Krueger, Berlin 1922.
79 Christian accounts of women, mothers and motherhood bear the stamp of the teachings of the church, and so diverge from the traditional, pagan Roman sources, so I have decided not to use them, even though literature on the subject is quite ample. See e.g. Brown 2008, with further reading. In this book I only cite a few excerpts from Tertullian and Augustine, but exclusively in the context of what they wrote on deities in charge of pregnancy, childbirth and the postpartum period, as well as Romans extracting dead foetuses.
80 Dixon 2001 (Introduction).
81 An aspect brought up by Richlin 2014.
82 In her commentary on the birth of Athena depicted on an Athenian amphora, M. Beard goes so far as to claim that 'The apparent madness of Greek myth has an important and awkward point here: in a perfect world you would not even need women to procreate' Beard 2017, fig. 21.

Chapter 1

1 Treggiari 1991: 5.
2 Dion. Hal. 2.15.2: πρῶτον μὲν εἰς ἀνάγκην κατέστησε τοὺς οἰκήτορας αὐτῆς ἅπασαν ἄρρενα γενεὰν ἐκτρέφειν καὶ θυγατέρων τὰς πρωτογόνους, ἀποκτιννύναι δὲ μηδὲν τῶν γεννωμένων νεώτερον τριετοῦς, πλὴν εἴ τι γένοιτο παιδίον ἀνάπηρον ἢ τέρας εὐθὺς ἀπὸ γονῆς. ταῦτα δ' οὐκ ἐκώλυσεν ἐκτιθέναι τοὺς γειναμένους ἐπιδείξαντας πρότερον πέντε ἀνδράσι τοῖς ἔγγιστα οἰκοῦσιν, ἐὰν κἀκείνοις συνδοκῇ. Gourevitch 1990: 139–51; Dixon 1992: 61; Treggiari 1991; Niczyporuk 2014: 195.
3 Dion. Hal. 2.25.7.
4 Gell. 4.3.2: Atque is Carvilius traditur uxorem, quam dimisit, egregie dilexisse carissimamque morum eius gratia habuisse, set iurisiurandi religionem animo atque amori praevertisse, quod iurare a censoribus coactus erat uxorem se liberorum quaerendorum gratia habiturum.

5 Leiwo, Halla-Aho 2002: 560–80. Sanders 1938: 104–16; http://papyri.info/ddbdp/chla;4;249.
6 Macrob., *Sat.* 1.16.18: uxorem liberum quaerendorum causa ducere religiosum est.
7 Suet., *Caes.* 52: quam Caesar ferre iussisset cum ipse abesset, uti uxores liberorum quaerendorum causa quas et quot vellet ducere liceret.
8 Tac., *Ann.* 11.27: Haud sum ignarus fabulosum visum iri tantum ullis mortalium securitatis fuisse in civitate omnium gnara et nihil reticente, nedum consulem designatum cum uxore principis, praedicta die, adhibitis qui obsignarent, velut suscipiendorum liberorum causa convenisse, atque illam audisse auspicum verba, subisse, sacrificasse apud deos; discubitum inter convivas, oscula complexus, noctem denique actam licentia coniugali. sed nihil compositum miraculi causa, verum audita scriptaque senioribus tradam.
9 Plaut., *Capt.* 888–9: At nunc Siculus non est, Boius est, Boiam terit: liberorum quaerundorum causa ei, credo, uxor datast.
10 Dig. 1.1.1.3: ius naturale est, quod natura omnia animalia docuit: . . . hinc descendit maris atque feminae coniunctio, quam nos matrimonium appellamus, hinc liberorum procreatio.
11 Lucr. 5.1011–14.
12 Cic. *Fin.* 3.68: Cum autem ad tuendos conservandosque homines hominem natum esse videamus, consentaneum est huic naturae, ut sapiens velit gerere et administrare rem publicam atque, ut e natura vivat, uxorem adiungere et velle ex ea liberos.
13 Cic. *Tusc.* 1.14.31: Quid procreatio liberorum, quid propagatio nominis, quid adoptationes filiorum, quid testamentorum diligentia, quid ipsa sepulcrorum monumenta, elogia significant nisi nos futura etiam cogitare?
14 Liv. Per. 59: Q. Metellus censor censuit ut cogerentur omnes ducere uxores liberorum creandorum causa. Extat oratio eius, quam Augustus Caesar, cum de maritandis ordinibus ageret, velut in haec tempora scriptam in senatu recitavit.
15 He had six children and eleven grandchildren; Plin. HN 7.13.59: Q. Metellus Macedonicus, cum sex liberos relinqueret, XI nepotes reliquit.
16 Suet. *Aug.* 89; the speech as quoted by Aulus Gellius: Gell. 1.6. However, in the *Attic Nights*, Gellius ascribes the speech to Quintus Metellus Numidicus, rather than Macedonicus. There is no agreement as to whether Gellius made an error, or two speeches were given on similar topics. For a discussion of that issue, see Tarwacka 2011: 359–75, esp. 360–1.
17 Suder 2005: 67; Suder 2007: 3–11.
18 Hor. *Od.* 3.6.17–20.
19 Suder 2004: 357–9.
20 Suder 2007: 4, with further reading.
21 Suder 2004: 364.
22 Suder 2007: 7.

23 Suder 2004: 365.
24 Tac. *Ann.* 3.25: Relatum deinde moderanda Papia Poppaea, quam senior Augustus post Iulias rogationes incitandis caelibum poenis et augendo aerario sanxerat. nec ideo coniugia et educationes liberum frequentabantur praevalida orbitate: ceterum multitudo periclitantium gliscebat, cum omnis domus delatorum interpretationibus subverteretur, utque antehac flagitiis ita tunc legibus laborabatur. ea res admonet ut de principiis iuris et quibus modis ad hanc multitudinem infinitam ac varietatem legum perventum sit altius disseram; Suet. *Aug.* 34: Leges retractavit et quasdam ex integro sanxit, ut sumptuariam et de adulteriis et de pudicitia ... de maritandis ordinibus.
25 E.g. Tac. *Ann.* 2.51: De praetore in locum Vipstani Galli, quem mors abstulerat, subrogando certamen incessit. Germanicus atque Drusus (nam etiam tum Romae erant) Haterium Agrippam propinquum Germanici fovebant: contra plerique nitebantur ut numerus liberorum in candidatis praepolleret, quod lex iubebat. laetabatur Tiberius, cum inter filios eius et leges senatus disceptaret. victa est sine dubio lex, sed neque statim et paucis suffragiis, quo modo etiam cum valerent leges vincebantur.; Plin. *Ep.* 7.16: Calestrium Tironem familiarissime diligo et privatis mihi et publicis necessitudinibus implicitum. Simul militavimus, simul quaestores Caesaris fuimus. Ille me in tribunatu liberorum iure praecessit, ego illum in praetura sum consecutus, cum mihi Caesar annum remisisset.
26 Plin. *Ep.* 7.16: Ille me in tribunatu liberorum iure praecessit, ego illum in praetura sum consecutus, cum mihi Caesar annum remisisset.
27 Cass. Dio 69.23.3: εἰ τέ τινα τῶν τέκνα ἐχόντων ὀφλῆσαι πάντως τι ἔδει, ἀλλ' οὖν πρός γε τὸν ἀριθμὸν τῶν παίδων καὶ τὰς τιμωρίας αὐτῶν ἐπεκούφιζεν.
28 Mart. 2.91: Rerum certa salus, terrarum gloria, Caesar,/ sospite quo magnos credimus esse deos,/ si festinatis totiens tibi lecta libellis / detinuere oculos carmina nostra tuos,/quod fortuna uetat fieri permitte uideri,/ natorum genitor credar ut esse trium./Haec, si displicui, fuerint solacia nobis;/haec fuerint nobis praemia, si placui; Mart. 2.92: Natorum mihi ius trium roganti/ Musarum pretium dedit mearum solus qui poterat / Valebis, uxor: / non debet domini perire munus.
29 Plin. *Ep.* 10.2.
30 Niczyporuk 2014: 218.
31 P. Oxy. 12 1467; From: Rowlandson 1998: no. 142.
32 Jońca, Szarek 2010.
33 Lambert 1982: 123–38; Tarwacka 2011: 361: even Metellus, the same Metellus mentioned by Aulus Gellius, said that 'if we could live without a wife, we would all of us shun the burden; however, since nature has ordained it so that it is impossible to live too comfortably with them or without them at all, one should attend to long-term good rather than brief pleasure' (Gell. 1.6.2: Si sine uxore possemus, Quirites, omnes ea molestia careremus; set quoniam ita natura tradidit, ut nec cum illis satis

commode, nec sine illis uno modo vivi possit, saluti perpetuae potius quam brevi voluptati consulendum est).
34 Iuv. 10.351–3.
35 Sen. *Controv.* 1.7.8: Infelix futura est etiam victoria mea: si non tenuero causam, fame moriar; si tenuero, hoc tantum consequar, ne fame moriar. Duxi uxorem nimium fecundam; peperit mihi tria nescioquae prodigia variis generibus inter se et iuditia furentia.
36 Tac. *Ann.* 2.37.
37 Although Suetonius records him as having four children, their genders are not mentioned: Suet. *Tib.* 47: Quinti Hortensi oratoris nepotem, qui permodica re familiari auctore Augusto quattuor liberos tulerat.
38 Plin. HN 10.83.172: In hominum genere maribus deverticula veneris excogitata omnia, scelera naturae, feminis vero abortus.
39 Dion. Hal. *Ant. Rom.* 2.15.2: πρῶτον μὲν εἰς ἀνάγκην κατέστησε τοὺς οἰκήτορας αὐτῆς ἅπασαν ἄρρενα γενεὰν ἐκτρέφειν καὶ θυγατέρων τὰς πρωτογόνους, ἀποκτιννύναι δὲ μηδὲν τῶν γεννωμένων νεώτερον τριετοῦς, πλὴν εἴ τι γένοιτο παιδίον ἀνάπηρον ἢ τέρας εὐθὺς ἀπὸ γονῆς. ταῦτα δ᾽ οὐκ ἐκώλυσεν ἐκτιθέναι τοὺς γειναμένους ἐπιδείξαντας πρότερον πέντε ἀνδράσι τοῖς ἔγγιστα οἰκοῦσιν, ἐὰν κἀκείνοις συνδοκῇ; see Eyben 1980: 26.
40 Milnor 2005: 140–54.
41 RGDA 8.5: Legibus novis me auctore latis multa exempla maiorum exolescentia iam ex nostro saeculo reduxi et ipse multarum rerum exempla imitanda posteris tradidi.
42 Sen. *Marc.* 19.2: minime probabili sed uero solacio utar, in ciuitate nostra plus gratiae orbitas confert quam eripit, adeoque senectutem solitudo, quae solebat destruere, ad potentiam ducit ut quidam odia filiorum simulent et liberos eiurent, orbitatem manu faciant. Sen. *Helv.* 16.3: Non te maximum saeculi malum, inpudicitia, in numerum plurium adduxit; non gemmae te, non margaritae flexerunt; non tibi diuitiae uelut maximum generis humani bonum refulserunt; non te, bene in antiqua et seuera institutam domo, periculosa etiam probis peiorum detorsit imitatio; numquam te fecunditatis tuae, quasi exprobraret aetatem, puduit, numquam more aliarum, quibus omnis commendatio ex forma petitur, tumescentem uterum abscondisti quasi indecens onus, nec intra uiscera tua conceptas spes liberorum elisisti; Ovid. *Nux.* 23–4: Nunc uterum vitiat, quae vult formosa videri: Raroque in hoc aevo est, quae velit esse parens.
43 Ovid. *Ars am.* 3.81–2: adde, quod et partus faciunt breviora iuventae tempora: continua messe senescit ager; Propert. 2.15.21–2: necdum inclinatae prohibent te ludere mammae: viderit haec, si quam iam peperisse pudet; Stat. *Silvae* 1.2.268–75: acceleret partu decimum bona Cynthia mensem, sed parcat Lucina precor; tuque ipse parenti parce, puer, ne mollem uterum, ne stantia laedas pectora; cumque tuos tacito natura recessu formarit vultus, multum de patre decoris, plus de matre feras. at

tu, pulcherrima forma Italidum, tandem merito possessa marito, vincla diu quaesita fove: sic damna decoris nulla tibi; longe virides sic flore iuventae perdurent vultus, tardeque haec forma senescat. Kapparis does not believe that an exaggeration, since if abortion for aesthetic reasons had never happened in imperial Rome, there would be no reason to preach against the practice; Kapparis 2002: 119.

44 Iuv. *Sat.* 6.594: sed iacet aurato vix ulla puerpera lecto.
45 See e.g. Suder 1994: 72–94, esp. 83–7.
46 Quint. *Decl. min.* 327.
47 Morgan 1991: 95–100; Watts 1973: 89–101.
48 Ov. *Fasti* 1.618–28.
49 Kapparis 2002: 128–30; Caldwell 2004: 1–17.
50 Cic. *Pro Cluentio* 11.32.
51 Although in this case there is the added relish of the abortion being due to the persuasion from heirs who intended to eliminate an as yet unborn child with a claim to the fortune they were after themselves (Cic. *Pro Cluentio* 11.32).
52 Ovid, *Amores* 2.14. 9–18; Kołosowski 2013: 251–62.
53 Dig. 47.11.4: Divus Severus et Antoninus rescripserunt eam, quae data opera abegit, a praeside in temporale exilium dandam: indignum enim videri potest impune eam maritum liberis fraudasse; see also Eyben 1980: 28.
54 Dig. 48.19.38.5: Qui abortionis aut amatorium poculum dant, etsi dolo non faciant, tamen quia mali exempli res est, humiliores in metallum, honestiores in insulam amissa parte bonorum relegantur. quod si eo mulier aut homo perierit, summo supplicio adficiuntur.
55 Eyben 1980: 9.
56 Soranus 1.19.60: Ἀτόκιον δὲ φθορίου διαφέρει, τὸ μὲν γὰρ οὐκ ἐᾷ γενέσθαι σύλληψιν, τὸ δὲ φθείρει τὸ συλληφθέν· εἴπωμεν οὖν ἄλλο 'φθόριον' καὶ ἄλλο 'ἀτόκιον'.
57 Soranus 1.19.61: εἰ γὰρ τοῦ [μὴ] φθείρειν τὸ συλληφθὲν πολὺ μᾶλλον συμφέρει τὸ μὴ συλλαβεῖν.
58 Soranus 1.19.61: κατέχειν χρὴ τὸ πνεῦμα καὶ μικρὸν ὑφέλκειν ἑαυτήν, ὡς μὴ πορρωτέρω ἐν τῷ κύτει τῆς μήτρας τὸ σπέρμα ἀκοντισθῆναι, καὶ διαναστᾶσαν εὐθέως καὶ ὀκλὰξ καθίσασαν πταρμὸν κινεῖν καὶ περιμάξασθαι τὸν κόλπον ἐπιμελῶς ἢ καὶ ψυχρὸν πίνειν.
59 Soranus 1.19.61: τὰ γὰρ τοιαῦτα, εἰ μὲν στυπτικὰ εἴη καὶ ἐμπλαστικὰ καὶ ψυκτικά, μύειν παρασκευάζει τὸ στόμα τῆς μήτρας πρὸ τοῦ καιροῦ τῆς συνουσίας καὶ οὐκ ἐᾷ παρελθεῖν εἰς τὸν πυθμένα αὐτῆς τὸ σπέρμα.
60 Soranus 1.19.61: [τὰ δὲ θερμὰ] καὶ ἐρεθίζοντα οὐ μόνον τὸ τοῦ ἀνδρὸς σπέρμα ἐναπομεῖναι [καὶ] ἐν τῷ κύτει τῆς μήτρας οὐ συγχωροῦσιν [ἐλθεῖν], ἀλλὰ καὶ ἑτέραν ὑγρότητα ἐξ αὐτῆς ἕλκουσιν.
61 Κιμωλία γῆ.

62 Soranus 1.19.62: ἢ σίδια μετὰ κόμμεως ἴσου καὶ ῥοδίνου ἴσου προστίθει. εἶτα μελίκρατον ἐπιρροφεῖν ὁμοίως, φυλάττεσθαι δὲ τὰ ἐπὶ πολὺ δριμέα διὰ τὰς ἀπ' αὐτῶν ἑλκώσεις.

63 Soranus 1.19.63.

64 Soranus 1.19.63: καθ' ἡμᾶς δὲ πλείων ἐστὶν ἡ ἀπὸ τούτων κάκωσις φθειρόντων μὲν καὶ ἀνατρεπόντων τὸν στόμαχον, πληρούντων δὲ τὴν κεφαλὴν καὶ συμπάθειαν ἐπιφερόντων. οἱ δὲ καὶ περιάπτοις ἐχρήσαντο πολλὰ τῷ τῆς ἀντιπαθείας λόγῳ ποιεῖν νομίζοντες, ἐν οἷς μήτρας ἡμιόνων καὶ τὸν ἐν τοῖς ὠσὶ ῥύπον αὐτῶν καὶ ἄλλα πλείονα τούτων, ἅπερ ἐπὶ τῶν ἀποτελεσμάτων φαίνονται ψευδῆ.

65 Vons 2000;Richlin 1997: 197-200.

66 *Cyranides* 2.15.

67 *Cyranides* 3.1a: ἐὰν δὲ γυνὴ τὸν μυελὸν τοῦ ζῴου πίῃ, ἐπιθήσῃ δὲ καὶ ὀλίγον ἐξ αὐτοῦ τῆς μήτρας στομίῳ, ἀσύλληπτος γίνεται.

68 *Cyranides* 5.5.

69 *Cyranides* 2.7: τοὺς δὲ ὄρχεις αὐτῆς ἀπότεμνε ἐν ἀποκρούσει, αὐτὴν δὲ ζῶσαν ἄφες. τοὺς δὲ ὄρχεις δὸς φορεῖν εἰς ἡμιόνου δέρμα· ἀσύλληπτον γάρ ἐστιν.

70 *Cyranides* 2.25 (appendix).

71 Lucr. 4.1269–75; childless prostitutes are often contrasted with fertile wives, whose lives ought to focus on producing offspring. Common sense dictates prostitutes got pregnant too, but the notion of a *meretrix* as a mother illustrates the conceptual separation between their respective duties. For more on the subject, see Strong 2016: 23–4.

72 Iuv. 6.367–8.

73 Soranus 1.19.64: γενομένης δὲ τῆς συλλήψεως τὸ μὲν πρῶτον ἕως τριάκοντα ἡμερῶν τὰ ἐναντία ποιεῖν οἷς ἔμπροσθεν εἰρήκαμεν, εἰς δὲ τὸ διαλυθῆναι τὸ συλληφθὲν [σφοδρότερον κινεῖσθαι] περιπατοῦσαν εὐτόνως καὶ διὰ ζευκτῶν κατασειομένην, εὐτόνως καὶ πηδᾶν καὶ βαστάζειν τὰ ὑπὲρ δύναμιν βάρη, ἀφεψήμασι δὲ διουρητικοῖς χρῆσθαι τοῖς δυναμένοις καὶ καταμήνια κινεῖν, καὶ τὴν γαστέρα λαπάττειν καὶ κλύζειν δριμυτέροις κλύσμασι, θερμῷ τε ἐλαίῳ καὶ γλυκεῖ ποτὲ μὲν ἐγχυματιζομένην, ποτὲ δὲ συναλειφομένην ὅλην καὶ τριβομένην εὐτόνως καὶ μάλιστα περὶ τὸ ἐφήβαιον καὶ τὸ ἐπιγάστριον.

74 Soranus 1.19.64: λουομένην καθ' ἡμέραν ἐν τῷ μὴ λίαν ζεστῷ ὕδατι γλυκεῖ καὶ τοῖς λουτροῖς ἐγχρονίζουσαν καὶ προπίνουσαν οἰνάριον καὶ δριμυφαγοῦσαν. εἰ δὲ μή, καὶ τοπικῶς ἐγκαθίζουσαν εἰς ἀφέψημα λινοσπέρμου, τήλεως, μαλάχης, ἀλθαίας, ἀρτεμισίας καὶ καταπλασσομένην τοῖς αὐτοῖς, ἐγχυματιζομένην δὲ τῷ παλαιῷ ἐλαίῳ κατ' ἰδίαν ἢ καὶ μετὰ πηγάνου χυλοῦ, ποτὲ δὲ καὶ μέλιτος, ἢ ἰρίνῳ ἢ ἀψινθίῳ σὺν μέλιτι ἢ ὀποπάνακι ἢ ἄλλως χόνδρῳ μετὰ πηγάνου καὶ μέλιτος ἢ μύρῳ Συριακῷ.

75 Soranus 1.19.64: κἂν ἐπιμένῃ, καταπλασσομένην μηκέτι τοῖς κοινοῖς καταπλάσμασιν, ἀλλὰ τοῖς διὰ θερμίνου ἀλεύρου μετὰ χολῆς ταυρείας καὶ ἀψινθίου, [καὶ τοῖς] ὁμοιογενέσιν τῶν ἐπιθεμάτων [χρωμένην].

76 Soranus 1.19.65: τὴν δὲ μέλλουσαν φθείρειν χρὴ πρὸ δύο ἢ καὶ τριῶν ἡμερῶν λουτροῖς συνεχέσι χρῆσθαι καὶ ὀλιγοτροφίᾳ καὶ πεσσοῖς μαλακτικοῖς, καὶ οἴνου ἀπέχεσθαι, εἶτα φλεβοτομεῖν καὶ πλεῖον ἀφαιρεῖν.
77 Soranus 1.19.65.
78 Soranus 1.19.65: ἐκ δὲ τῶν πραϋτέρων οἱ τοιοῦτοι καθεστᾶσιν οἷον·· μυρσίνης, λευκοΐου σπέρματος, θέρμων πικρῶν ἐξ ἴσου μετὰ ὕδατος ἀναπλάττειν τροχοὺς ὡς κυάμου μέγεθος. ἢ φύλλων πηγάνου [γ, μυρσίνης [β, δάφνης ἴσας ὁμοίως διιέναι μετ' οἴνου, καὶ πότιζε. ἄλλος πεσσὸς ἀκινδυνότερον ἐκβάλλων· λευκοΐου, καρδαμώμου, θείου, ἀψινθίου, σμύρνης, ἑκάστου ἴσον, δι' ὕδατος ἀνάπλασσε.
79 *Cyranides* 2.25 (appendix).
80 Garg. 5.9 (ed. V. Rose, Garg. 5.11): Olympias Thebana abortivas putat esse malvas cum adipe anseris genitali parti subiectas.
81 Garg 13.5: (ed. V. Rose, Garg. 13.11): seminis maior effectus adeo ut etiam partus necet.
82 *Cyranides* 5.1: τὸ δὲ ἀφέψημα αὐτῆς (scil. ἀργεμώνης) πινόμενον ἔμβρυα ἀποβάλλει.
83 *Cyranides* 5.2: λεῖος δὲ προστιθέμενος ἔμβρυα κατασπᾷ καὶ ἔμμηνα ἄγει.
84 López Eire, Cortés Gabaudan 2006; Pedanii Dioscuridis Anazarbei, *De materia medica*, ed. M. Wellmann, Berlin 1907; Pedanius Dioscorides of Anazarbus, *De materia medica*, transl. L. Y. Beck, Hildesheim 2005.
85 See Riddle 1992, although some authors disagree with his opinions (e.g. Scheidel 2001: 39); so also Kapparis 2002: 16), who does, however, stress that 'faith in the potential of abortifacients would have eventually faded, had they brought no effects'.
86 Soranus 1.19.65: πολλὰ δὲ καὶ ἄλλα παρ' ἄλλοις εἴρηται, φυλάσσεσθαι δὲ δεῖ τὰ λίαν πληκτικὰ καὶ τὸ καταλύειν τὸ ἔμβρυον διά τινος ἐπάκμου, κίνδυνος γὰρ τρωθῆναί τι τῶν παρακειμένων.
87 Kapparis 2002: 12–31.
88 Ovid. 2.13: Dum labefactat onus gravidi temeraria ventris, / in dubio vitae lassa Corinna iacet . . . illa quidem clam me tantum molita pericli / ira digna mea; sed cadit ira metu.
89 Iuv. *Sat.* 2.32–3: Cum tot abortivis fecundam Iulia vulvam solveret.
90 Suet. *Dom.* 22.
91 Plin. *Ep.* 4.11.6.
92 Tac. *Ann.* 14.63: At Nero praefectum in spem sociandae classis corruptum et incusatae paulo ante sterilitatis oblitus, abactos partus conscientia libidinum, eaque sibi comperta edicto memorat insulaque Pandateria Octaviam claudit.
93 Kapparis 2002: 143.
94 Dixon, 2003: 121 and Evans Grubbs 1995: 87 both believe the present-day interest in contraception and abortion in Rome is excessive and ignores how the societies of the time were themselves more concerned with fertility and efforts to have children.

95 Based on: López Eire, Cortés Gabaudan 2006. I am very grateful to Dr Łukasz Skrzypczak from the Section of Medical Biology and Parasitology of the Poznań University of Medical Sciences for letting me consult him on the terminology.

Chapter 2

1. Verg. *Aen.* 7.53: Iam matura viro, iam plenis nubilis annis. = Ausonius, Cento Nuptialis 17. 3.
2. For a book on Roman marriage which will for many years continue to be regarded as a classic, see Treggiari 1991.
3. Harlow, Laurence 2002: 62.
4. Hindermann 2013: 143–61; Watson 1983: 119–43.
5. Cic. *Att.*13.21a.4: quod autem de illa nostra cogitatione scribis, in qua nihil tibi cedo, ea quae novi valde probo, hominem, domum, facultates. quod caput est, ipsum non novi sed audio laudabilia, de [S]crofa etiam proxime. accedit, si quid hoc ad rem, εὐγενέστερος est etiam quam pater. coram igitur, et quidem propenso animo ad probandum. accedit enim quod patrem, ut scire te puto, plus etiam quam non modo tu sed quam ipse scit, amo, idque et merito et iam diu.
6. Harlow, Laurence 2002: 58.
7. Plin. *Ep.* 5.16.2: Nondum annos xiiii impleverat, et iam illi anilis prudentia, matronalis gravitas erat et tamen suavitas puellaris cum virginali verecundia.
8. Lelis, Percy, Verstraete 2003: 103–25.
9. Harlow, Laurence 2002: 59.
10. The Roman families' demand for the would-be bride's virginity may have been due not just to tradition and the widely accepted social norms, but also the fear of a cuckoo's egg. Dig. 2.4.5: Quia semper certa est, etiam si volgo conceperit: pater vero is est, quem nuptiae demonstrant (for [the mother] is always certain, even if she has conceived out of wedlock, but the father is he whom the marriage points to). In the light of the Roman law, the child whose paternity was in question had to be born no earlier than in the seventh month from the marriage ceremony (or 182 days after it), and no later than in the tenth month after the marriage ended (within 300 days), but only provided the parents lived, or had lived, in a *iustum matrimonium*: see Jurewicz 2006: 95–119.
11. Macrob. *Sat.* 6.6: Nec hoc tacebo quod, cum calor semper generationis causa sit, feminae ideo celerius quam pueri fiunt idoneae ad generandum quia calent amplius. nam et secundum iura publica duodecimus annus in femina et quartus decimus in puero definit pubertatis aetate; see also Dig. 23.2.4: Minorem annis duodecim nuptam tunc legitimam uxorem fore, cum apud virum explesset duodecim anno.

12 W. Suder writes that in the provinces of Africa, Gaul and Spain, the most female deaths can be observed for the age range of fifteen to twenty, which was also the cohort with the highest female fertility. Hopkins believed that in the light of Latin sepulchral inscriptions, the mean age of marriage in ancient Rome was fifteen years for women and twenty-four for men. The average age women married corresponds to the period of their greatest fertility (fifteen to twenty), which explains the high mortality rate, likely childbirth-related. This could also explain why the rates of birth, number of children per person and population replacement did reach the high levels necessary to compensate for the enormous mortality of the time: Suder 1987: 621–8, esp. 626–7.

13 Eyben 1972: 677–97; Durry 1955: 84–91.

14 Pomeroy 2002:154.

15 Cass. Dio 54.16.7: ὡς δ᾽ οὖν βρέφη τινὲς ἐγγυώμενοι τὰς μὲν τιμὰς τῶν γεγαμηκότων ἐκαρποῦντο, τὸ δὲ ἔργον αὐτῶν οὐ παρείχοντο, προσέταξε μηδεμίαν ἐγγύην ἰσχύειν μεθ᾽ ἣν οὐδὲ δυοῖν ἐτοῖν διελθόντων γαμήσει τις, τοῦτ᾽ ἔστι δεκέτιν πάντως ἐγγυᾶσθαι τόν γέ τι ἀπ᾽ αὐτῆς ἀπολαύσοντα· δώδεκα γὰρ ταῖς κόραις ἐς τὴν τοῦ γάμου ὥραν ἔτη πλήρη, καθάπερ εἶπον, νομίζεται.

16 Tac. Ger. 20: Sera iuvenum venus, eoque inexhausta pubertas.

17 Shaw 2002: 195–242, McGinn 2015:107–55. Hopkins 1965a: 309–27: the minimum age at which Roman girls could be married was twelve, but the law prescribed no sanctions for breaking that regulation. Based on 287 tombstones, it is possible to compare the ages of pagan and Christian girls as they married. The median range was from twelve to fifteen years for the former (represented by 43 per cent), and from fifteen to eighteen for the latter (42 per cent), although it should be remembered inscriptions are representative of relatively wealthy families from larger towns.

18 Laes 2012: 93–111.

19 Inscr It 3,1,113; ILS 9390; AE 1910, 191: C(aio) Utiano C(ai) f(ilio) Pom(ptina) Rufo / Latiniano IIII vir(o)i(ure) d(icundo) iter(um) /Insteia M(arci) f(ilia) Polla sacerd(os) Iuliae / Augustae Volceis et Atinae / optimo et indulgentissimo viro, qui / eam pupillam annorum VII in domum/ receptam per annos LV cum summo / honore uxorem habuit. / hunc decuriones Volceiani inpensa /publica funerandum et statua eque/stri hnorandumcensuerunt/ Latiniae M(arci) f(iliae) Posillae [sor]ori Latiniani.

20 CIL X 155: D(is) M(anibus) / Cisatiae Pollae quae bixit ann(os) / XXXVIII me(n)s(es) VIIII Figelius / Atimetus co(n)iugi cum quo vixit / a(nnos) XXVII m(enses) XI et Figellia / Procula filia matri b(ene) m(erenti).

21 AE 1985, 355: D(is) M(anibus) / Herennia L(uci) f (ilia) Cervilla/ uxor vixi annis XVIII et diem trecesimum/ Liberis tribus relictis/ vita(m) finivi dolens / Co(n)iux karus ut memoriaeposuit hoc vivos mihi / ut prodesset in suppre/mis talem titulum consequi. C(aius) Carrenas / Verecundus coniugi/ incomprabili b(ene) m(erenti); for

other, sometimes very early marriages in the light of inscriptions, see Laes 2012: 93–111, esp. 108–10; Musca 1988: 176–81. Musca analysed inscriptions indicative of marriage age, and listed more than ten where the twelve-years-old rule was violated and people married earlier: CIL VI 21562 (married at seven); CIL VI 28257 (married at the age of nine years, eleven months); CIL VI 22765 9 (married at ten); CIL VI 29299 (died, married, at eleven); CIL VI 18412 (married at eleven); CIL VI 22820 (died, married, at twelve). Several other inscriptions are dated to late antiquity and considered Christian. See also Frier 2015: 652–65.
22 Plin. HN 7.13.63: Solum autem animal menstruale mulier est.
23 Plut. *De amore prolis* 3.495e.
24 For a history of menstruation, see e.g. Shail, Howie 2005; Hufnagel 2012 (esp. 15–20).
25 Papadimitrou 2016: 527–30; So Soranus 1.4.20, whereas Pliny writes that in most cases menstruation only lasts until the age of 40: Plin. HN 7.14.61: Mulier post quinquagensimum annum non gignit, maiorque pars XL profluvium genitale sistit.
26 Soranus 1.4.23: ἢ διὰ σύλληψιν ἀναλισκομένου τοῦ αἵματος εἰς τὴν τοῦ ἐμβρύου διατροφήν.
27 Garg. 4.8 [ed. V. Rose, 4.15]. Gargilius' source here is Pliny the Elder, HN 20.82.218: si vera est, menstrua contineri uno die, si unum granum biberint feminae, biduo, si duo, et totidem diebus quot grana sumpserint.
28 Garg. 9.3: Hippocrates praecepit ad sistenda nimia menstrua feminarum in cibo dandos; The information from a passage from Pliny the Elder that Gargilius used (HN 20.93.252): Hippocrates mestrua sisti eo cibo putat.
29 Plin. HN 20.4.9: purgat eas elaterium.
30 Soranus 1.5.26: αἱ μὲν γὰρ συνήθως ἠρεμοῦσιν, αἱ δὲ ἐπὶ μετρίας προΐασιν κινήσεις. ἀσφαλέστερον δὲ τὸ ἠρεμεῖν καὶ ἀλουτεῖν καὶ μάλιστα τῇ πρώτῃ τῶν ἡμερῶν.
31 Soranus 1.4.21: συμμέτρως οὖν κεκαθάρθαι λεκτέον τὰς μετὰ τὴν ἀπόκρισιν εὐσταθεῖς, εὔπνους, ἀταράχους τήν τε δύναμιν ἀκαθαιρέτους, τὰς δὲ μὴ τοιαύτας ἀσυμμέτρως.
32 Lucr. 6.794.
33 Soranus 1.6.29. There was some awareness of the fact that menstruation and fertility are related: Cuius ea castitas fuisse dicitur ut ne virum suum quidem scierit nisi temptandis conceptionibus. nam cum semel concubuisset, exspectatis menstruis continebat se, si praegnans esset, sin minus, iterum potestatem quaerendis liberis dabat. *HA, List of Thirty Tyrants* 30: 'Such was her continence, it is said, that she would not know even her own husband save for the purpose of conception. For when once she had lain with him, she would refrain until the time of menstruation to see if she were pregnant; if not, she would again grant him an opportunity of begetting children.'
34 Soranus 1.7.31: κίνδυνος οὖν δι' ὅλου τῆς συμπλοκῆς ἀπεχομένων αὐτῶν παραπολέσθαι τὴν τῆς ὑστέρας ἐνέργειαν. πρὸς δὲ τὸ τὰς μὴ συνουσιαζούσας

ἀπαλλάσσεσθαι τῆς ἐκ τοῦ τίκτειν κακώσεώς φασιν, ὅτι πρὸς ἕτερα πολλῷ χείρονα διὰ τὸ μὴ συνουσιάζειν βλάπτονται παραποδιζομένης τῆς ἐμμήνου καθάρσεως.

35 Soranus 1.4.22: παρὰ δὲ τὰς συγκρίσεις· καταπιμέλοις μὲν γὰρ καὶ παχείαις ὀλιγώτερον, ὡς ἂν τῆς ὕλης διὰ τὴν εὐτροφίαν τοῦ συγκρίματος ἀναλισκομένης, ταῖς ἰσχνοτέραις δὲ καὶ ἀσάρκοις πλεῖον· ὃ γὰρ οὐκ ἐδαπάνησεν εἰς εὐτροφίαν ἡ φύσις, τοῦτο ἐπλεόνασεν εἰς ἔκκρισιν. παρὰ δὲ τὸ ἐπιτήδευμα καὶ τὴν ἀγωγήν· ταῖς μὲν [γὰρ] ἀργῷ βίῳ χρωμέναις πλεῖον, ταῖς δὲ γυμναστικῷ καθ' ὁνδήποτε τρόπον ἔλαττον.

36 πρὸς δὲ τῷ διδασκαλικῷ καὶ ἐπ' ἄκρον ἀναβᾶσα τῆς πρακτικῆς ἀρετῆς, δικαία τε καὶ σώφρων γεγονυῖα, διετέλει παρθένος, οὕτω σφόδρα καλή τε οὖσα καὶ εὐειδής, ὥστε καὶ ἐρασθῆναί τινα αὐτῆς τῶν προσφοιτώντων. ὁ δὲ οὐχ οἷός τε ἦν κρατεῖν τοῦ ἔρωτος, ἀλλ' αἴσθησιν ἤδη παρείχετο καὶ αὐτῇ τοῦ παθήματος. οἱ μὲν οὖν ἀπαίδευτοι λόγοι φασί, διὰ μουσικῆς αὐτὸν ἀπαλλάξαι τῆς νόσου τὴν Ὑπατίαν· ἡ δὲ ἀλήθεια διαγγέλλει πάλαι μὲν διεφθορέναι τὰ μουσικῆς, αὐτὴν δὲ προενεγκαμένην τι τῶν γυναικείων ῥακῶν αἵματι βεβαμμένον καὶ τὸ σύμβολον ἐπιδείξασαν τῆς ἀκαθάρτου γενέσεως, 'τούτου μέντοι', φάναι, 'ἐρᾷς, ὦ νεανίσκε, καλοῦ δὲ οὐδενός', τὸν δὲ ὑπ' αἰσχύνης καὶ θάμβους τῆς ἀσχήμονος ἐπιδείξεως διατραπῆναί τε τὴν ψυχὴν καὶ διατεθῆναι σωφρονέστερον; Suidae Lexicon, ed. A. Adler, 4.644.12, Leipzig 2001.

37 Plin. HN 28.23.82: multi vero inesse etiam remedia tanto malo: podagris inlini, strumas et parotidas et panos, sacros ignes, furunculos, epiphoras tractatu mulierum earum leniri; Lais et Salpe canum rabiosorum morsus et tertianas quartanasque febres menstruo in lana arietis nigri argenteo bracchiali incluso.

38 Plin. HN 28.23.83: Diotimus Thebanus vel omnino vestis ita infectae portiuncula ac vel licio bracchiali inserto.

39 Plin. HN 28.23.83: Sotira obstetrix tertianis quartanisque efficacissimum dixit plantas aegri subterlini, multoque efficacius ab ipsa muliere et ignorantis; sic et comitiales excitari.

40 Plin. HN 28.23.83: Icatidas medicus quartanas finiri coitu, incipientibus dumtaxat menstruis, spopondit.

41 Plin. HN 28.23.84: inter omnes vero convenit, si aqua potusque formidetur a morsu canis.

42 Plin. HN 28.23.78: quocumque autem alio menstruo si nudatae segetem ambiant, urucas et vermiculos scarabaeosque ac noxia alia decidere ... ire ergo per media arva retectis super clunes vestibus. alibi servatur ut nudis pedibus eant capillo cinctuque dissoluto.

43 Solinus 1.54–5; cf. Pliny: 'I have already said the asphalt arising in Judaea yields only to that force [sc. menstruation], adheres to the thread of stained clothing and is not even conquered by fire itself' (Plin. HN 28.23.80: Bitumen in Iudaea nascens sola hac vi superari filo vestis contactae docuimus. ne igni quidem vincitur).

44 Plin. HN 7.15.65: quin et bituminum sequax alioqui ac lenta natura in lacu Iudaeae, qui vocatur Asphaltites, certo tempore anni supernatans non quit sibi avelli, ad omnem contactum adhaerens praeterquam filo ... quem tale virus infecerit. etiam formicis, animali minimo, inesse sensum eius ferunt abicique gustatas fruges nec postea repeti.

45 Plin. HN 28.23.79.

46 Plin. HN 28.23.80: ipsis quidem feminis malo suo inter se inmunibus: abortus facit inlitu aut si omnino praegnas supergradiatur.

47 Plin. HN 28.23.81: Lais et Elephantis inter se contraria prodidere de abortivo carbone e radice brassicae vel myrti vel tamaricis in eo sanguine extincto.

48 Plin. HN 28.23.81: itemque asinas tot annis non concipere, quot grana hordei contacta ederint, quaeque alia nuncupavere monstrifica aut inter ipsa pugnantia, cum haec fecunditatem fieri isdem modis, quibus sterilitatem illa, praenuntiaret, melius est non credere.

49 Plin. HN 28.23.82.

50 Plin. HN 28.23.79: quamvis procul visas, si purgatio illa post virginitatem prima sit aut in virgine aetatis sponte manet.

51 Plin. HN 28.24.87.

52 Moraw, Kieburg 2014: 14.

53 Amundsen, Diers 1969: 125–32; Tan, Haththotuwa, Fraser 2017: 121–33.

54 Soranus 1.6.29: ἔδει δὲ καὶ τὰς μήπω καθαιρομένας τῶν παρθένων ἧττον ὑγιαίνειν· εἰ δὲ τῆς ὑγείας μετέχουσιν ἀνελλιπῶς, μὴ δήποτε μὲν πρὸς τὸ ὑγιαίνειν ἡ κάθαρσις οὐ συμβάλλεται, πρὸς μόνον δὲ τὸ παιδοποιεῖν· χωρὶς γὰρ τῆς καθάρσεως σύλληψις οὐ γίνεται.

55 Soranus 1.4.20: τὸ δὲ ἔμμηνον ἐπιφαίνεται πρῶτον περὶ τὸ τεσσαρεσκαιδέκατον ἔτος κατὰ τὸ πλεῖστον, ὅτε καὶ τὸ ἡβᾶν καὶ τὸ διογκοῦσθαι τοὺς μαστούς. 1.5.24: Μέλλουσαν δὲ γίνεσθαι κάθαρσιν σημειωτέον ἐκ τοῦ κατὰ τὴν προθεσμίαν τοῦ συνήθους καιροῦ δυσκινησίαν παρακολουθεῖν καὶ βάρος ὀσφύος; Based on osteological analysis of thirty-eight skeletons of people who died between the ages of eight and twenty (found in the cemeteries of Roman Britain), it was established menarche occurred between the ages of fifteen and seventeen. For the methodology and results of the research, see Arthur, Gowland, Redfern 2016: 698–713.

56 Soranus 1.5.25: τῆς δὲ ἐπιμελείας χάριν πρὸ μὲν τοῦ ἐκκρίνεσθαι τὸ ἔμμηνον πειρᾶσθαι δεῖ συνεργεῖν ἀπὸ τῆς τρισκαιδεκαετοῦς ἡλικίας, ὅπως δι' ἑαυτοῦ καὶ πρὸ διακορήσεως ἐνεχθῇ. πρὸς γὰρ τὴν συνουσίαν τῆς ὕλης ἐπὶ τὰ μέρη φερομένης ὡς ἐπὶ ἀρρένων οὕτως καὶ ἐπὶ θηλειῶν, φόβος μή πως τῇ ἀποκρίσει καθυπηρετουμένου τοῦ ζῴου διάτασις γένηται καὶ φλεγμονή.

57 Soranus 1.5.25.

58 Soranus 1.8.33: κίνδυνος [γὰρ] τὸ καταβληθὲν σπέρμα συλληφθῆναι μικρομεγέθους ἔτι τῆς μήτρας ὑπαρχούσης καὶ διὰ τοῦτο θλιβησομένου μετὰ τὴν ὄγκωσιν τοῦ

ἐμβρύου καὶ οὕτως ἤτοι φθαρησομένου παντελῶς ἢ τοὺς χαρακτῆρας ἀπολέσαντος ἢ πάντως ἐν τῷ καιρῷ τῆς ἀποτέξεως κίνδυνον παρεξομένου τῇ κυοφορούσῃ τῷ διὰ στενῶν ἔτι καὶ ἀτελειώτων ἀκμὴν τῶν περὶ τὸ στόμιον τῆς ὑστέρας μερῶν διέρχεσθαι.

59 Laes 2011: 51.
60 Soranus emphasizes that girls brought up immodestly want to have affairs earlier: Soranus 1.8.33. For a discussion of the definition of virginity, see Mastrocinque 2014; Sissa 2013: 67–123; Pinault 1992: 123–39.
61 Soranus 1.8.33.
62 Plin. *Ep.* 4.21: Tristem et acerbum casum Helvidiarum sororum! Utraque a partu, utraque filiam enixa decessit.
63 For the time of entering into adulthood, rites of passage, changes in an adolescent girl's behaviour and that of others towards her, changes to her diet and daily rhythm, see Alberici, Harlow 2007: 193–203.
64 Plin. *Ep.* 8.10: dum se praegnantem esse puellariter nescit, ac per hoc quaedam custodienda praegnantibus omittit, facit omittenda.
65 For marriage rituals, symbolism and their interpretations, see e.g. the excellent book by Hersch 2010 with further reading.
66 Caldwell 2015: 100.
67 Dolansky 2012: 256–92.
68 Caldwell 2015: 101; Gourevitch 2009: 120–2.
69 In Lacan's theory, a girl playing with and taking care of a doll mirrors motherhood as a typical behaviour of women. For more on the subject, see Lacan 2007; Ambrosini, Stanghellini 2012: 277–86.
70 Pers. 2.69–71.
71 Kuryłowicz 2011: 42.
72 Tac. *Ann.* 2.37: patres conscripti, hos, quorum numerum et pueritiam videtis, non sponte sustuli sed quia princeps monebat; simul maiores mei meruerant ut posteros haberent. nam ego, qui non pecuniam, non studia populi neque eloquentiam, gentile domus nostrae bonum, varietate temporum accipere vel parare potuissem, satis habebam, si tenues res meae nec mihi pudori nec cuiquam oneri forent. iussus ab imperatore uxorem duxi. en stirps et progenies tot consulum, tot dictatorum.
73 Plin. *Ep.* 1.14: Petis ut fratris tui filiae prospiciam maritum; quod merito mihi potissimum iniungis. Scis enim quanto opere summum illum virum suspexerim dilexerimque, quibus ille adulescentiam meam exhortationibus foverit, quibus etiam laudibus ut laudandus viderer effecerit. Nihil est quod a te mandari mihi aut maius aut gratius, nihil quod honestius a me suscipi possit, quam ut eligam iuvenem, ex quo nasci nepotes Aruleno Rustico deceat. Qui quidem diu quaerendus fuisset, nisi paratus et quasi provisus esset Minicius Acilianus, qui me ut iuvenis iuvenem – est enim minor pauculis annis – familiarissime diligit, reveretur ut senem. Nam ita

formari a me et institui cupit, ut ego a vobis solebam. Patria est ei Brixia, ex illa nostra Italia quae multum adhuc verecundiae frugalitatis, atque etiam rusticitatis antiquae, retinet ac servat. Pater Minicius Macrinus, equestris ordinis princeps, quia nihil altius volvit; allectus enim a Divo Vespasiano inter praetorios honestam quietem huic nostrae – ambitioni dicam an dignitati? – constantissime praetulit. Habet aviam maternam Serranam Proculam e municipio Patavio. Nosti loci mores: Serrana tamen Patavinis quoque severitatis exemplum est. Contigit et avunculus ei P. Acilius gravitate prudentia fide prope singulari. In summa nihil erit in domo tota, quod non tibi tamquam in tua placeat.

74 For more on the subject, see Golden 1998: 152–63; Dyjakowska 2014: 7–22, esp. 16–18.
75 Stat. *Silvae* 4.8.25–7.
76 Kelley 2013: 65–72 and appendix p. 93; Tatarkiewicz 2021: 407–12.
77 CIL VI 16631: D. M. Miniciae Marcellae Fundani f(ilia) v(ixit) a(nnis) XII m(enses) XI d(ei) VII; Bodel 1995: 453–60.
78 Plin. *Ep.* 5.16.
79 AE 1974, 00260: Trebia C(ai) f(ilia) Sa/turnina vi/xit annis XIII / mutatum officium est alium sper[ave]rat usum / fax infelicis virginis heu superi / quae thalamis aetas fuerat iam nubilis apta / destituit sponsum flebilis et soceros.
80 A wedding turned into a funeral is a common motif in ancient literature. One example is to be found in Heliodorus' *Aethiopica*, where Charicles speaks of his daughter, dead in a fire on her wedding night: the nuptial hymn changed into a lament, his daughter was carried from the bridal chamber to her grave, and the torches which had illuminated the festivities were now used to light the pyre (Heliodorus, 2.29.3). Still, in that tale the girl had formally become a wife already.
81 Burning torches were a common feature of celebrations, processions, feasts and funerals, and not just in ancient Rome. Wedding torches were used to decorate the groom's house, but also accompanied the bride on her way to her future husband's house. Their role in the marriage ceremony is not quite clear. It used to be believed that the fire was meant to protect the newly-weds and the wedding guests from evil spirits. It may have symbolized the unbreakable bond between the spouses, or perhaps the presence of torches had a connection to the goddess Vesta. For the symbolism of torches, see Hersch 2010: 164–75.
82 AE 1905, 107 D(is) M(anibus) / memoriae / Iulia Sidonia felix / de nomine tantum / cui nefas ante diem / ruperunt stemina (sic) Par/cae quam procus heu / nuptiis hymen(a)eos con/tigit ignes ingemuere / omnes Dryades doluere puellae / et Lucina facis demerso lumi/ne flevit virgo quod et so/lum pignus fueratque paren/tum Memphidos haec fu/erat divae sistratae sacer/dos hic tumulata silet / aeterno munere somni / v(ixit) a(nnos) XVIIII m(enses) IIII d(ies) XIIII / h(ic) s(ita) e(st); Hemelrijk 2020: 230–1.

83 CIL VI 18937: D(is) M(anibus) / Gaviae C(ai) f(iliae) Qua/dratillae vixit /annis XVII /mensibus VI /C(aius) Gavius Da/phnus pater infelicissimus /qui pos(uit) dies XX despepondit.
84 CIL III 2875: Opiniae M(arci) f(iliae) Neptil[l=I]ae/annor(um) XIIII virg(ini) desp(eratae)/ prope diem nuptiar(um) def(unctae)/M(arcus) Op[i]n[i]us Rufus et/ Gellia Neptil[l=I]a parentes.
85 BCTH-1910-CCIII: D(is) M(anibus) s(acrum) / Calliste vixit / annis XVI me(n) s(ibus) III hor(is) / VI et s(emis) nuptura Idibus O[ct(obribus)] / moritur IIII Idus Oct(obres) PV/AIS mater pia kar(issimae) fil(iae) fe[cit].
86 For a detailed inventory of items found in such tombs, see e.g. Stawowska-Jundziłł 2011: 49–83.
87 Hersch 2010: 65–114.
88 Harlow 2012: 155.
89 Newby 2018.
90 Bettini 1999: 213–27.
91 See also D'Ambra 2014: 312–19.
92 Newby 2018.
93 Carroll 2014: 167–73.
94 Hoepken 2007: 298–9.
95 Carroll 2001: 91.
96 Bellae Von/uci F(iliae) Remae / Longinus / vir Illaeius / fecit pie.
97 Mancini 1930: 353–69.
98 Borg 2013: 234–5.
99 Bordenache Battaglia 1983: 124–38; Dolansky 2012: 256–92.
100 ILS 8393: Fuerunt optati liberii, quos aliquamdiu sors inviderat.
101 See Morice, Chapron, Dubuisson 1995: 497-504; For more see this chapter 4.3. Male infertility.
102 Plut. *Rom.* 22,3: ἔθηκε δὲ καὶ νόμους τινάς, ὧν σφοδρὸς μέν ἐστιν ὁ γυναικὶ μὴ διδοὺς ἀπολείπειν ἄνδρα, γυναῖκα δὲ διδοὺς ἐκβάλλειν ἐπὶ φαρμακείᾳ τέκνων ἢ κλειδῶν ὑποβολῇ καὶ μοιχευθεῖσαν· εἰ δ᾽ ἄλλως τις ἀποπέμψαιτο, τῆς οὐσίας αὐτοῦ τὸ μὲν τῆς γυναικὸς εἶναι, τὸ δὲ τῆς Δήμητρος ἱερὸν κελεύων· τὸν δ᾽ ἀποδόμενον γυναῖκα θύεσθαι χθονίοις θεοῖς.
103 Tarwacka 2014: 235–40.
104 Gell. 4.3.1–2.
105 Tarwacka 2013: 187–201.
106 Cass. Dio 59: καὶ τοῦτο μὲν ὕστερον ἐγένετο· τότε δὲ ἐκβαλὼν τὴν Παυλῖναν, προφάσει μὲν ὡς μὴ τίκτουσαν, τὸ δ᾽ ἀληθὲς ὅτι διακορὴς αὐτῆς ἐγεγόνει, Μιλωνίαν Καισωνίαν ἔγημεν, ἣν πρότερον μὲν ἐμοίχευε, τότε δὲ καὶ γαμετὴν ποιήσασθαι ἠθέλησεν, ἐπειδὴ ἐν γαστρὶ ἔσχεν, ἵν᾽ αὐτῷ παιδίον τριακονθήμερον τέκῃ.

107 Tac. *Ann.* 14.60: itur accepto patrum consulto, postquam cuncta scelerum suorum pro egregiis accipi videt, exturbat Octaviam, sterilem dictitans; Suet. *Ner.* 35.2: Eandem mox saepe frustra strangulare meditatus dimisit ut sterilem, sed improbante divortium populo nec parcente conviciis etiam relegavit, denique occidit sub crimine adulteriorum adeo impudenti falsoque, ut in quaestione pernegantibus cunctis Anicetum paedagogum suum indicem subiecerit, qui fingeret et dolo stupratam a se fateretur.
108 For more on the subject, see Tarwacka 2009: 171–5.
109 Val. Max. 2.1.4: Repudium inter uxorem et virum a condita urbe usque ad centesimum et quinquagesimum annum nullum intercessit. Primus autem Sp. Carvilius uxorem sterilitatis causa dimisit. qui, quamquam tolerabili ratione motus videbatur, reprehensione tamen non caruit, quia ne cupiditatem quidem liberorum coniugali fidei praeponi debuisse arbitrabantur. Sed quo matronale decus verecundiae munimento tutius esset, in ius vocanti matronam corpus eius adtingere non permiserunt, ut inviolata manus alienae tactu stola relinqueretur.
110 *Laud. Turiae* 2.25–30: pacato orbe terrarum res[titut]a re publica quieta/ deinde n[obis et felicia] / tempora contigerunt fue[ru]nt / optati liberi quos aliqua[mdiu sors nobis invi]/derat si fortuna procede[re e]sset passa sollemnis inservie[ns quid / utrique no]/strum defuit(?) procedens a[li]as spem finiebat.
111 *Laud. Turiae* 2.31–7: diffidens fecunditati tuae [et do]lens orbitate mea ne tenen[do in matrimonio] / te spem habendi liberos [dep]onerem atque eius caussa ess[em infelix de divertio] / elocuta es vocuamque [do]mum alterius fecunditati t[e tradituram non alia] / mente nisi ut nota con[co]rdia nostra tu ipsa mihi di[gnam et aptam con]/dicionem quaereres p[ara]resque ac futuros liberos t[e communes pro]/que tuis habituram adf[irm]ares.
112 *Laud. Turiae* 2.48–50.
113 Soranus 1.9.34: Ἐπεὶ τέκνων ἕνεκα καὶ διαδοχῆς, ἀλλ' οὐχὶ ψιλῆς ἡδυπαθείας, αἱ πολλαὶ γάμοις συγκαταζεύγνυνται, παντελῶς [δ']ἐστιν ἄτοπον περὶ μὲν τῆς προγονικῆς αὐτῶν εὐγενείας ἐξετάζειν καὶ τῆς τῶν χρημάτων περιουσίας, περὶ δὲ τοῦ πότερον δύνανται συλλαμβάνειν ἢ μή, καὶ εἰ πρὸς τὸ τίκτειν εὐφυῶς ἔχουσιν ἢ οὔ, ἀνεξέταστον ἀπολιπεῖν· δεόντως τὸν περὶ τοῦ προκειμένου ποιούμεθα λόγον. Although for social reasons, the other opinion was held. See e.g. 'And so noble birth is a great treasure. Those who enjoy it may openly and freely express themselves on every topic, which should be of special importance for people aiming at producing legitimate children. Indeed, the pride of those whose lineage is suspicious or prevaricated is destroyed and humiliated' (Pseudo-Plutarch, *The Education of Children*, retransl. from the Polish translation by T. Krynicka).
114 Soranus 1.9.35; Bradley 2011: 1–41 (on depicting the body as a fertility symbol, see esp. p. 12).
115 Soranus 1.10.36.

116 Soranus 1.10.36.
117 Soranus 1.10.37: προσεθήκαμεν δὲ ὅτι καὶ ὁρμῆς καὶ ὀρέξεως πρὸς συνουσίαν ὑπαρχούσης. ὡς γὰρ χωρὶς ὀρέξεως οὐκ ἐνδεχόμενον ὑπὸ τῶν ἀρρένων τὸ σπέρμα καταβληθῆναι, τὸν αὐτὸν τρόπον χωρὶς ὀρέξεως ὑπὸ τῶν θηλειῶν οὐκ ἐνδεχόμενον αὐτὸ συλληφθῆναι; A third-century-CE Oxyrrhynchus papyrus contains a spell intended to help with fertilization, and the woman's sexual satisfaction comes up as conducive to that effect: 'a good [spell to say] over the excretion [i.e. semen]: during the intercourse, say: 'I have spilled blood (αἷμα) ABRATHIAOU in the vagina of so-and-so; I have granted you my pleasure, so-and-so. Into your womb (κοιλία) I have spilled the blood BABRAOTH'. P. Oxy. LVI 3834 (retransl. from the English transl. by A. Wypustek).
118 'When the body neither wants nor is full, nor heavy from excessive drinking or indigestion.'
119 Soranus 1.10.36: καὶ τοῦ σώματος μήτ' ἐνδεοῦς ὄντος μήτ' ἄγαν πλήρους καὶ βαρέος ἐκ μέθης καὶ ἀπεψίας, καὶ ὁ μετὰ τὴν ἀποθεραπείαν τοῦ σώματος ἐμβρωματίου ληφθέντος ὀλίγου καὶ κατὰ πᾶν εὐαρέστου τοῦ καταστήματος ὑπάρχοντος.
120 Abel 1999: 868–72.
121 Soranus 1.10.38.
122 Ps.-Plut. 3.
123 Cael. Aurel. 2.64.
124 Soranus is quoting Euenor and Euryphon, but himself regards that as a superstition. Soranus 1.9.35: μάλιστα δὲ προσέχει σημειώσει τῇ διὰ τῶν προσθέτων, οἷον ῥητίνης, πηγάνου, σκόρδου, καρδάμου, καριάνδρου·· εἰ μὲν γὰρ ἡ ποιότης προστεθέντων αὐτῶν μέχρι τοῦ στόματος ἀναφέροιτο, δύνασθαί φησιν συλλαμβάνειν αὐτάς, εἰ δὲ μή, τοὐναντίον, Εὐήνωρ δὲ καὶ Εὐρυφῶν ἐπὶ δίφρου μαιωτικοῦ καθίσαντες τοῖς αὐτοῖς ὑπεθυμίασαν. Fumigating the genitals and the smell 'passing' through the mouth may have had a connection to beliefs concerning female anatomy. A woman's body was described as having upper and lower positions. An analogy was observed by Greek medicine: lips and neck were found in both the head and the genital parts. The terminology is still in use, in its Latin guise (since *labia* means lips, and *cervix*, neck). See Hawkins 2015: 43–68, esp. 48–9.
125 Lucr. 4.1264–1267.
126 Richlin 1997: 197–220.
127 *Orphei Lithica* 16.12.
128 Plin. HN 20.22.
129 Plin. HN 30.43.125: cavendum et ne in terra ponantur. conceptus quoque causa dantur in potu quini aut septeni.
130 Aet. 16.34. 38–41, cited from Kokoszko 2014: 296.

131 *Cyranides* 2.24: σὺν δὲ σατυρίῳ ἥ τε χολὴ καὶ ἡ πυτία καὶ ὁ ἐγκέφαλος προστιθέμενα ἐν πεσσῷ σὺν χυλῷ ἀλθαίας ἢ μαλάχης καὶ ἐλαίῳ σύλληψιν ἐργάζεται.
132 *Cyranides* 2.28: ἐὰν δέ τις τὸ αἷμα αὐτῆς κροκύδι δεξάμενος ἀποθῆται πρὸς κεφαλὴν γυναικὸς ἀγνοούσης καὶ συγγένηται αὐτῇ, εὐθέως συλλήψεται.
133 *Cyranides* 2.2: ἡ δὲ κόπρος αὐτοῦ σὺν ῥοδίνῳ ἐν πεσσῷ σύλληψιν ποιεῖ.
134 Plin. HN 7.13.57: Est quaedam privatim dissociatio corporum, et inter se sterilis ubi cum aliis iunxere se, gignunt, sicut Augustus et Livia; item alii. aliaeque feminas tantum generant aut mares, plerumque et alternant, sicut Gracchorum mater duodeciens, Agrippina Germanici noviens; aliis sterilis est iuventa, aliis semel in vita datur gignere; quaedam non perferunt partus, quales, si quando medicina naturam vicere, feminam fere gignunt.
135 Suet. *Aug.* 63: Ex Scribonia Iuliam, ex Livia nihil liberorum tulit, cum maxime cuperet. Infans, qui conceptus erat, immaturus est editus.
136 Lucr. 4.1248–56.
137 Plin. HN, 7.11.48: Praeter mulierem pauca animalia coitum novere gravida; unum quidem omnino aut alterum superfetat. extat in monimentis et medicorum et quibus talia consectari curae fuit uno abortu duodecim puerperia egesta. sed ubi paululum temporis inter duos conceptus intercessit, utrumque perfertur.
138 Solinus 1.59: Mulierum aliae in aeternum steriles sunt, aliae mutatis coniugiis exuunt sterilitatem, nonnullae tantum semel pariunt, quaedam aut feminas aut mares semper.
139 Soranus 1.10.40.
140 Solinus 1.62: Ante omnia subolem cogitantibus sternutatio post coitus cavenda, ne prius semen excutiat inpulsus repentinus, quam penetralibus se matris insinuet umor paternus.
141 Dig. 28.2.6: sed est quaesitum, an is, qui generare facile non possit, postumum heredem facere possit, et scribit Cassius et Iavolenus posse: nam et uxorem ducere et adoptare potest: spadonem quoque posse postumum heredem scribere et Labeo et Cassius scribunt: quoniam nec aetas nec sterilitas ei rei impedimento est.
142 Lucr. 4.1233–47.
143 Devine 1985: 313–17, believes one of the reasons behind the low birthrate could have been the easy availability and popularity of baths, or, to be precise, hot baths which, as we know today, do degrade the sperm.
144 Lucr. 4.1237–47.
145 Soranus 1.10.41.
146 It is possible that *crassum* should be read rather than *grassum*. Cf. Lucr. 4.1237–47.
147 Cael. Aurel. 2.64.
148 Laes 2016.

149 Cod. Iust. 5.17.10: In causis iam dudum specialiter definitis, ex quibus recte mittuntur repudia, illam addimus, ut, si maritus uxori ab initio matrimonii usque ad duos continuos annos computandos coire minime propter naturalem imbecillitatem valeat, possit mulier vel eius parentes sine periculo dotis amittendae repudium marito mittere, ita tamen, ut ante nuptias donatio eidem marito servetur.
150 Mart. 10.91.
151 Mart. 10.102.
152 Iuv. 9.70–89.
153 Plin. HN 20.21.47: inponitur et vulneribus, venerem stimulat; the beneficial effects of leeks are also mentioned in Gargilius (Garg. 21.7; 21.21).
154 Plin. HN 24.28.43: medetur et attritis partibus sive oleo e semine eius facto ceraeque mixto sive foliis ex oleo decoctis, si hae cum aqua ita foveantur.
155 Plin. HN 20.42.108: venerem stimulant; 20.43.111: item veneri, vesicae quoque nisi decoctum.
156 Plin. HN 24.28.43: eadem recens trita et in vino pota venerem concitat.
157 Plin. HN 24.89.140: actis quoque ubertatem faciunt in cibis et infantibus inlita capillum aiunt, ex aceto edentium venerem stimulant.
158 Plin. HN 20.23.57: venerem quoque stimulare cum coriandro viridi tritum potumque e mero.
159 Garg. 25.13 [ed. V. Rose 25.20]: simili modo temperatum venerem stimulat.
160 Garg. 31.10 [ed. V. Rose 31.10] semen eorum tritum cum vino potum venerem stimulat; Garg 33.7 [ed. V. Rose 33.16]: venerem stimulat copiosior in cibo sumpta.
161 Garg. 35.5 [ed. V. Rose 35.5] venerem stimulant, eo validius si cum eruca condiantur.
162 Plin. HN 22.38: peculiaris laus eius, quod fatigato venere corpori succurrit marcentesque iam senio coitus excitat; age was seen as a major cause of impotence. E.g. Iuv. 10.206–9.
163 Plin. HN 22.39.82: Et iasine olus silvestre habetur, in terra repens, cum lacte multo, florem fert candidum; conchylium vocant. et huius eadem commendatio ad stimulandos coitus.
164 *Cyranides* 2.2: ὁ δὲ ὄρχις ὁ δεξιὸς ξηρός, λεῖος ἐπιπασθεὶς ἐν ποτῷ, φιλτροπόσιμόν ἐστιν ἐπὶ γυναικῶν, ὁ δὲ εὐώνυμος ἐπὶ ἀνδρῶν. τὸ δὲ ἄκρον αὐτοῦ περιαφθὲν μεγίστην ἔντασιν ποιεῖ. ὁμοίως καὶ λεῖον ἐπιπασθὲν ἐν ποτῷ λάθρα. καὶ οἱ ὄρχεις πινόμενοι ξηροὶ τὸ αὐτὸ δρῶσιν. δίδου δὲ ὅσον κοχλιαρίου πλῆθος. τοσοῦτον δέ ἐστιν ἀνυτικὸν ὥστε ἀβλαβῆ τὴν ἔντασιν ποιεῖν καὶ τὴν πύρωσιν ἀδιάψευστον τηρεῖν. // τοὺς ὄρχεις τούτου ζῶντος τοῦ ζῴου ἔκκοψον· εἶτα ζῶντα μὲν αὐτὸν ἀπόλυσον, θεραπεύσας δὲ περίαψον. ἐὰν γὰρ αὐτῶν τοὺς διδύμους ὡς εἴρηται περιάψῃς, πάραυτα ἐντείνει. τινὲς δὲ αὐτοὺς βάλλουσιν εἰς τὰ ἰσχία τοῦ τράγου. // ἐὰν δὲ τοῦ αἰδοίου αὐτοῦ τὸ ἄκρον ἐν κύστει ἢ ἐν δέρματι ἐνδήσῃς, ἐν ᾧ ἐπιγράψεις τὸ ὄνομα τοῦτο διὰ σμυρνομέλανος 'τιν βιβ ηλιθι' καὶ περιάψῃς,

ἀβλαβῶς συνουσιάσεις. // . . . οἱ δὲ νεφροὶ αὐτοῦ ἐσθιόμενοι ἢ πινόμενοι ἀφροδίσια παρορμῶσιν.

165 Emotions a person could have while reading a novel were so intense that Theodorus Priscianus prescribed reading erotic novels as treatment of impotence: ad delicias animum pertrahentibus . . . ceteris suauiter amatorias fabulas describentibus (Diosc. Ped. *Euporista* 2.11.34).

166 Plin. HN 7.13.58: quaedam non perferunt partus, quales, si quando medicina et cura vicere, feminam fere gignunt. Although Pliny may also have counted on a remark made by his uncle, who had written that in some cases miscarriage would cause the woman to go through a period of greater fertility.

167 Plut. *Mor. Coniugalia praecepta* 145d: παιδίον μὲν γὰρ οὐδεμία ποτὲ γυνὴ λέγεται ποιῆσαι δίχα κοινωνίας ἀνδρός, τὰ δ᾽ ἄμορφα κυήματα καὶ σαρκοειδῆ καὶ σύστασιν ἐν ἑαυτοῖς ἐκ διαφθορᾶς λαμβάνοντα μύλας καλοῦσι.

168 Kursa 201: 60–80, esp. 71–3. The Justinian code, here modelled on earlier solutions, allowed for unilateral divorce if the reason was just. In the *Digest*, *sterilitas* is listed as one such reason (Dig. 24.1.60.1).

169 Women returning into the care of their father or guardian had generally poor chances of marrying again. That remained true even if the dismissal was merely part of an intrigue, as in the case of Sulla's third wife (Plut., *Sulla* 6.11); there were rumours in Rome that him accusing Cloelia of infertility was only an excuse for the divorce, since a few days later he married Caecilia Metella.

170 J.-N. Corvisier thinks infertility afflicted around 10 per cent of women in antiquity, which was partly due to poorer hygiene and lack of specialized medical knowledge regarding women's ailments (Corvisier 1985: 163).

171 Tatarkiewicz 2015: 57–70.

172 Aubert 2004: 259–76.

173 In *Ad nationes* (2.11), dated to the final years of the second century CE, Tertullian criticizes the earliest, traditional Roman religion, saying in it, a human being was subordinate to the workings of supernatural forces which were present and affected their whole life and all its aspects. He then lists the names and responsibilities of the several deities.

174 Aug. *De Civitate Dei* 7.2: Nam ipse primum Ianus, cum puerperium concipitur, unde illa cuncta opera sumunt exordium minutatim minutis distributa numinibus, aditum aperit recipiendo semini. Ibi est et Saturnus propter ipsum semen; ibi Liber, qui marem effuso semine liberat; ibi Libera, quam et Venerem uolunt, quae hoc idem beneficium conferat feminae, ut etiam ipsa emisso semine liberetur. Omnes hi ex illis sunt, qui selecti appellantur. Sed ibi est et dea Mena, quae menstruis fluoribus praeest, quamuis Iouis filia, tamen ignobilis. Et hanc prouinciam fluorum menstruorum in libro selectorum deorum ipsi Iunoni idem auctor adsignat, quae in diis selectis etiam regina est et hic tamquam Iuno Lucina cum eadem Mena

priuigna sua eidem cruori praesidet. Ibi sunt et duo nescio qui obscurissimi, Vitumnus et Sentinus, quorum alter uitam, alter sensus puerperio largiuntur.

175 Tert. *Ad nat.* 2.11.1: Non tamen contenti eos deos asseuerare, qui uisi retro, auditi contrectatique sunt, quorum effigies descriptae, negotia digesta, memoria propagata est, umbras aliquas incorporales, inanimales et nomina de rebus efflagitantes deos sanciunt, diuidentes omnem statum hominis singulis potestatibus ab ipso quidem uteri conceptu, ut sit deus Conseuius quidam, qui con[...]nibus concubitalibus praesit, et Fluuionia, quae infantem in utero nutriat; hinc Vitumnus et Sentinus, per quem uiuiscat infans et sentiat primum; dehinc Diespiter qui puerum perducat ad partum cum primig[...] et Candelifera, quoniam ad candelae lumina pariebant.
176 Cid López 2007: 357–72.
177 Flambar 1987: 191–210. It mentions the theory that this Juno's shrine was located at the site now occupied by the church of S. Lorenzo (St Lawrence) in Lucina.
178 Ovid. *Fasti* 2.429–34.
179 Ovid. *Fasti* 2.435–8.
180 Duval 1989: 1163–73.
181 Ducaté-Paarmann 2005: 33–4.
182 Turfa 1986: 205–13.
183 Oberhelman 2014: 47–62, esp. 57–8.
184 Baggieri 1998: 790 confirms that some of the clay models even contained two balls, which could mean twins. Although twin pregnancy was very risky for both the mother and the children, it was regarded as singled out by the gods (cf. e.g. Dasen 2005). Doubling the number of balls might also mean strengthening the prayer for numerous offspring. That is one theory. Others put forward that a model of a uterus may point to a request to be healed of some illness or unusual affliction, but most often it is assumed to be a call upon the gods to let the petitioner become pregnant shortly.
185 Nissen 2006: 804–9; Durand, Finon 2000: 9–91; Ehmig 2013: 111–29.
186 Deyts 2004: 227–37; Nissen 2006: 804–9.
187 Cic. *De div.* 2.145: Parere quaedam matrona cupiens, dubitans essetne praegnans, visa est in quiete obsignatam habere naturam. Rettulit. Negavit eam, quoniam obsignata fuisset, concipere potuisse. At alter praegnantem esse dixit; nam inane obsignari nihil solere. Quae est ars coniectoris eludentis ingenio? An ea quae dixi et innumerabilia quae conlecta habent Stoici quicquam significant nisi acumen hominum ex similitudine aliqua coniecturam modo huc, modo illuc ducentium? Medici signa quaedam habent ex venis et ex spiritu aegroti multisque ex aliis futura praesentiunt; gubernatores, cum exsultantis lolligines viderunt aut delphinos se in portum conicientes, tempestatem significari putant. Haec ratione explicari et ad naturam revocari facile possunt, ea vero, quae paulo ante dixi, nullo modo.
188 CIL XI 1129c.

189 Soranus 1.12.44.
190 Plin. HN 7.6.41.

Chapter 3

1. Ter. *Adel.* 3.2.56: Canthara, curre, obstetricem accerse, ut quom opus sit ne in moranobis siet.
2. It is worth noting that only 5 per cent (or should one say, as many as 5 per cent) of all known inscriptions dealing with physicians relate to women who practised medicine in any way; see e.g. Flemming, 2007: 259, n. 14.
3. According to Lewis and Short, *A Latin Dictionary*, *obstetrix* (or, *opstetrix*, *obstitrix* or *opstitrix*) means 'a midwife' (*s. v.*), that is, 'a person, usually a woman, who is trained to assist women in childbirth, but who is not a physician'.
4. In both literary and epigraphical sources, one also encounters terms such as *iatromea* (= *medica*) and *maia* (= *obstetrix*). Those tend to be rendered and understood as Greek terminology carried over into Latin. For more on the terminology of medical professions, see e.g. Flemming 2007: 257–9; Dasen 2016: 9–15. Dasen 2016a, Korpela 1987 groups all the women the sources call *obstetrix*, *medica*, *maia* and *iatromea* as midwives (die Hebamme).
5. Wainwright 2006; Pomeroy 1987: 496–500; For lists of *medicae*, see Parker 1997: 140–6; Alonso Alonso 2011: 283–4. The discrepancies between those stem from the authors having adopted different criteria.
6. Parker 1997: 143.
7. Due to the wider context of the inscription, that interpretation is suggested, among other authors, by U. Gehn: 'The honorand, Geminius Dativus, was curator of the city of Avitta Bibba (lines 2–3), on the office see LSA-2406. He was possibly a doctor (lines 1–2)' (http://laststatues.classics.ox.ac.uk/database/discussion.php?id=2723, accessed on 5 October 2019). Gehn reads the inscription as follows: Salus omnium / medicine Gemini ---/ Dativi cur(atoris) [r(ei) p(ublicae)] /iter[um ---] / univ [ers] --- /--- / ---/---; ('The well of all through the medicine of Geminius ... Dativus, curator of the city for the second time ... all ...'. Generally, it bears noting the text does not pose great difficulties in terms of reconstruction. The database Epigraphische Datenbank Clauss – Slaby (http://db.edcs.eu/epigr/edcs_id.php?s_sprache=en&p_edcs_id=EDCS-15600905, accessed on 25 September 2016), for instance, quotes the inscription as per CIL (http://arachne.uni-koeln.de/Tei-Viewer/cgi-bin /teiviewer.php?manifest=BOOK-ZID1314679, accessed on 25 September 2019), but without the emendations and commentary from CIL VIII,1,12269 (http://arachne.uni-koeln.de/Tei-Viewer/cgi-bin/teiviewer.php?manifest=BOOK-ZID1315261, accessed on 25 September 2019).

8 CIL VIII 24679: Asyllia L(ucii) f(ilia) Polla / medica h(ic) s(ita) e(st) / vixs(it) a(nnos) LXV / Euscius l(ibertus) d(e) s(uo) f(ecit).
9 CIL VI 7581: Deae sanctae meae / Primillae medicae / L(ucii) Vibi(i) Metilonis f(iliae) / vixit annis XXXXIIII / ex eis cum L(ucio) Cocceio / Apthoro XXX sine / querella fecit / Apthorus coniug(i) / optimae castae / et sibi.
10 CIL XIII 2019: Metilia Donata medic[a] / de sua pecunia dedi[t] / l(oco) d(ato) d(ecreto) d(ecurionum).
11 CIL XIII 5919: Boruoni / et Damo/nae / [Se]xtilia / [S]exti fil(ia) / med(ica) / - - - -.
12 CIL X 3980: Scantiae Redemptae in/comparabilissimae feminae que/ius de vitae documenta non sufficit / mediocritas hominum at cumulum laudis /pervenire fuit namque iuvenis ista / omni genere laudis condigna primo deificae / sanctitatis pudicitiae vallata honestate morum /[in]nata pietas in parentibus procliva castitate inlustris /[t]enacitatis magistra (v)er(e)cundiae antistis disclipin[ae] / [in] medicina fuit et innocentiae singularis / [t]alis fuit ut esset exemplum matrimoni fuit t[alis] / ut contemneret iuventutem nam maritus am[isit ?] / co(n)iugem familiarem salutis et vitae suae nut[ric(em)] / haec vixit annis XXII mensibus X / Fl(avius) Tarentinus et Scantia Redempta / parentes filiae dulcissimae / sibique fecerunt.
13 CIL VI 9615: Minucia / (mulieris) l(iberta) Asste / medica.
14 CIL VI 9617: Venuleia / (mulieris) l(iberta) Sosis / medica.
15 AE 1972, 83: Iulia Sophia / Isidori Ti(berii) Caesaris / Augusti l(iberti) l(iberta) medic(a) / vixit annos XXII.
16 IG XIV 1751: Τι(βερίῳ) · Κλαυδίῳ Ἀλκίμῳ · ἰατρῷ Καίσαρος · ἐποίησε Ῥεστιτοῦτα · πάτρωνι · καὶ · καθηγητῇ ἀγαθῷ καὶ ἀξίῳ ἔζη(σε) ἔτη πβ.
17 CIL IX 5861: Deis Manib(us) / Iuliae Q(uinti) l(ibertae) / Sabinae / medicae / Q(uintus) Iulius Atimetus / coniugi / bene merenti.
18 CIL V 3461: C(aius) Cornelius / Meliboeus / sibi et / Sentiai / Elidi medicai / contuber(nali) / Sentiai Aste; although Alonso clearly regards her as a freedwoman (Alonso Alonso, 2011: 284, no. 15), Parker is not so sure, allowing for the possibility of her having been born free (Parker 1997: 142, no. 15).
19 AE 1937,17: Hic iacet Sarman /na medica vixit / pl(us) m(inus) an(nis) LXX Pientius / Pientinus fili(i) et / Honorata norus / titolum posuerunt /in pace.
20 CIL VI 9616: D(iis) M(anibus) / Terentiae / Niceni Terentiae / Primaes medicas li/bertae fecerunt / Mussius Antiochus / et Mussia Dionysia / fil(ii) m(atri) b(ene) m(erenti).
21 CIL II 497: D(iis) M(anibus) s(acrum) / Iuliae Saturni[nae] / a[nn(orum)] XXXXV / uxori [inco]mpara/bili m[edica]e optimae / mulie[risan]ctissimae / Cassius Philippus / maritus ob meritis / h(ic) s(ita) e(st) s(it) t(ibi) t(erra) l(evis).
22 CIL VI 9477: Valeriae Berecundae Iatromeae regionis suae primae q(uae) v(ixit) ann(os) XXXIII m(enses) VIIII d(ies) XXVIII Valeria Bitalis filia matri dulcissimae et Publius) Gellius Bitalio coiugi sanctissimae b(ene) m(erenti) f(e)c(e)r(unt) et sibi

et Gellio Chresimo fratrii et Iuliae Chreste sorori et ego Bitalio Chresten s(upra) s(criptam) quem vice filiae attendo et liberis eorum. Hoc monimentum et loci sca lare cubiculi superioris f(aciendum) c(uravi) et lib(ertis) lib(ertabus) q(ue) p(os)t(e) r(is)q(ue) eorum. Petrei bibas.

23 CIL VI 9478: Valiae (=Valeriae?) Calliste iatromeae Caecilius Lusimacii chus (sic) Coiugi suae fec(it).
24 Parker 1997: 284, no. 23).
25 CIL VI 9614: Iulia / Pye / medica.
26 CIL XII 3343.
27 CIL VI 6851: Melitine / medica Appulei.
28 CIL VI 8711: Secunda / Livillaes / medica // Ti(berius) Claudius / Caesaris l(ibertus) / Celer aeditu(u)s / a Vesta.
29 CIPRBu 379: Ambat(a)e Me/dicae Placi/di f(iliae) an(norum) LXXV.
30 Parker 1997: 135; Flemming 2007: 259, n. 14.
31 E.g. CIL XIII 4334 (18) (a tomb stele from Metz); Todman 2008: 108.
32 Retief 2005: 179; Kollesch: 1979: 507–13; Nickel 1979: 515–18; Drabkin 1957: 286–96.
33 E.g. Drabkin 1944: 333–51; Cilliers, Retief 2006: 34–40; Turgut 2011: 197–200.
34 Naevia Clara AE 2001, 263: C(aius) Naevius C(aii) l(ibertus) Phi[lippus] / medicus chirurg(us) / Naevia C(aii) l(iberta) Clara / medica philolog(a) / in fro(nte) ped(es) XI s(emis) / in agr(o) ped(es) XVI.
35 Scantia Redempta CIL X 3980: Scantiae Redemptae in/ comparabilissimae feminae que/ ius de vitae documenta non sufficit / mediocritas hominum at cumulum laudis / pervenire fuit namque iuvenis ista / omni genere laudis condigna primo deificae / sanctitatis pudicitiae vallata honestate morum / [in]nata pietatas in parentibus procliva castitate inlustris / [t]enacitatis magistra (v)er(e)cundiae antistis disciplin[ae] / [in] medicina fuit et innocentiae singularis / [t]alis fuit ut esset exemplum matrimoni fuit t[alis] / ut contemneret iuventutem nam maritus am[isit ?] / co(n)iugem familiarem salutis et vitae suae nut[ric(em)] / haec vixit annis XXII mensibus X / Fl(avius) Tarentinus et Scantia Redempta / parentes filiae dulcissimae / sibique fecerunt.
36 Restituta IG XIV 1751: Τι(βερίῳ) · Κλαυδίῳ Ἀλκίμῳ · ἰατρῷ Καίσαρος · ἐποίησε Ῥεστιτοῦτα · πάτρωνι · καὶ · καθηγητῇ ἀγαθῷ καὶ ἀξίῳ ἔζη(σε) ἔτη πβ; Irving 2012: 45–56.
37 Parker 1997: 141, no. 5.
38 Iulia Saturnina CIL II, 497: D(iis) M(anibus) s(acrum) / Iuliae Saturni[nae] / a[nn(orum)] XXXXV / uxori [inco]mpara/bili m[edica]e optimae / mulie[risan]ctissimae / Cassius Philippus / maritus ob meritis / h(ic) s(ita) e(st) s(it) t(ibi) t(erra) l(evis).
39 French 1986: 69–84; Tatarkiewicz 2013: 127–51.

40 Soranus 1.1.4; see also Cael. *Aurel.* 5: Obstetrix est femina omnium mulierum causarum docta, medicinali eruditione perita, que possit universaliter valitudines competenter curare, ita ut non sit turbulenta, nec avara, nec verbosa, sed sapiens et sobria et taciturna nec superstitiosa, que sua sollicitudine mulieres in partu gubernet. sit etiam obstetrix compatiens, solida, pudica, arguta, quieta, prudens.

41 Soranus 1.1.3: τίς ἐστιν ἐπιτήδειος πρὸς τὸ γενέσθαι μαῖα. εὔχρηστος μὲν ὁ λόγος πρὸς τὸ μὴ διὰ κενῆς πονεῖν καὶ τὰς ἀνεπιτηδείους διδάξαι προσδεχομένως. ἐπιτήδειος δέ ἐστιν ἡ γραμμάτων ἐντός, ἀγχίνους, μνήμων, φιλόπονος, κόσμιος καὶ κατὰ τὸ κοινὸν ἀπαρεμπόδιστος ταῖς αἰσθήσεσιν, ἀρτιμελής, εὔτονος, ὡς δ' ἔνιοι λέγουσιν καὶ μακροὺς καὶ λεπτοὺς ἔχουσα καὶ τοὺς τῶν χειρῶν δακτύλους καὶ ὑπεσταλκότας ταῖς ῥαξὶν τοὺς ὄνυχας. γραμμάτων μὲν ἐντός [εἶναι], ἵνα καὶ διὰ θεωρίας τὴν τέχνην ἰσχύσῃ παραλαβεῖν· ἀγχίνους δέ πρὸς τὸ ῥᾳδίως τοῖς λεγομένοις καὶ γινομένοις παρακολουθεῖν· μνήμων δέ, ἵνα καὶ τῶν παραδιδομένων ἀποκρατῇ μαθημάτων (μάθησις γὰρ ἐκ μνήμης γίνεται [καὶ] καταλήψεως)· φιλόπονος δὲ πρὸς τὸ ἐπιμένειν τοῖς συμβεβηκόσι (δεῖ γὰρ ἀνδρώδους τληπαθείας τῇ βουλομένῃ τοσοῦτον μάθημα παραλαβεῖν)· κόσμιος δὲ διὰ τὸ μέλλειν οἰκίας πιστεύεσθαι καὶ μυστήρια βίου, καὶ ὅτι ταῖς φαύλαις τὸ ἦθος εἰς τὸ ἐπιβουλεύειν ἐφόδιόν ἐστι τὸ δοκεῖν ἰατρικὰς ἔχειν κατηχήσεις· ἀπαρεμπόδιστος δὲ ταῖς αἰσθήσεσιν, ἐπεὶ τὰ μὲν ὁρᾶν δεῖ, τῶν δὲ ἐξ ἀνακρίσεως ἀκούειν, τὰ δὲ διὰ τῆς ἁφῆς καταλαμβάνειν· ἀρτιμελὴς δὲ πρὸς τὸ τῆς ἐν τοῖς ἔργοις ὑπηρεσίας ἀπαρεμπόδιστος εἶναι· εὔτονος δέ, διὰ γὰρ τῆς ἐν τῷ περιοδεύειν κακοπαθείας δισσὴν τὴν πρᾶξιν παραλαμβάνειν· μακροὺς δὲ καὶ λεπτοὺς ἔχουσα τοὺς δακτύλους καὶ ὑπεσταλκότας τοὺς ὄνυχας, εἰς τό τῆς ἐν βάθει φλεγμονῆς ἀσκυλτότερον ἅπτεσθαι. τοῦτο μέντοι γε καὶ δι' αὐτῆς ἐπιτυγχάνεται τῆς ἐν τοῖς ἔργοις σπουδαιοτέρας τριβῆς καὶ συγγυμνασίας.

42 The whole passage listing the virtues of the perfect midwife, complete with justifications for the several skills: Soranus 1.1.4.

43 Soranus 2.(2)21.69 (see the Greek text quoted in Chapter 5 this volume, section 2.2. The second stage of labour).

44 Gourevitch 2004: 135–61; Galanakis 1998: 2012–13.

45 Soranus 2.(6)26.79: εἶτα λοιπὸν ἐκ τοῦ τεθὲν ἐπὶ γῆς εὐθέως αὐτὸ κλαυθμυρίσαι μετὰ τόνου τοῦ προσήκοντος· τὸ γὰρ ἕως πλείονος ἀκλαυστὶ διάγον ἢ καὶ παρέργως κλαυθμυρίζον ἐνύποπτον ὡς διά τινα περίστασιν τοῦτο πάσχον. ἔκ τε τοῦ πᾶσιν τοῖς μέρεσι καὶ μορίοις καὶ ταῖς αἰσθήσεσιν ἄρτιον ὑπάρχειν καὶ τοὺς πόρους ἔχειν ἀπαρεμποδίστους, οἷον ὤτων, ῥινῶν, φάρυγγος, οὐρήθρας, δακτυλίου, καὶ τὰς ἑκάστου [μορίου] φυσικὰς κινήσεις μὴ νωθρὰς [καὶ] μηδὲ ἐκλύτους καὶ τὰς τῶν ἄρθρων κάμψεις τε καὶ ἐκτάσεις μεγέθη τε καὶ σχήματα καὶ τὴν πᾶσαν ἐπιβάλλουσαν εὐαισθησίαν, ἣν γνωρίζομεν κἀκ τῆς ἐπιφανείας ἐπερείδοντες τούς δακτύλους· κατὰ φύσιν γάρ ἐστιν τὸ πρὸς ἕκαστον ἀλγεῖν τῶν νυσσόντων ἢ θλιβόντων.

46 It is from the eastern Mediterranean that well-educated midwives hailed. Obstetrics was a high-prestige profession in the East, for which women earned money and enjoyed respect. See Laes 2010: 261–86.
47 For more on depictions of midwives delivering children, see e.g. Tatarkiewicz 2015: 175–90.
48 Museo Nazionale, Naples, No. 109905A.
49 Thylander 1952, A 222.
50 CIL VIII 4896: Diis M(anibus) sac(rum) / Irene ops(t)e/trix Fausti / D(- - -) S(- - -) S(- - -) medici / v(ixit) a(nnis) XXXIII.
51 Schumacher 2001.
52 Many inscriptions only contain a name and the information that the person commemorated was an *obstetrix*; e.g. AE 1980, 936: D(is) M(anibus) s(acrum) / Aurelia Ma/[c]ula p(ia) vixit / annis LVI / obs(t)etrix; AE 1903, 107: O(ssa) t(ibi) b(ene) q(uiescant)] / [D(is)] M(anibus) s(acrum) / [---]inia Victoria / [obst]etrix(?) p(ia) v(ixit) a(nnos) XLVIIII / [m(enses)] VI d(ies) XIIII / h(ic) s(itus) e(st) // t(erra) t(ibi) l(evis) s(it); AE 1991, 126: Helena/Lucretia/ opstetrix; CIL XI 3391: [V]olusia [---]/opstetrix/vixit annos.
53 CIL VI 9724 : [- - -]antiv [- - -V]aleriae Syre/[- - -] qu(a)e vixit annis XXXI / [- - -q]uo fecit annos VIIII et / [- - - - de]posita pri(die) idus novem(bres) /[- - -]a filia obs(t)etricis i CILVI 8207: Sallustia Q(uinti) l(iberta) Imerita opstetrix / Q(uintus) Sallustius Q(uinti) l(ibertus) Artimidorus / p(atronus ?).
54 CIL VI 8948: Prima Liviae opstetrix Asterope Maximi (servus) / Epicharis Maximi (servus) mater i CIL VI 9720: Claudiae Trophim(e) / obs(t)etrici / T(itus) Cassius Trophimus f(ilius) / matri pientissimae et / Ti(berius) Cassius Trophimianus /aviae et posterisque suis / fecerunt / vix(it) ann(os) LXXV m(enses) V.
55 CIL VI 6647: Hygiae / Flaviae Sabinae / opstetr(ici) vixit ann(os) XXX / Marius Orthrus et / Apollonius contubernali / carissimae.
56 AE 2005, 328: Secunda / Aug(ustae) l(iberta) opste/trix vix(it) ann(is) / XXIV.
57 AE 1926, 52, AE 1991 127: Taxis Ionidis, Iulia[e Aug(ustae)]/opstetrix, v(ixit) a(nnis) XXX[---]/Hesper et Epitync[hanus]/vicari de suo [fec(erunt)?].
58 PIR A 885; CIL VI 8947: Antoniae Aug(ustae) l(ibertae) / Thallusae / opstetric(i).
59 PIR C 1102; CIL VI 4458: Hygia / Marcellae l(iberta) / obstetrix.
60 CIL VI 6832: Sempronia Peloris / Atratinae opstetrix / [- - -]ris v(ixit) a(nnos) [- -] / - - - - - -, and CIL VI 6836.
61 PIR S 858; CIL VI 6325: Secunda / opstetrix / Statiliae maioris.
62 PIR2 F 440; CIL VI 6647: Hygiae / Flaviae Sabinae / opstetr(ici) vixit ann(os) XXX / Marius Orthrus et / Apollonius contubernali / carissimae.
63 CIL VI 8192: Q(uintus) Sallustius / Diogae l(ibertus) / Dioges / Sallustia / Artemidori l(iberta) / Athen[ai]s / opstetrix.
64 CIL VI 8207: Sallustia Q(uinti) l(iberta) Imerita opstetrix / Q(uintus) Sallustius Q(uinti) l(ibertus) Artimidorus / p(atronus?).

65 PIR2 S 83.
66 Alonso Alonso 2011: 279.
67 CIL VI 6836.
68 CIL VI 6320.
69 CIL VI 8174.
70 As in CIL VI, 9723: Poblicia ((mulieris)) l(iberta) Aphe / opstetrix /ossa tibi bene quiescant / Vixit annos XXI; VI 37810 Sex(tus) Teidiu[s Sex(ti) l(ibertus)] / Ánte[ros] Teidia/ Sex(ti) [l(iberta) ---] /opstetri[x ---].
71 AE 1914, 240: [C]aeliae / Victori/ae obste/trici ra/rissimae /piae quae / vixit an/nis XXVI / h(ic) s(ita) // [C]ae[l]i[u]s Nori/[cus] coniugi et / [so]ror[i] caris/[si]mis.
72 Alonso Alonso 2011: 273.
73 Soranus 1.2.4.
74 Dig. 50.13.1.2: Sed et obstetricem audiant, quae utique medicinam exhibere videtur.
75 Dig. 9.2.9: Item si obstetrix medicamentum dederit et inde mulier perierit, Labeo distinguit, ut, si quidem suis manibus supposuit, videatur occidisse: sin vero dedit, ut sibi mulier offerret, in factum actionem dandam, quae sententia vera est: magis enim causam mortis praestitit quam occidit.
76 Tatarkiewicz 2013: 127–51.
77 Dig. 25.4.1.4: Quid ergo, si interrogata dixerit se praegnatem? ordo senatus consultis expositus sequetur. quod si negaverit, tunc secundum hoc rescriptum praetor debebit obstetrices adhibere; Dig. 25.4.1.5: Et notandum, quod non permittitur marito vel mulieri obstetricem adhibere, sed omnes a praetore adhibendae sunt.
78 Plin. HN 28.20: quaeque alia non obstetrices modo, verum etiam ipsae meretrices.
79 Plin. HN 28.18.66: Salpe fovet illa (sc. urina) cum oculos firmitatis causa, inlinit sole usta cum ovi albo, efficacius struthocameli, binis horis.
80 Plin. HN 32.47.135: Psilotrum est thynni sanguis, fel, iocur, sive recentia sive servata, iocur etiam tritum mixtoque cedrio plumbea pyxide adservatum. ita pueros mangonicavit Salpe obstetrix.
81 Plin. HN 32.51.140: Salpe negat canes latrare, quibus in offa rana viva data sit.
82 Plin. HN 28.7.38: Salpe torporem sedari quocumque membro stupente, si quis in sinum expuat aut si superiores palpebras saliva tangat.
83 Plin. HN 28.80.261: Salpe genitale id in oleum fervens mergi iubet septies eoque perungui pertinentes partes.
84 Plin. HN 28.23.82: canum rabiosorum morsus et tertianas quartanasque febres menstruo in lana arietis nigri argenteo bracchiali inclus.
85 Plin. HN 28.23.83: Sotira obstetrix tertianis quartanisque efficacissimum dixit plantas aegri subterlini, multoque efficacius ab ipsa muliere et ignorantis; sic et comitiales excitari. Icatidas medicus quartanas finiri coitu, incipientibus dumtaxat menstruis, spopondit.
86 Plin. HN 28.23.81: Lais et Elephantis.

87 Suet. *Tib.* 43.2: Cubicula plurifariam disposita tabellis ac sigillis lascivissimarum picturarum et figurarum adornavit librisque Elephantidis instruxit, ne cui in opera edenda exemplar impe[t]ratae schemae deesset.
88 Vons 2000: 74–5.
89 Plin. HN 28.23.81.
90 'Furthermore, whereas it usually happens that children at birth are provided by nature with a caul, which the midwives seize and sell to credulous lawyers (for it is said that this brings luck to those who plead)'; HA, *Diadoumenianus Antoninus* 4.2: Solent deinde pueri pilleo insigniri naturali, quod obstetrices rapiunt et advocatis credulis vendunt, si quidem causidici hoc iuvari dicuntur.
91 Dig. 9.2.9 pr. For more on responsibility for medical errors, see Tadajczyk 2014: 102–28, esp. 108.
92 Ter. *Andr.* 228–30: 'Audivi, Archylis, iamdudum: Lesbiam adduci iubes. / sane pol illa temulentast mulier et temeraria / nec sati' digna quoi committas primo partu mulierem.'
93 Amm. Marc. 16.10.19.
94 For a discussion of this, see Parker 1997: 132–3 and 147–9; Barragán Nieto 2009: 84.
95 Pauli sententiarum interpretatio 2.25.8.
96 Dig. 50.13.1.2.
97 For a discussion of the passage, see Parker 1997: 149, n. 29.
98 Künzl, Engelmann 1997: 375–9.
99 Apul., *Met.* 5.10: nec uxoris officiosam faciem sed medicae laboriosam personam sustinens.
100 Alonso Alonso 2011: 267–96; Barragán Nieto 2009: 82–8; Retief 2005: 179–91; Flemming 2013: 271–95; Flemming 2007: 257–79; Parker 1997: 131–50.
101 Often, but not always. For a discussion of the legal aspects and verification of the qualifications of members of broadly understood medical professions in Rome, see Tadajczyk 2014.
102 Even though Soranus' work clearly does mention it.
103 Alonso Alonso 2011: 294–6.
104 Publicia Sp(uri) f(ilia) / Procula / medica idem opstetrìx / fecit sibi et suis libertìs/ libertábusq(ue) posterisq(ue) eorûm. Unfortunately, I only know the inscription from the EDR database, which lists it as coming from Puteoli and published in Marcone 2018: 270–2.
105 More information on male physicians (caring for women) can be found in Chapter 5 this volume, section 5 on difficult births.
106 Galen, Περὶ φυσικῶν δυνάμεων, 3.3: καὶ μέντοι καὶ αἱ μαῖαι τὰς τικτούσας οὐκ εὐθὺς ἀνιστᾶσιν οὐδ᾽ ἐπὶ τὸν δίφρον καθίζουσιν, ἀλλ᾽ ἅπτονται πρότερον ἀνοιγομένου τοῦ στόματος κατὰ βραχὺ καὶ πρῶτον μέν, ὥστε τὸν μικρὸν

δάκτυλον καθιέναι, διεστηκέναι φασίν, ἔπειτ' ἤδη καὶ μεῖζον καὶ κατὰ βραχὺ δὴ πυνθανομένοις ἡμῖν ἀποκρίνονται τὸ μέγεθος τῆς διαστάσεως ἐπαυξανόμενον.

107 On specializations of Roman doctors, see e.g. Dasen 2016: 9–15, Dasen 2016a with further reading.

108 Soranus 3.1.3: γυναικείους τινὰς λέγομεν ἰατρούς, ὅτι τὰ γυναικῶν θεραπεύουσι πάθη. Unfortunately, although very many medical specializations are known and mentioned in medical texts and inscriptions, this is the only one to confirm the existence of 'women's doctors'.

109 Green 2008: 32–4.

110 While it is not the primary focus of this book, it is still worth referencing a find unique on the global scale: a fragment of a Spanish lamp found in the late 1970s in a garbage dump made during the construction of a car park in León. The lamp came to be the property of a private collector, but was later handed over to a museum in León for research. It was a clay oil lamp with remains of a pink glaze. In A. Morillo's opinion, part of it depicts a gynaecological examination of an ill woman. The doctor performing the procedure, a man, has his eyes averted. Of course, that could be conventional; the idea may be that the person examining the patient is the main character in the image, and so looks at the potential viewer. However, it is possible one other reason was to respect the woman giving birth and her right to privacy; Morillo Cerdán 1999: 446; fig. 51.

111 Soranus 2.(6)21.70b: φυλασσέσθω δὲ ἡ μαῖα τὸ εἰς τούς γυναικείους κόλπους τῆς τικτούσης τὸ πρόσωπον ἐνατενίζειν, ὅπως μὴ αἰδουμένης συσταλῇ τὸ σῶμα.

112 King 1986: 53–77.

113 Identified with the physician Herophilus of Chalcedon; see Moog 2004: 575–9.

114 Hyginus, *Fabulae* 274.

115 The trope of shame as an obstacle preventing one from getting proper gynaecological care is also found in Hippocrates, who observes that female patients are reluctant to see a doctor and unable to communicate with him to describe their condition. Still, his writings do not mention female doctors as a potential solution. See Green 2008: 31–2.

116 Cael. Aurel. 1: Quoniam specialia quedam nature officia feminarum corporibus videntur esse concessa, virorum communitate carentia, ut purgatio, conceptio, partus, et morbi sequentes ex ipsis, qui sepe exigunt diligentiam medicine, veteres secretas eorum tradere curationes principaliter providerunt, quas genecias appellarunt, eo quod feminarum gratia sint specialiter ordinate, maxime cum in illis, ceteris communibus irruentibus morbis, pudendorum loca tangantur. sunt enim corporis condicione †illorum eorum corpora† omnium capacia vitiorum, que sepe femine pudore tangendi gravia reddiderunt, et nimietate coacte sera sunt necessitate confesse. Hinc denique consultum est ut medicas instituere antiquitas providisset, ne femine pudendorum vitia virilibus offerrentur oculis perscrutanda.

117 Green 2008: 32–4. Soranus, for instance, clearly said his book could be used not only by midwives, being also addressed to people who wanted to know how to choose 'the best midwife'. Those people could have been women, although M. Green thinks men were more likely, as masters of the house hiring midwives to care for their pregnant wives.

Chapter 4

1. Sen. QN 3.27.2: Quam longo tempore opus est ut conceptus ad puerperium perduret infans.
2. Soranus 1.11.42.
3. Plin. HN 7.6.41: A conceptu decimo die dolores capitis, oculorum vertigines tenebraeque, fastidium in cibis, redundatio stomachi indices sunt hominis inchoati.
4. Solinus 1.62.
5. Soranus 1.12.43.
6. Plut. *De amore prolis* 3.
7. Soranus 1.12.44.
8. P. Oxy. 744 (1 BCE); P. Oxy. 4.744 = HGV P. Oxy. 4.744 = Trismegistos 20442 (papyri.info)].
9. The problem of children being abandoned because of their gender has long been present in many studies. A few of those are: Harris 1994: 1–22; Scott 2000: 143–51; Corbier 2001: 53–7; Engels 1980: 112–20; Haentjens 2000: 261–4. Hallet thinks matters were different for girls born in upper-class families: Hallet 1984.
10. Plin. HN 7.13.57.
11. Cens. 6.8: Ceterum Parmenidis sententia est, cum dexterae partes semina dederint, tunc filios esse patri consimiles, cum laevae, tunc matri.
12. Soranus 1.13.45: τὴν δὲ δύσχροιαν ἐπὶ τῶν θηλυτόκων διὰ τὴν περὶ τὸ κυούμενον ἀργίαν.
13. Plin. HN 7.6.41: A conceptu decimo die dolores capitis, oculorum vertigines tenebraeque, fastidium in cibis, redundatio stomachi indices sunt hominis inchoati. melior color marem ferenti et facilior partus, motus in utero quadragensimo die. contraria omnia in altero sexu, ingestabile onus, crurum et inguinis levis tumor, primus autem XC die motus.
14. Solinus 1.63.
15. Garg. 17. 5–8.
16. Ehmig 2013: 111–29.
17. Shelton 2013: 125–7; Denooz 2010: 163–72.
18. Plin. *Ep.* 8.10; see also: Carlon 2009: 172–4; Shelton 2013: 125–7.

19 Garsney 1999, esp. 101–7. Much more information can be found on methods of contraception and abortion. See e.g. Kapparis 2002; Hopkins 1965: 124–51; Krenkel 1978: 197–203.
20 Soranus 1.14.47: διότι, κἂν παραβαινούσης τινὸς ἔνια τῶν εἰρημένων ἢ πάντα μὴ γίνηται τοῦ συλληφθέντος ἔκτρωσις, οὐχὶ πάντως ἠδίκηται τὸ συλληφθέν. βέβλαπται γὰρ ὥστε καὶ ἀτονώτερον γίνεσθαι καὶ ἀναυξητότερον καὶ δυστροφώτερον καὶ τὸ κοινὸν εὐαδίκητον εὐάλωτόν τε τοῖς βλάπτουσιν καὶ κακόμορφον καὶ κατὰ ψυχὴν ἀγενές. χωρὶς εἰ μὴ τῶν μὲν οἰκοδομουμένων ὅστις ἂν πεπηγόσι ἐποικοδομῆται τοῖς θεμελίοις οἶκος, δυσπερίτρεπτος μένει πλείοσιν χρόνοις, ὅσα δὲ σαθροῖς καὶ ἀπήκτοις, ῥαδίως καὶ πρὸς ὀλίγην ἀφορμὴν ἀπορρίπτεται, τῶν δὲ ζῴων ἡ γέννησις οὐκ ἂν εἴη διάφορος παρὰ τὸ τοῖς πρώτοις ὡσανεὶ στοιχείοις καὶ θεμελίοις διαφόροις ἐξερεισθῆναι.
21 Soranus 1.14.46: Ἡ τῶν συνειληφυιῶν ἐπιμέλεια τρίχρονός ἐστιν. ἡ μὲν γάρ ἐστι τῶν πρώτων χρόνων εἰς τήρησιν τοῦ καταβληθέντος σπέρματος, ἡ δὲ τῶν δευτέρων πρὸς παρηγορίαν τῶν ἐπιγινομένων συμπτωμάτων, καθάπερ ἡ τῆς ἐπιγινομένης κίσσης, ἡ δὲ τῶν τελευταίων καὶ πλησίον ἤδη τῆς ἀποκυήσεως εἰς τὴν τοῦ ἐμβρύου τελείωσιν καὶ εἰς εὐχερῆ τῆς ἀποτέξεως ὑπομονήν. That division is not the same as the modern concept of trimesters.
22 And has been composed to oppose the later chapter on contraception and abortion. Soranus remarks that women who want to miscarry ought to disregard the advice listed in chapter 1.14., and adds a list of plant-based agents considered dangerous to pregnant women, that is, abortifacient: Soranus 1.14. especially paragraphs 64–5; see also Riddle 1992: 46–56; more in the section entitled 'Abortion'.
23 Soranus 1.14.46.
24 Soranus 1.14.46: φυλάττεσθαι δὲ καὶ συνουσίαν· καὶ γὰρ αὕτη κίνησιν ἐμποιεῖ κοινότερον μὲν τοῖς ὅλοις σώμασιν, μάλιστα δὲ τοῖς περὶ τὴν ὑστέραν τόποις ἠρεμίας δεομένοις.
25 Soranus 1.14.48: ἐπιγίνεται δὲ ταῖς πλείσταις τῶν κυοφορουσῶν περὶ [τὴν] τεσσαρακοστὴν κατὰ τὸ πλεῖστον ἡμέραν, ἔτι δὲ μέχρι τεσσάρων μηνῶν ὡς ἐπὶ τὸ πλεῖστον ἔπεται. ἐνίαις δὲ καὶ τάχιον καὶ βράδιον ἔρχεται, καὶ παραμένει πάλιν τισὶ μὲν ὀλιγωτέρως, τισὶ δὲ μέχρι πλείονος, σπανίως δέ τισι μέχρι τῆς ἀποτέξεως, τισὶ δ᾿ οὐδ᾿ ὅλως ἐπηκολούθησεν. παρέπεται δὲ ταῖς ἐν τῷ [συμ]πτώματι τυγχανούσαις ἀνατροπὴ στομάχου, ἤτοι πλάδος, ναυτία τε καὶ ἀνορεξία, ποτὲ μὲν πρὸς πάντα, ποτὲ δὲ πρὸς τινά, καὶ τῶν ἀσυνήθων ὄρεξις οἷον γῆς, ἀνθράκων, ἑλίκων ἀμπέλου καὶ ὀπώρας ἀώρου τε καὶ ὀξώδους, σιέλου ῥοῦς καὶ δυσαρεστήσεις, ὀξυρεγμία, βραδυπεψία καὶ ταχεῖα διαφθορὰ σιτίων; for a discussion on choosing the right food and its potential consequences for both the mother and the child, see Gourevitch 2003: 219–23.
26 Soranus 1.14.50: καὶ ῥόδινον δὲ καὶ μήλινον καὶ μύρσινον καὶ μαστίχινον καὶ νάρδινον ἐπισυστροφεῖ τὸν στόμαχον ὑπτιωμένον.

27 Soranus 1.15.50: εἰ δὲ εὐτονωτέρας χρεία στύψεως γένοιτο διὰ τοὺς ἐμέτους, ἐπιθέμασι χρηστέον, ἐξ ὧν εἰσι φοίνικες ξηροὶ προβρεχθέντες ἢ ἑψηθέντες ἐν οἴνῳ αὐστηρῷ ἢ ὀξυκράτῳ, καὶ μῆλα καὶ κυδώνια παραπλησίως ἑφθά, κατ' ἰδίαν ἢ μετὰ τῆς πρὸς τοὺς φοίνικας συμπλοκῆς ἢ μετά τινος τῶν εἰρημένων κηρωταρίων.

28 Soranus 1.15.50: κατὰ δὲ τοῦ στόματος τῆς κοιλίας πλατύστομον σικύαν μεθ' ὑποβολῆς πλείονος φλογὸς κολλᾶν, εἰ δὲ μή, καὶ δευτέραν κατὰ μεταφρένου.

29 Ancient doctors often considered food and its preparation methods medicinal. See e.g. Kokoszko, Jagusiak, Rzeźnicka 2014: 5–26.

30 Soranus 1.15.51: καὶ τῶν πτηνῶν τὰ μὴ καταπίμελα, ψαφαρωτέραν δὲ ἔχοντα τὴν σάρκα (καθάπερ ἀτταγῆνα, φάσσαν, πέρδικα, νήσσας ἀγρίας, κίχλας, κοσσύφους, περιστεράς, ὄρνεις κατοικητηρίους), καὶ τούτων μάλιστα τὰ στήθη· καὶ τῶν ἀγριμαίων κρέας λάγειον ἢ δορκάδειον, τῶν δὲ ἄλλων τὰ ἐρίφεια καὶ τῶν τρυφερῶν χοιρείων ῥύγχη, πόδας, ὦτα, κοιλίας, μήτρας·· τῶν δὲ ἀπὸ θαλάττης ὁμοίως τὰ στερεόσαρκα (τούτων δέ εἰσι τρίγλαι, κάραβοι, καρίδες, κήρυκες, σφόνδυλοι, πελωρίδες, πορφύραι). For more on eating meat while pregnant, see also Gourevitch 1995: 283–93.

31 Soranus 1.15.51: λαχάνων δὲ σέριν ὠμήν τε καὶ ἑφθήν, σίσαρον, ἀνδράχνην, ἀρνόγλωσσον, ἀσπάραγον ἄγριον·· τῶν δὲ ἀπὸ ταμείου ἐλαίας κολυμβάδας.

32 Soranus 1.15.51: ἢ κρεμαστήν (πνευματοῖ γὰρ ἡ πρόσφατος) καὶ ἀμύγδαλα.

33 Soranus 1.15.52: οἱ δ' αὐτοί φασιν δριμέος μὲν καὶ πυρώδους πλεονάσαντος ὑγροῦ καὶ διὰ τοῦτο τὸν στόμαχον ἀναδάκνοντος καὶ πυροῦντος ἀνδράχνης ἀπόβρεγμα ἢ ἀπόζεμα διδόναι πίνειν ἢ καὶ αὐτὴν ἐσθίειν πέπονά τε καὶ σικύων σπέρμα μεθ' ὕδατος καὶ γλυκὺν Κρητικὸν ἢ ἀβρότονον ἢ ἀψίνθιον ἢ Συριακῆς νάρδου ἀπόβρεγμα ἢ Κρητικῆς τραγοριγάνου.

34 Plin. HN 28.77.247: inveniuntur et ossicula in corde et in vulva perquam utilia gravidis parturientibusque. nam de pumice, qui in vaccarum utero simili modo invenitur, diximus in natura bovum.

35 Plin. HN 23.56.105: Citrea ... faciunt oris suavitatem decocto eorum volluti aut suco expresso. Horum semen edendum praecipiunt in malacia praegnantibus, ipsa vero contra infirmitatem stomachi, sed non nisi ex aceto facillime manduntur.

36 Plut. QN. 7: ὡς δῆλόν ἐστιν ἐπὶ τῶν γυναικῶν, ὅταν κύωσι, καὶ λίθους καὶ γῆν προσφερομένων· διὸ καὶ τῶν νοσούντων ταῖς ὀρέξεσιν.

37 Solinus 1.64: Cum salsiores escas edit gravida, unguiculis caret partus.

38 Soranus 1.15.53: ταῖς δὲ πρὸς τὰ βλαβερὰ τῶν κυουσῶν ἐπιθυμίαις τὸ μὲν πρῶτον ἐνστατέον διὰ λόγων, ὡς τῆς ἀπ' αὐτῶν βλάβης [καὶ] τῶν τὰς ἐπιθυμίας πληρούντων παραλόγως ᾗ καὶ τὸν στόμαχον κακούσης, οὕτως δὲ καὶ τὸ κατὰ γαστρός, διὰ τὸ μήτε καθαρὰν μήθ' ἁρμοδίαν ἐπισπᾶσθαι τροφήν, ἀλλὰ τοιαύτην ὁποίαν ἐπιπέμψαι δύναται τὸ σῶμα κακῶς διακείμενον.

39 Soranus 2.34(27).96: μὴ δὲ ἀπορήσῃ τις, πῶς οὖν ἁπάσας [ἐντὸς] ὑστέρας ὑπάρχον πρὸ τῆς ἀποτέξεως ἔφερεν τὰς εἰρημένας ποιότητας τῆς μητρὸς αὐτοῦ καὶ οἶνον καὶ ποικίλην τροφὴν προσφερομένης. πρὸς ὃν λεκτέον, ὅτι ταῖς τῆς μητρὸς δυνάμεσι τότε διοικούμενον ὡσπερεὶ μέρος οὐκ ἔκαμνεν; Censorinus knew two theories on

how the child was nourished in the womb. One of them had food filtered through the navel; proponents of the other, such as Diogenes and Hippo, believed there was a mound in the mother's body where the child attached with its mouth and drew food from the way it would from her breasts once born (Cens. 6.3).

40 This theombrotium should probably be identified with amaranth (*Amaranthus tricolor*). 'Amaranthus tricolor ... Alijs Bitum maculatum peregrinum; Theombrotium Plinj. Quibusdam': Ambrosini 1666: 41.

41 Plin. HN 24.102.166.

42 Soranus 4.(1)17.(1)53: καὶ τὰς τὰ ἤθη ὀξεί[ας οὔσας ἢ τρυ]φερῶς ἢ ἀργῶς βιού[σας] φησὶ δυστοκεῖν· ἡ γὰρ ἀργία δυστοκίας αἰτία, τὰ δὲ γυμνάσια εὐτοκίας καὶ τῶν κατὰ γαστρὸς εὐτροφίας. Soranus adduces the opinion of Cleophantus, a Greek physician from the third century BCE, who believed lack of exercise could affect the course of labour and lead to a so-called difficult birth.

43 Soranus 1.16.55.

44 Soranus 1.16.55.

45 Soranus 1.16.56.

46 While the *Cyranides*, a treatise on magic and medicine, has this to advise on avoiding stretch marks: 'once you stew it [the conger] until it dissolves completely, drain the oil and add wax to it, you will obtain ointment for pregnant women which prevents stretch marks on the belly' (οὗτος σὺν ἐλαίῳ ἑψηθεὶς καὶ τακεὶς καὶ διηθουμένου τοῦ ἐλαίου καὶ κηροῦ ἐπιβαλλομένου, ἐὰν ἐπιπλάσσῃς τὴν κηρωτὴν γυναιξὶν ἐγκύοις, οὐκ ἐᾷ ῥήγνυσθαι τὰς κοιλίας αὐτῶν; *Cyranides* 4.10).

47 Reiss, Ask 1988: 270–3; Hanson 1987: 589–602. For superstitions to do with the eighth month of pregnancy, see the fragment on the length of pregnancy.

48 Soranus 1.14.56: καὶ αὐτὴ δὲ ἡ μαῖα συνεχῶς τῷ δακτύλῳ περιαλείφουσα τὸ στόμιον τῆς ὑστέρας διαστελλέτω.

49 It was the midwife who took care of a woman when pregnant or in preparation for giving birth. For more on the midwife's role, see Chapter 3 this volume.

50 Dasen 1998: 183–204; Lewandowska 2021.

51 Dasen 2005; Treggiari 1991: 60–80.

52 Dasen 1997: 125–40.

53 Tac. *Ann.* 2.84.

54 The Curiatii triplets are also mentioned in the context of unusual fertility in Columella (Col. 3.8): ed i Italici generis esse voluit eximiae fecunditatis Albanas Curiatiae familiae trigeminorum matres.

55 Dion. Hal. *Ant. Rom.* 3.22.10: ἔστι δὲ καὶ νόμος παρ' αὐτοῖς δι' ἐκεῖνο κυρωθεὶς τὸ πάθος, ᾧ καὶ εἰς ἐμὲ χρῶνται, τιμὴν καὶ δόξαν ἀθάνατον τοῖς ἀνδράσιν ἐκείνοις περιτιθεὶς ὁ κελεύων, οἷς ἂν γένωνται τρίδυμοι παῖδες ἐκ τοῦ δημοσίου τὰς τροφὰς τῶν παίδων χορηγεῖσθαι μέχρις ἥβης. τὰ μὲν δὴ περὶ τὴν Ὁρατίων οἰκίαν γενόμενα θαυμαστὰς καὶ παραδόξους περιπετείας λαβόντα τοιούτου τέλους ἔτυχεν.

56 Gell. 10.2.2: Sed et divo Augusto imperante, qui temporum eius historiam scripserunt, ancillam Caesaris Augusti in agro Laurente peperisse quinque pueros dicunt eosque pauculos dies vixisse; matrem quoque eorum non multo, postquam peperit, mortuam, monumentumque ei factum iussu Augusti in via Laurentina, inque eo scriptum esse numerum puerperii eius, de quo diximus.
57 Strabo 15.1.22.695C; Plin. HN 7.33. In his *Historia animalium*, Aristotle mentions the extremely unusual case of a miscarriage of twelve infants (Arist. *Hist. an.* 7.4.585a), a matter which can be invoked thanks to an eleventh-century manuscript now located in Brussels. There are also images accompanying a work by Mustio, an African physician from the sixth century CE; their sources may be much older, since Mustio was adapting Soranus' gynaecological treatise, possibly illustrated with similar diagrams. Among the figures there are triplets in a number of cross-sections, quadruplets and the amazing eleven or twelve foetuses, perhaps mentioned in Aristotle; Bonnet-Cadilhac 1995: 339–50, fig. 9.
58 Obseq. 14, but elsewhere (Obseq. 40), he writes of 'monstrous' twins: Nursiae gemini ex muliere ingenua nati, puella integris omnibus membris, puer a parte priore alvo aperto ita ut nudum intestinum conspiceretur, idem posteriore natura solidus natus, qui voce missa.
59 Cicero recounted that according to the Roman law a crippled or deformed infant ought to be killed (Cic. *De leg.* 3.3.8). Seneca confirms it was customary to drown children right after birth if they were feeble or physically disabled (Sen. *De ira* 1.15.2). Dionysius of Halicarnassus reports a law existed which allowed the killing of a deformed child, who had to be inspected by five people from the neighbourhood (Dion. Hal. 2.15). It seems no law required that quadruplets or quintuplets be killed, most likely because such laws were in place dealing with children with deformities. Their short life expectancy can also be explained by a lack of regulations. More: Allély 2003, 2004.
60 HA. *Pius* 9.3.
61 Plin. HN 7.3.33.
62 Artem. 5.12.
63 As well as the babies. Pliny informs the reader that '*Vopiscus* was the word used for the twin held up in the womb who is only born once the other twin dies in a miscarriage' (Plin. HN 7.10). Following him, Solinus (1.69) writes: 'The name Vopiscus used to be given to cases of a twin born after being retained in the womb when the other twin had been killed by premature delivery — for extremely remarkable though infrequent cases of this occur'.
64 Plin. HN 7.4.37: editis geminis raram esse aut puerperae aut puerperio praeterquam alteri vitam; si vero utriusque sexus editi sint gemini, rariorem utrique salutem.
65 Sexti Pompei Festi, De verborum significatu quae supersunt cum Pauli epitome, 124–5 L (ed. W. M. Lindsay, Leipzig 1913). As indicated by the text above, when explaining the meaning of the word *molucrum*, Festus draws on a work by Afranius; see Suder 1993: 89–94.

66 Plin. HN 7.63: 'consequently she alone has what are called moles in her womb. This mole is a shapeless and inanimate mass of flesh that resists the point and the edge of a knife; it moves about, and it checks menstruation, as it also checks births: in some cases causing death, in others growing old with the patient, sometimes when the bowels are violently moved being ejected.'
67 Plut. Mor. Coniugalia praecepta 145d: παιδίον μὲν γὰρ οὐδεμία ποτὲ γυνὴ λέγεται ποιῆσαι δίχα κοινωνίας ἀνδρός, τὰ δ᾽ ἄμορφα κυήματα καὶ σαρκοειδῆ καὶ σύστασιν ἐν ἑαυτοῖς ἐκ διαφθορᾶς λαμβάνοντα μύλας καλοῦσι.
68 Suder, Stankiewicz 1994: 163–75.
69 Winsbury 2013: 126–33, believes that interpretation incorrect and instead thinks Pliny had two wives, of whom Calpurnia was the second (p. 128).
70 Sherwin-White 1966: 459.
71 Still, Calpurnia's young age, which Pliny does mention, implies the marriage took place in the year 104.
72 Plin. Ep. 8.10; Tatarkiewicz 2017: 23–33; Gourevitch 1990: 139–51; Frier 1994: 318–33; Hänninen, 2005: 49–59; Gourevitch 2009: 115–25.
73 But in letter 8.11 (to Hispulla) a different tone can be heard. They were friends and Hispulla was like a mother to Calpurnia. That latter clearly emphasizes not the miscarriage itself, but rather Pliny's young wife's improving health.
74 Plin. HN 30.47.135: Postea harundini inligata suspenditur in fumo, traduntque pariter cum expirante ea sanari infantem.
75 Plin. HN 36.40.152: lapis Samius ... volunt et partus contineri adalligato eo.
76 Plin. HN 30.44.130: lapis aëtites in aquilae repertus nido custodit partus contra omnes abortuum insidias. See also: Richlin 1997: 213–14.
77 Garg. 21.11–12; Dioscorides [2.178]: ad eandem causam profluvii septem seminis scripulos cum myrti bacis pari pondere in potione dandos putat.
78 Plin. HN 7.13.58: quaedam non perferunt partus, quales, si quando medicina et cura vicere, feminam fere gignunt.
79 Sherwin-White 1966: 459.
80 CIL VI 3499: D(is) M(anibus) / Q(uintus) Tineius Q(uinti) f(ilius) Sab(atina) Her[mes(?)] / domo Nicomedia mi/litiarum IIII pater in/felix Tineiae Hiero/pis quae et matron[a] / cuius corpus con[di]/tum a patre cum pa[rtu] / inmaturo hic po[si]/tum [est].
81 Soranus 1.18.59; see also: Denooz 2010: 171.
82 Celsus, De medicina 2.8.41: Mulieri gravidae si subito mammae emacuerunt, abortus periculum est.
83 Soranus 1.18.59: καθώς φησιν Ἱπποκράτης, παράλογος μαστῶν ἴσχνωσις, ὡς δὲ Διοκλῆς φησι, ψύξις μηρῶν [καὶ] βάρος ἐγκαθιζόμενον ὀσφύι περὶ τὸν καιρὸν τῆς ἀποτέξεως.
84 Plin. HN 7.5.40.

85 Celsus, *De medicina* 2.1.14: Si vero austri pluviaeque hiemem occuparunt, ver autem frigidum et siccum est, gravidae quidem feminae, quibus tum adest partus, abortu periclitantur; eae vero, quae gignunt, inbecillos vixque vitales edunt.
86 Celsus, *De medicina* 2.8.30: Mulier quoque gravida eiusmodi casu rapi potest; atque, etiamsi ipsa convaluit, tamen partum perdit.
87 Plin. HN 27.80: neutra danda mulieribus, quoniam gravidis abortum, ceteris sterilitatem facit.
88 Garg. 36.2: Thymum ... menstrua feminis provocat, uteri reliquias vulvae inhaerentes vel ipsos partus emortuos extrahit.
89 *Cyranides* 2.17: ὄνυξ δὲ αὐτῆς θυμιώμενος νεκρὰ ἔμβρυα ἐκβάλλει.
90 *Cyranides* 2.24: σὺν δὲ χυλῷ πράσου καὶ εἰρηνομύρῳ (but rather: ἰρίνῳ μύρῳ) προστιθεῖσα νεκρὰ ἔμβρυα καθέλκει.
91 *Cyranides* 2.39: σὺν δὲ ἀμαρακίνῳ μύρῳ καὶ ἐλλεβόρῳ προστιθεῖσα νεκρὰ ἔμβρυα καθέλκει.
92 *Cyranides* 2.22 (appendix).
93 Garg. 20.2–4: Satureiae ... ideo et gravidae prohibentur eam in cibo sumere. nam trita et ventri superposita partus etiam mortuos pellit.
94 Garg. 30.18: Catapotia ... partus etiam mortuos pellit.
95 Plin. HN 2.52.137. This is about Marcia, wife of Cato and a grandmother of Julius Caesar. As P. Tansey writes, Marcia's true identity is revealed in this excerpt from *De ostentis* by John the Lydian: ὁ γὰρ ἐν αὐτοῖς λεγόμενος ἀργής, ὃν καὶ λαμπρὸν ἐξαιρέτως καλοῦσιν οἱ ἀρχαῖοι, πολλάκις ἐμπεσὼν ἐπὶ πίθον ἢ ἄγγος ἁπλῶς ἢ οἴνου ἢ ὕδατος, τὸ μὲν περιέχον ἀπήμαντον τὸ δὲ ἐμπεριεχόμενον ἄφαντον ἐποίησεν. οὐχ ἥκιστα δὲ καὶ ἐν σκεύεσι χρυσίον ἢ ἀργύριον φέρουσιν ἐμπεσὼν τῷ ἴσῳ τρόπῳ τὰ μὲν ἔνδον ἔτηξε, τὰ δὲ ἔξωθεν ἔσωσε. καὶ τὸ δὴ πάντων θαυμασιώτατον ἐπὶ γυναικὸς ἐγκύμονος συμβῆναί φησιν ὁ μέγας Ἀπουλήιος, καὶ γυναικὸς οὐκ ἠγνοημένης, Μαρκίας δὴ ἐκείνης τῆς Κάτωνι τῷ τελευταίῳ συνοικησάσης. ἐμπεσὼν γὰρ αὐτῇ κεραυνὸς ὁ λεγόμενος ἀργὴς ἤτοι λαμπρὸς αὐτὴν μὲν παντελῶς ἐφύλαξεν ἀβλαβῆ, τὸ δὲ ἐν αὐτῇ διεφόρησεν οὕτως ἀνεπαισθήτως, ὡς μηδὲ αὐτὴν συνιδεῖν ὅ τι γέγονε τὸ ἐν αὐτῇ, καίτοι πρὸς ἔξοδον ἔχον (*De ostentis* § 44 = C. Wachsmuth, I*oannis Laurentii Lydi liber de ostentis et calendaria Graeca omnia* (Leipzig 1897), 97.18–98.13); for the complete argument, see Tansey 2013: 423–6.
96 Cantarella 2002: 269.
97 CIL VI 28753; English translation foll. Hug 2014: 277.
98 Naturally pregnant women were not only ever the victims of those closest to them, or of men. An analysis of interesting legal sources from Graeco-Roman Egypt was carried out by Danielle Gourevitch and Antonio Ricciardetto. Having investigated complaints preserved on papyri, the authors concluded that mentioning pregnancy was only supposed to make the fines heavier; there was never any mention of punishment or compesation for causing the death of an unborn child. See Gourevitch, Ricciardetto 2018: 690–4.

99 Philostratus VS 2.555.
100 Cass. Dio 62.28: καὶ ἡ Σαβῖνα ὑπὸ τοῦ Νέρωνος τότε ἀπέθανε· κυούσῃ γὰρ αὐτῇ λάξ, εἴτε ἑκὼν εἴτε καὶ ἄκων, ἐνέθορεν.
101 Pomeroy 2007: 125.
102 Pawlak 2015: 94.
103 Deacy 2013: 994–1010.
104 Pomeroy 2007: 12–129.
105 Philostratus VS 2.556.
106 Pawlak 2015: 95–6.
107 Pawlak 2015: 96.
108 Cass. Dio 48.45: τοῖς εὐτυχοῦσι τρίμηνα παιδία γεννᾶσθαι ἔλεγεν.
109 Wołodkiewicz, Zabłocka 1996: 117.
110 Hanson 1987: 589–602; Bruun 2010: 758–77; Cilliers 2004: 343–67; Dasen 2013: 23–5.
111 Cic. *Att* 10.18.
112 Zabłocki 1992: 197–210, esp. 199, n. 11.
113 This is about lunar months, which could lead to differences in the reported length of pregnancy, with nine calendar months corresponding to ten lunar ones.
114 Dig. 38.16.3.12: De eo autem, qui centensimo octogensimo secundo die natus est, Hippocrates scripsit et divus pius pontificibus rescripsit iusto tempore videri natum, nec videri in servitutem conceptum, cum mater ipsius ante centensimum octogensimum secundum diem esset manumissa. In Hippocrates and a rescript of Antoninus Pius addressed at the pontifices, it is actually 182 days. In Dig. 1.5.12 more generally the seventh month. Children born in the seventh and nine months were considered viable, unlike those born in the eighth month. It was believed that seventh-month children would live under certain conditions: they had to be born after at least 185.5 days, but no later than 204 days (when they became eighth-month children). In Galen, one month of pregnancy is 29.5 days. A seven-month foetus has spent full five months in the womb, that is, 147.5 days. To this, the author adds 23 days of the first month and at least 15 days of the seventh, and so 23 + 5 × 29.5 + 15 = 185.5.
115 Gell. 3.10.7–8: Ad homines quoque nascendos vim numeri istius ... 'Nam cum in uterum', inquit, 'mulieris genitale semen datum est, primis septem diebus conglobatur coagulaturque fitque ad capiendam figuram idoneum. Post deinde quarta hebdomade, quod eius virile secus futurum est, caput et spina, quae est in dorso, informatur. Septima autem fere hebdomade, id est nono et quadragesimo die, totus,' inquit, 'homo in utero absolvitur.' Illam quoque vim num eri huius observatam refert, quod ante mensem septimum neque mas neque femina salubriter ac secundum naturam nasci potest, et quod hi qui iustissime in utero sunt, post ducentos septuaginta tres dies postquam sunt concepti, quadragesima denique hebdomade inita nascuntur.

116 Gell. 3.16.1: Multa opinio est eaque iam pro vero recepta, postquam mulieris uterum semen conceperit, gigni hominem septimo rarenter.

117 Gell. 3.16.9–11: Antiquos autem Romanos Varro dicit non recepisse huiuscemodi quasi monstruosas raritates, sed nono mense aut decimo, neque praeter hos aliis partionem mulieris secundum naturam fieri existimasse, idcircoque eos nomina Fatis tribus fecisse a pariendo et a nono atque decimo mense. Nam 'Parca', inquit, 'in mutata una littera a partu nominata, item 'Nona' et 'Decima' a partus tempestivi tempore.

118 Gell. 3.16.1: Et medici et philosophi inlustres de tempore humani partus quaesiverunt. Multa opinio est eaque iam pro vero recepta, postquam mulieris uterum semen conceperit, gigni hominem septimo rarenter, numquam octavo, saepe nono, saepius numero decimo mense, eumque esse hominum gignendi summum finem: decem menses non inceptos, sed exactos. Below, Gellius cites Plautus' *Cistellaria*, where a baby is born after ten full months, to confirm ten complete months were in fact meant rather than nine (and the tenth begun): Gell. 3.16.2: Idque Plautum, veterem poetam, dicere videmus in comoedia *Cistellaria* his verbis: tum illa, quam compresserat, decumo post mense exacto hic peperit filiam.

119 Cens. 7.2: Iam primum quoto post conceptionem mense infantes edi soleant, frequenter inter veteres agitatum, non convenit. Hippon Metapontinus a septimo ad decimum mensem nasci posse aestimavit: nam septimo partum iam esse maturum, eo quod in omnibus numerus septenarius plurimum possit.

120 Cens. 7.5: Nam septimo mense parere mulierem posse, plurimi affirmant, ut Theano Pythagorica, Aristoteles Peripateticus, Diocles, Euenor, Straton, Empedocles, Epigenes multique praeterea, quorum omnium consensus Euthyphronem Cnidium non deterret, id ipsum intrepide pernegantem. Contra eum ferme omnes, Epicharmum sequti octavo mense nasci negaverunt.

121 Gell. 3.16.7–8: Sed huius de mense octavo dissensionis causa cognosci potest in libro Hippocratis qui inscriptus est περί τροφῆς, ex quo libro verba haec sunt: ἔστιν δέ καί οὐκ ἔστιν τὰ ὀκτάμηνα. Id tam obscure atque praecise et tamquam adverse dictum Sabinus medicus, qui Hippocratem commodissime commentatus est, verbis [his] enarravit: ἔστιν μέν, φαινόμενα ὡς ζῷα μετὰ τὴν ἔκπτωσιν· οὐκ ἔστιν δέ, θνήσκοντα μετὰ ταῦτα· καὶ ἔστιν οὖν καὶ οὐκ ἔστιν, φαντασίᾳ μέν παραυτίκα ὄντα, δυνάμει δέ οὐκέτι.

122 Cens. 7; on seven as a magical number, see e.g. Szram 2001: 134–8.

123 Gell. 3.16.21: Memini ego Romae accurate hoc atque sollicite quaesitum negotio non rei tunc parvae postulante, an octavo mense infans ex utero vivus editus et statim mortuus ius trium liberorum supplevisset, cum abortio quibusdam, non partus, videretur mensis octavi intempestivitas.

124 Zabłocki 1992: 204.

125 Plin. HN 7.5.38–40: Ceteris animantibus statum et pariendi et partus gerendi tempus est: homo toto anno et incerto gignitur spatio, alius septimo mense, alius octavo et usque ad initium undecimi; ante septimum mensem haut umquam vitalis est. septimo non nisi pridie posterove plenilunii die aut interlunio concepti nascuntur. tralaticium in Aegypto est et octavo gigni, iam quidem et in Italia tales partus esse vitales contra priscorum opiniones. variant haec pluribus modis: Vistilia Gliti ac postea Pomponi atque Orfiti clarissimorum civium coniunx ex his quattuor partus enixa, septimo semper mense, genuit Suillium Rufum undecimo, Corbulonem septumo, utrumque consulem, postea Caesoniam Gai principis coniugem octavo. in quo mensium numero genitis intra quadragensimum diem maximus labor, gravidis autem quarto et octavo mense, letalesque in his abortus. Masurius auctor est L. Papirium praetorem secundo herede lege agente bonorum possessionem contra eum dedisse, cum mater partum se tredecim mensibus diceret tulisse, quoniam nullum certum tempus pariendi statutum videretur.

126 Jurewicz 1997: 255–62.

127 Gell. 3.16.13–14: Hodie quoque in satura forte M. Varronis legimus, quae inscribitur Testamentum, verba haec: 'Si quis mihi filius unus pluresve in decem mensibus gignantur, ii si erunt ὄνοι λύρας, exheredes sunto; quod si quis undecimo mense κατ' Ἀριστοτέλην natus est, Attio idem, quod Tettio, ius esto apud me.' Per hoc vetus proverbium Varro significat, sicuti vulgo dici solitum erat de rebus nihil inter sese distantibus: 'idem Atti, quod Tetti', ita pari eodemque iure esse in decem mensibus natos et in undecim.

128 Gell. 3.16.15: Quod si ita neque ultra decimum mensem fetura m ulierum protolli potest, quaeri oportet cur Homerus scripserit, Neptunum dixisse puellae a se recens compressae: χαῖρε, γυναί, φιλότητι,·περιπλομένου δ'ἐνιαυτοῦ / τέξεις ἀγλαὰ τέκν', ἐπεὶ οὐκ ἀποφώλιοι εὐναί / ἀθανάτων (Hom. Od. 11, 248).

129 Gell. 3.16.16–18: Id cum ego ad complures grammaticos attulissem, partim eorum disputabant Homeri quoque aetate, sicuti Romuli annum fuisse non duodecim mensium, sed decem; alii convenisse Neptuno maiestatique eius dicebant, ut longiori tempore fetus ex eo grandesceret; alii alia quaedam nugalia. Sed Favorinus mihi ait περιπλομένου ἐνιαυτοῦ non 'confecto' esse 'anno', sed 'adfecto'.

130 Gell. 3.16.12: Praeterea ego de partu humano, praeterquam quae scripta in libris legi, hoc quoque usu venisse Romae comperi: feminam bonis atque honestis moribus, non ambigua pudicitia, in undecimo mense post mariti mortem peperisse factumque esse negotium propter rationem temporis, quasi marito mortuo postea concepisset, quoniam decemviri in decem mensibus gigni hominem, non in undecimo scripsissent; sed divum Hadrianum, causa cognita, decrevisse in undecimo quoque mense partum edi posse; idque ipsum eius rei decretum nos legimus. In eo decreto Hadrianus id statuere se dicit requisitis veterum philosophorum et medicorum sententiis.

131 Gell. 3.16.22–4: Sed quoniam de Homerico annuo partu ac de undecimo mense diximus quae cognoveramus, visum est non praetereundum quod in Plinii Secundi libro septimo Naturalis Historiae legimus. Id autem quia extra fidem esse videri potest, verba ipsius Plinii posuimus: 'Masurius auctor est, L. Papirium praetorem, secundo herede lege agente, bonorum possessionem contra eum dedisse, cum mater partum se tredecim mensibus tulisse diceret, quoniam nullum certum tempus pariendi statutum ei videretur'. In eodem libro Plini Secundi verba haec scripta sunt: 'Oscitatio in nixu letalis est, sicut sternuisse a coitu abortivum'.

132 Dig. 38.16.3.9/11: Utique et ex lege duodecim tabularum ad legitimam hereditatem is qui in uterofuit admittitur ... Post decem menses mortis natus non admittetur ad legitimam hereditatem; Jan Zabłocki thinks that the discrepancy between the Law of the Twelve Tables and later decisions can be explained as follows: the Law of the Twelve Tables prescribed that a *postumus* was an heir *ab intestato* if born no later than in the tenth month. 'Such a posthumous child was treated by that law the same as children born within the father's lifetime, that is, was a statutory heir, and all that can be told from praetor Lucius Papirius' ruling is that he refused inheritance to a more distant relative, arguing that a child born after the father's death does deserve *hereditas*, even if born in the thirteenth month' (Gell. 3.16.23). That solution was probably a result of applying a new, so-called praetorial order of inheritance, in which all of a man's children inherited, rather than just those who were in his paternal power, one which placed the children's interest higher than the rigid principles of civil law (transl. from J. Zabłocki 1992: 209–10.

133 Seneca, *De consolatione ad Helviam matrem* 16.3.

134 They will be discussed in more detail in Chapter 5 this volume.

135 Discovered in 1999, now in a museum in Senlis; A.99.3.14: https://musees.ville-senlis.fr/Collections/Explorer-les-collections/Rechercher-une-oeuvre/Musee-d-Art-et-d-Archeologie/Ex-voto-du-temple-de-la-foret-de-Halatte-divinite-enceinte-sans-tete (accessed on 16 July 2022).

136 Also found in Halatte, France, during a 1987 excavation. Now in a museum in Senlis; A.97.4.8: https://www.pop.culture.gouv.fr/notice/joconde/M0809007015 (accessed on 16 July 2022)..

137 The exact dimensions and origin of the images are not available. Wellcome Collection does not have this data.

138 Oria Segura 2016: 99–115.

139 For that reason most of the photographs in this book are meant as illustrations only rather than as material for extra interpretation.

140 Kampen 1994: 117.

141 Kampen 1994: 111–37, with further reading.

Chapter 5

1 Ovid. *Fasti* 3.257–8: Si qua tamen gravida est, resoluto crine precetur / ut solvat partus molliter illa suos.
2 Soranus 2.(1)20.66: παρέπεται δὲ ταῖς μελλούσαις ἀποτίκτειν περὶ τὸν ἕβδομον ἢ τὸν ἔννατον ἢ τὸν δέκατον μῆνα βάρος ἤτρου καὶ ἐπιγαστρίου μετὰ πυρώσεως τοῦ γυναικείου αἰδοίου [καὶ] ἄλγημα βουβώνων καὶ ὀσφύος καὶ ἰξύος πρὸς τὸ ὑποκείμενον τῆς ὑστέρας· ἥ τε ὑστέρα προσχωρεῖ τῷ αἰδοίῳ, ὥστε ῥᾳδίως τὴν μαῖαν σημειουμένην ἅψασθαι αὐτῆς [καὶ διέστηκεν αὐτῆς τὸ στόμα μετὰ εὐαφίας [καὶ] καθυγρασμοῦ], τὸ δὲ στόμιον αὐτῆς μετὰ τρυφερίας ἀναπετάννυται καὶ διέστηκε μετὰ τοῦ ἐπινοτίζεσθαι, πρὸς λόγον δὲ τοῦ συνεγγισμοῦ τῆς ἀποτέξεως συμπίπτει μὲν τὰ ἰσχία καὶ τὸ ἐπιγάστριον, συνογκοῦται δὲ μετὰ βουβώνων [τὸ] ἐφήβαιον, καὶ συνεχὴς γίνεται πρὸς ἀπούρησιν προθυμία. φέρεται δὲ ὑγρὸν γλίσχρον, εἶτα καὶ αἷμα ταῖς πλείσταις ῥηγνυμένων τῶν ἐν τῷ χορίῳ λεπτῶν ἀγγείων, τῷ δὲ καθιεμένῳ δακτύλῳ εἰς τὸ γυναικεῖον αἰδοῖον περιφερὴς ὄγκος ὑποπίπτει [γὰρ] παρόμοιος ᾠῷ.
3 For the role and significance of the midwife, see e.g. French 1986: 69–86; Laes 2010: 261–268; Tatarkiewicz 2013: 127–51.
4 Soranus 2.(2)21.68: *** [κατακλιτέον δὲ αὐτὴν] ἐν ὑπτίῳ τῷ σχήματι, συνηγμένων μὲν τῶν ποδῶν, διεστώτων δὲ τῶν μηρῶν, προϋποκειμένου δὲ τοῖς ἰσχίοις τινός, ὥστε κατωφερὲς γενέσθαι τὸ γυναικεῖον αἰδοῖον.
5 Soranus 2.(2)21.69: ἡ μαῖα θερμῷ ἐλαίῳ προλιπάνασα τὰς χεῖρας τὸν τῆς εὐωνύμου χειρὸς λιχανὸν δάκτυλον ἀπωνυχισμένον καθιείτω, πράως τῇ προσαγωγῇ προδιαστέλλουσα τὸ στόμιον.
6 Soranus 2.(2)21.68: if the cervix does not dilate, Soranus advises to douche it with warm olive oil, a decoction of mallow or linseed, or egg white, as well as poultices and bathing in water with oil added. He recommends against sudden movements or being shaken about; Soranus 4.(2)18.(7)59. There is more about moving the parturient to a chair in Galen (Περὶ φυσικῶν δυνάμεων 3.3.152: καὶ μέντοι καὶ αἱ μαῖαι τὰς τικτούσας οὐκ εὐθὺς ἀνιστᾶσιν οὐδ᾽ ἐπὶ τὸν δίφρον καθίζουσιν, ἀλλ᾽ ἅπτονται πρότερον ἀνοιγομένου τοῦ στόματος κατὰ βραχὺ καὶ πρῶτον μέν, ὥστε τὸν μικρὸν δάκτυλον καθιέναι, διεστηκέναι φασίν, ἔπειτ᾽ ἤδη καὶ μεῖζον καὶ κατὰ βραχὺ δὴ πυνθανομένοις ἡμῖν ἀποκρίνονται τὸ μέγεθος τῆς διαστάσεως ἐπαυξανόμενον. ὅταν δ᾽ ἱκανὸν ᾖ πρὸς τὴν τοῦ κυουμένου δίοδον, ἀνιστᾶσιν αὐτὰς καὶ καθίζουσι καὶ προθυμεῖσθαι κελεύουσιν ἀπώσασθαι τὸ παιδίον. ἔστι δ᾽ ἤδη τοῦτο τὸ ἔργον, ὃ παρ᾽ ἑαυτῶν αἱ κύουσαι προστιθέασιν, οὐκέτι τῶν ὑστερῶν, ἀλλὰ τῶν κατ᾽ ἐπιγάστριον μυῶν, οἳ πρὸς τὴν ἀποπάτησίν τε καὶ τὴν οὔρησιν ἡμῖν συνεργοῦσιν).
7 Soranus 2.(2)21.69: τοῦ προχείρου δὲ τὸ μέγεθος [ᾠοῦ] λαμβάνοντος ὑπὸ τὸ στόμιον τῆς ὑστέρας, εἰ μὲν ἀσθενὴς εἴη ἡ κυοφοροῦσα καὶ ἄτονος, τὴν μαίωσιν ἐπὶ

κατακειμένης αὐτῆς ποιητέον, ὅτι ἀσκυλτότερος οὗτος ὁ τρόπος καὶ ἀφοβώτερος, εἰ δ' εὔτονος τυγχάνει, διαναστατέον αὐτὴν [καὶ] κατὰ τοῦ μαιωτικοῦ λεγομένου δίφρου καθιστέον * * * θερμῷ ἐλαίῳ καὶ καταχλιαστέον καὶ ἐγχυματιστέον πρὸς τὸ τῆς κυοφορούσης εὔψυκτον.

8 Soranus 4.(2)18.(7)59: εἰ μὲν οὖν διὰ τὸ κοίλην ἔχειν τὴν ὀσφὺν τὴν τίκτουσαν ἡ δυστοκία γίγνοιτο, σχηματίζειν αὐτὴν χρὴ ἐπὶ τὰ γόνατα, ἵνα ἡ ὑστέρα μεταπεσοῦσα εἰς τὸν κατὰ τὸ ἐπιγάστριον τόπον κατ' εὐθὺ σχηματισθῇ τῷ τραχήλῳ··ὁμοίως δὲ καὶ τὰς πιμελώδεις καὶ κατασάρκους σχηματιστέον.

9 Soranus 2.(3)21.68.

10 Soranus 2.(2)21.68: κλίνας δὲ δύο, τὴν μὲν τρυφερῶς ἐστρωμένην πρὸς [τὸ] τὴν μετὰ τὸ τεκεῖν ἀνάπαυλαν, τὴν δὲ σκληρὰν πρὸς τὴν ἐν ταῖς ἀποτέξεσιν κατάκλισιν, ὥστε μὴ κατὰ τετρυμένης κλίνης [πρὸς τὸ εἶκον ἐνδιδόναι τὴν ὀσφύν] * * *.

11 Soranus explains that they were meant to calm down the patient, since it was believed her state of mind was vital for the course of the delivery. He advises the people delivering the baby to put a lot of effort into preparing the parturient psychologically, reassuring her, calming her nerves and dispelling fears (Soranus 2.(2)21.70): τρεῖς δὲ γυναῖκες ὑπηρέτιδες ἔστωσαν προσηνῶς δυνάμεναι τὸ δειλὸν παραμυθεῖσθαι τῆς κυοφορούσης, κἂν μὴ πεπειραμέναι τῶν τοκετῶν τυγχάνωσιν, ὧν δύο μὲν ἑκατέρωθεν, μία δὲ ἐξόπισθεν διακρατοῦσα πρὸς τὸ μὴ διὰ [τοὺς] πόνους τὴν κύουσαν παρεγκλίνειν. μὴ παρόντος δὲ τοῦ μαιωτικοῦ δίφρου καὶ ἐπὶ μηροῖς γυναικὸς καθεζομένης ὁ αὐτὸς δύναται γενέσθαι σχηματισμός· δεῖ δὲ τὴν γυναῖκα τυγχάνειν εὔτονον, ἵνα καὶ τὸ βάρος ἐνέγκη τῆς ἐφεδραζομένης γυναικὸς καὶ παρὰ τὰς ὠδῖνας κατέχειν αὐτὴν δύνηται.

12 Soranus 2.(2)21.69: διισταμένου δὲ τοῦ στόματος τῆς ὑστέρας ἡ μαῖα θερμῷ ἐλαίῳ προλιπάνασα τὰς χεῖρας τὸν τῆς εὐωνύμου χειρὸς λιχανὸν δάκτυλον ἀπωνυχισμένον καθείτω, πράως τῇ προσαγωγῇ προδιαστέλλουσα τὸ στόμιον, ὥστε τὸ πρόχειρον τοῦ χορίου μέρος ἐπιπροπίπτειν, τῇ δεξιᾷ δὲ χειρὶ τούς τόπους ἐλαιοχυτείτω φυλασσομένη τὸ ἐκ τῆς ἑψήσεως κεκνισμένον ἔλαιον … [70a] λοιπὸν δὲ ἡ μαῖα περιζωσαμένη κοσμίως ἄνωθεν καὶ κάτωθεν καθεζέσθω μὲν ἄντικρυς τῆς ἀποτικτούσης ταπεινοτέρα··δεῖ γὰρ ἐξ ὑπερκειμένων εἰς τὰ ὑποκείμενα τὴν ἐξολκὴν γίνεσθαι τοῦ ἐμβρύου. τὸ δὲ εἰς τὸ γόνυ καθίζειν αὐτήν, ὡς ἐδοκίμασάν τινες, μετὰ τοῦ δυσεργοῦς καὶ ἄσχημον· ὡσαύτως δὲ καὶ τὸ ἑστῶσαν ἐν βόθρῳ χάριν τοῦ μὴ ἐξ ὑπερκειμένου τὰς χεῖρας ἐπιβαλεῖν, ὡς ἠξίωσεν Ἥρων, τοῦτο γὰρ οὐ μόνον ἀπρεπές, ἀλλὰ καὶ ἀδύνατον ἐπὶ τῶν διστέγων οἴκων. καθεζέσθω τοίνυν ἡ μαῖα, διεστῶτας τούς μηρούς ἔχουσα καὶ μικρὸν τὸν εὐώνυμον προκλίνουσα πρὸς τὸ εὐεργὲς τῆς εὐωνύμου χειρός, ἔμπροσθεν, ὡς εἴρηται, τῆς ἀποτικτούσης … [70b] *** καὶ ἀνατρέχει τὸ στόμιον αὐτῆς, ποτὲ δὲ καὶ προκύπτει. πειθηνίως οὖν δεῖ καθιέναι τούς δακτύλους ἐν τῷ καιρῷ τῆς διαστολῆς καὶ τὸ ἔμβρυον ἐπισπᾶσθαι, προσενδιδοῦσαν μέν, ὅτε εἰς αὐτὴν ἡ μήτρα συνέλκεται, προσηνῶς δὲ ἐπισπωμένην, [ὅ]τε διαστέλλεται· τὸ γὰρ ἐν τῷ καιρῷ τῆς συστολῆς τοῦτο ποιεῖν

φλεγμονῆς ἢ αἱμορραγίας ἢ κατασπασμοῦ τῆς μήτρας ἀποτελεστικόν. For abnormal and difficult births, on the other hand, see below in the same chapter, and Soranus 4.(1)17(1) 53–(5)57; on abnormal presentation, Soranus 4.(2)18.(8)60; on the size of the baby threatening the mother's life, on the child dying during delivery, and on the actions to take then to save the mother's life, Soranus 4.(3)19.(9)61–(13)65.

13 During the excavation, a fairly small, free-standing, uncased grave was found, with terracotta relief sculptures placed on both sides of the inscription. One of those shows a seated surgeon bent over a patient's leg. Right next to the patient, surgical instruments can be seen. Above the burial chamber, there is a marble plaque, 35 × 42 cm in size, which reads: H(uic) m(onumento) d(olus) m(alus) a(besto) / D(iis) M(anibus) / Scribonia Attice / fecit sibi et M(arco) Ulpio Amerimno / coniugi et Scriboniae Calli/tyche matri et Diocli et suis / et libertis libertabusque poste/risque eorum praeter Panara/tum et Prosdocia(m) h(oc) m(onumentum) h(eredem) e(xterum) n(on) s(equetur): Thylander 1952: 162, A222; Ostia, Museo Ostiense inventory no. 5204; Kampen 1981, Kat. I, 6; fig. 58.

14 N. Kampen emphasizes that the subject of the sculpture is not delivery, but rather Scribonia's profession. The composition of the image showcases the heroine's social standing, and the heroine is the midwife, not the woman giving birth. The composition itself is rather primitive and clichéd, with the characters depicted in profile, the midwife's assistant(s) in the back and the midwife herself facing the patient. Kampen 1981: 71; Coulon 2004: 209–25.

15 Additionally, they were sometimes forged, as antiquity has always been a source of fascination also to forgers, who copied, or part-copied/part-forged, various works of art. Inevitably, there were among them some depictions of birth. One of the most infamous forgeries was a marble relief found in Rome, supposedly originating in the second century CE. It featured rich visual detail, a unique birthing chair and two physicians, both male, one of them holding obstetrical forceps – except that obstetrical instrument was only introduced in the seventeenth century. All those elements were fascinating at first, but also clearly indicated the sculpture could have been forged. It was demonstrated it had been made in 1937, having been commissioned by a professor of the Medical Faculty of the University of Rome. But although the forgery had been proven and the relief destroyed, the depiction would for a long time be used in various publications as an illustration of Roman birth (Hibbard 2001: 1); On the difficulties of interpreting iconography and ancient archeology, see: Perkins 2012: 146–201.

16 Museo Nazionale, Naples, no. 109905A; a relief sculpture in ivory 7 × 11 cm.

17 Coulon 1994: 210.

18 Soranus 4.(2)18.(7)59: τὴν δὲ ἄτονον μὲν διὰ μακρᾶς ἀσθενείας βραχέος κουφισμοῦ παρεμπεσόντος θρεπτέον ὀλίγῃ καὶ ἁπλῇ τροφῇ (οἷον ἄρτῳ, σικύῳ πέπονι, ἀλφίτῳ νενοτισμένῳ, μήλῳ, πᾶσι τοῖς παραπλησίοις).

19 Soranus 2.(2)21.70: εἶτα καλὸν καὶ τὴν ὄψιν τῆς κυοφορούσης φαίνεσθαι τῇ μαίᾳ, ἥτις παραμυθείσθω τὸ δειλὸν αὐτῆς εὐαγγελιζομένη τὸ ἄφοβον καὶ τὴν εὐτοκίαν.
20 Soranus 2.(2)21.70b: δακτύλῳ δὲ κυκλοτερῶς διαστελλέτω τό τε στόμιον τῆς ὑστέρας [καὶ] τὰ πτερυγώματα *** καὶ ἀνατρέχει τὸ στόμιον αὐτῆς, ποτὲ δὲ καὶ προκύπτει. πειθηνίως οὖν δεῖ καθιέναι τοὺς δακτύλους ἐν τῷ καιρῷ τῆς διαστολῆς, καὶ τὸ ἔμβρυον ἐπισπᾶσθαι, προσενδιδοῦσαν μὲν, ὅτε εἰς αὐτὴν ἡ μήτρα συνέλκεται, προσηνῶς δὲ ἐπισπωμένην [ὅ]τε διαστέλλεται· τὸ γὰρ ἐν τῷ καιρῷ τῆς συστολῆς τοῦτο ποιεῖν φλεγμονῆς ἢ αἱμορραγίας ἢ κατασπασμοῦ τῆς μήτρας ἀποτελεστικόν. χερσὶ δὲ τὸν ὄγκον ἐκ πλαγίων ὑπηρέτιδες ἐστῶσαι πρὸς τοὺς κάτω τόπους πρᾴως ἐρειδέτωσαν.
21 Soranus 2.(2)21.70b: λοιπὸν δὲ ἡ μαῖα δι' ἑαυτῆς ἀποδεχέσθω τὸ ἔμβρυον, προϋποβεβλημένου ῥάκους κατὰ τῶν χειρῶν ἤ, ὡς αἱ ἐν Αἰγύπτῳ ποιοῦσιν, λεπτῆς παπύρου ξεσμάτων πρὸς τὸ μήτε ἀπολισθάνειν αὐτὸ μήτε θλίβεσθαι, τρυφερῶς δὲ ἐφηδράθαι. συναποκριθέντων μὲν οὖν καὶ τῶν δευτέρων, τὰ ἑξῆς ποιητέον· εἰ δ' ὑπομένοι τὸ χόριον, κατακειμένης μὲν τῆς τικτούσης πλησίον θετέον τὸ βρέφος.
22 Soranus 4.(4)20.(16,1)73: τὸ δὲ χόριον ἐμπεφυκὸς κατηγγειωμένως σπλάγχνῳ μετὰ βίας ἀποσπάσαι δεῖ καὶ μὴ καταλείπειν τῷ χαλασμῷ δυνάμενον πειθηνίως περιμυδῆσαι.
23 Soranus 4.(4)20.(16,1)73: εἶτα διὰ τοῦ συμπεφυκότος οὐραχοειδοῦς ἐντέρου τῷ ὀμφαλῷ τρόπον τινὰ ὁδηγούμενον ἐπικαθιέναι δεῖ τὴν χεῖρα πειθηνίως [τε] διὰ τῆς ἐφ' ἑκάτερα τὰ μέρη παραφορᾶς, συνεντεινομένης ἅμα τῆς κυούσης ἄνευ σπαραγμοῦ τε καὶ ἀποσπασμοῦ κομίζεσθαι τὸ χόριον.
24 See below.
25 Soranus 4.(4)20.(16,1)73: καὶ μηδενὸς προκύπτοντος μέρους, ἐν διαστάσει δὲ τοῦ στομίου μένοντος, λελιπασμένην τὴν χεῖρα καθιέναι, καὶ εἰ μὲν ἀπολελυμένον τῆς πρὸς τὴν μήτραν συμφύσεως τὸ χόριον καὶ εἰς αὐτὸ συνεστραμμένον εἴη, ἐπισπᾶσθαι λαβόμενον, εἰ δὲ συμπεφυκός, ἁπλώσαντα τοὺς δακτύλους ἔνδοθεν πειρᾶσθαι διὰ τῆς ἐξ ἑκατέρου μέρους ἀντιπεριαγωγῆς ἀπολύειν αὐτὸ πειθηνίως.
26 Sage or wood sage.
27 Soranus 4.(4)20.(14, 1).71.
28 Soranus 4.(4)20.(14, 1).71: Μαντίας δὲ παρακατακλίνει τὸ βρέφος τοῖς μηροῖς τῆς κυούσης, ἵνα διὰ τῆς οἰκείας φύσεως καὶ κινήσεως οὕτως ἐφέλκηται τὸ χόριον· μὴ σῳζομένης δὲ τῆς πρὸς τὸ βρέφος τοῦ χορίου συνεχείας μολίβδου μέγεθος ἐκ τοῦ προέχοντος ἀποκρίμνησιν, ἵνα τῷ βάρει κατασπασθῇ τὸ χόριον.
29 Garg. 36.2: uteri reliquias vulvae inhaerentes vel ipsos partus emortues extrahit.
30 See e.g. Tatarkiewicz 2013a: 49–62.
31 Musée de l'Abbaye de Saint-Germain d'Auxerre; inv. 1861.3.2.
32 Coulon 1994: 212–13.
33 Dig. 25.4.1.4–6 and 37.9–10.
34 Catull. 57.45–8.

35 Klęczar 2013: 131–2.
36 Dig. 25.4.1.10: mulier in domu honestissimae feminae pariat, quam ego constituam. mulier ante dies triginta, quam parituram se putat, denuntiet his ad quos ea res pertinet procuratoribusve eorum, ut mittant, si velint, qui ventrem custodiant. in quo conclavi mulier paritura erit, ibi ne plures aditus sint quam unus: si erunt, ex utraque parte tabulis praefigantur. ante ostium eius conclavis liberi tres et tres liberae cum binis comitibus custodiant. quotienscumque ea mulier in id conclave aliudve quod sive in balineum ibit, custodes, si volent, id ante prospiciant et eos qui introierint excutiant. custodes, qui ante conclave positi erunt, si volunt, omnes qui conclave aut domum introierint excutiant. mulier cum parturire incipiat, his ad quos ea res pertinet procuratoribusve eorum denuntiet, ut mittant, quibus praesentibus pariat. mittantur mulieres liberae dumtaxat quinque, ita ut praeter obstetrices duas in eo conclavi ne plures mulieres liberae sint quam decem, ancillae quam sex. hae quae intus futurae erunt excutiantur omnes in eo conclavi, ne qua praegnas sit. 'tria lumina ne minus ibi sint', scilicet quia tenebrae ad subiciendum aptiores sunt. Quod natum erit, his ad quos ea res pertinet procuratoribusve eorum, si inspicere volent, ostendatur. apud eum educatur, apud quem parens iusserit. D. 25.4.1.12: Denuntiare igitur mulierem oportet his scilicet, quorum interest partum non edi, vel totam habituris hereditatem vel partem eius sive ab intestato sive ex testamento; Dig. 25.4.2.1: Sed hoc aliquando remittere praetor debet, si non malitia, sed imperitia mulieris factum fuerit, ne venter inspiceretur aut partus custodiretur.
37 Tac. *Ann.* 3.22–3: At Romae Lepida, cui super Aemiliorum decus L. Sulla et Cn. Pompeius proavi erant, defertur simulavisse partum ex P. Quirinio divite atque orbo. adiciebantur adulteria venena quaesitumque per Chaldaeos in domum Caesaris, defendente ream Manio Lepido fratre.
38 Aemilia was charged with (and convicted of) not merely procuring a child, but also adultery, poisoning and asking astrologers questions about the future of the imperial family. One source for the list of charges and the course the trial took is Shotter 1966: 312–17.
39 Soranus 4.(2)18.(7)59: εἰ δὲ τὸ στόμιον τῆς ὑστέρας μέμυκε, τοῖς λιπάσμασι μαλάσσειν καὶ ἀναχαλᾶν, ἤγουν ἐγχυματίζειν συνεχῶς ἐλαίῳ γλυκεῖ τε καὶ θερμῷ ἢ σὺν ἀφεψήματι τήλεως ἢ μολόχης ἢ λινοσπέρμου, ποτὲ δὲ καὶ τῶν ᾠῶν [τῷ λευκῷ]· οὕτω γὰρ παρηγορεῖται εἰς ἄνεσιν μὲν τὸ θλῖβον, νοτίζεται δὲ εἰς ὄλισθον τὸ δυσοδοῦν.
40 *Cyranides* 2.40: στέαρ δὲ ἐκ τῶν ὀστῶν τῆς ὀσφύος αὐτῆς ὑποκαπνιζόμενον ταῖς δυστοκούσαις ὠκυτόκιόν ἐστιν μέγιστον.
41 Plin. HN 28.27.103: sinistrum pedeum superlatum parturienti letalem esse, dextro inlato facile eniti.
42 *Cyranides* 3.6.
43 *Cyranides* 3.9: ἰᾶται καὶ ὑστερικὴν πνίγα, ἐκβάλλει καὶ τὰ ἔμβρυα.

44 *Cyranides* 2.17: ὄνυξ δὲ αὐτῆς ... καὶ ὑποκαπνιζόμενος ὠκυτόκιός ἐστιν.
45 *Cyranides* 2.47: εἰσὶ δὲ καὶ ᾠὰ [ἀράχνης] ὠκυτόκια ὑποθυμιώμενα καὶ περιαπτόμενα.
46 *Cyranides* 2.47a: τὰ δὲ ἀράχνια ᾠὰ ὑποθυμιώμενα ἢ περιαπτόμενα ὠκυτόκια γίνεται.
47 *Cyranides* 3.38: καὶ ὠκύτοκά εἰσιν.
48 *Cyranides* 3.1: τῆς δὲ εὐωνύμου χειρὸς πτερὸν ἐὰν λάβῃ καὶ βάψῃ εἰς ἔλαιον καὶ ἀλείψῃ ἀπὸ τοῦ τένοντος μέχρι τοῦ ἱεροῦ ὀστοῦ δυστοκούσῃ γυναικί, πάραυτα τέξεται.
49 *Cyranides* 3.1: ἀετίτης δὲ λίθος ὁ κρουόμενος καὶ εὐειδής, πυρρὸς τῇ χρόᾳ, φορούμενος φυλάττει τὰ ἐν τῇ κοιλίᾳ βρέφη καὶ οὐκ ἐᾷ ἐκτιτρώσκεσθαι αὐτά. ἔστι δὲ καὶ εὐτόκιον.
50 *Cyranides* 3.25: τούτου [= λάρου] τὴν καρδίαν κρατῶν, εἴσελθε πρὸς δυστοκοῦσαν γυναῖκα, καὶ εὐθέως τέξεται.
51 *Cyranides* 3.50: τὰ δὲ τῶν πτερύγων πτίλα σὺν ὠκίμου ῥίζῃ περιαπτόμενα γυναικὶ δυστοκούσῃ ὠκυτόκιά εἰσιν.
52 Garg. 40.16–17.
53 Soranus 4.(3)19.(13)65.
54 For more on patrurition pain, see Tatarkiewicz 2021a: 49–64.
55 Soranus 4.(2)18.(7)59: τὴν δὲ ἄπειρον ὠδίνων διδακτέον ἐντόνως μάλιστα τὸ πνεῦμα κατέχειν καὶ πρὸς τὴν λαγόνα συνωθεῖν.
56 Soranus 2.(2)21.69.
57 Soranus 4.(2)18.(7)59.
58 Soranus 2.(2)21.70a: εἶτα καλὸν καὶ τὴν ὄψιν τῆς κυοφορούσης φαίνεσθαι τῇ μαίᾳ, ἥτις παραμυθείσθω τὸ δειλὸν αὐτῆς, εὐαγγελιζομένη τὸ ἄφοβον καὶ τὴν εὐτοκίαν. [70b] εἶτα δὲ ἐγκόπτειν εἰς τὴν λαγόνα τὸ πνεῦμα παραινεῖν δεῖ δίχα κραυγῆς, μετὰ στεναγμοῦ δὲ μᾶλλον καὶ κατοχῆς πνεύματος, ἔνιαι γὰρ τῶν ἀπείρων τοῖς ἄνω μέρεσιν ἐντεινόμεναι καὶ μὴ ἀπωθούμεναι τὸ πνεῦμα πρὸς κάτω βρογχοκήλας ἐποίησαν ... παραινετέον οὖν αὐταῖς συνεντείνειν τὸ πνεῦμα καὶ μὴ ἀποφεύγειν τὰς ὠδῖνας, ἀλλ' ὅτε πάρεισιν αὗται, τότε μάλιστα προσβιάζεσθαι; see also: Soranus 4.(2)18. (7)59 (in a previous footnote).
59 Plin. HN 20.73.191: Dalion herbarius parturientibus ex eo cataplasma inposuit cum apio, item vulvarum dolori deditque bibendum cum aneto parturientibus ... [194] Vertigines a partu cum semine cucumeris et lini pari mensura ternum digitorum, vini albi tribus cyathis discutit.
60 CIL III 2267: D(is) M(anibus) / Candidae coniugi bene me/renti ann(orum) p(lus) m(inus) XXX qu(a)e me/cum uixit ann(os) p(lus) m(inus) VII / qu(a)e est cruciata ut pari/ret diebus IIII et non pe/periit et est ita uita fu/ncta Iustus conser(uus) p(osuit).
61 Gourevitch 1987: 187–93; Suder 1998: 161–6.

62 Soranus 4.(1)18.(1)53: ἐπιλιπεῖς δέ μοι δοκοῦσιν οἱ ὅροι εἶναι, ὅθεν αὐτός φησιν δυστοκίαν εἶναι δυσχέρειαν τῶν κυουμένων παρά τινα αἰτίαν γινομένην.
63 Soranus 4.(2)18.(7)59: ἐπί τῶν δυστοκουσῶν χρὴ τὸν ἰατρὸν ἐπερωτᾶν τὴν μαῖαν.
64 Soranus 4.(1)17.(5)57: ἤγουν παρὰ τὸ κατάσαρκον καὶ καταπίμελον εἶναι τὴν τίκτουσαν.
65 Soranus 4.(1)17.(2)54: ὅταν [ἢ] ἐν ψυχικῇ δυνάμει ᾖ τὸ αἴτιον ἢ ἐν τῇ ζωτικῇ, ἤγουν τοῖς σώμασι. καὶ [ἐν] ψυχικῇ μὲν δυνάμει γίνεται, ὅταν λύπη, χαρά, φόβος, δειλία, ἔκλυσις, ὀργὴ γένηται [ἢ] τρυφὴ ὑπερτεταμένη (ἔνιαι γάρ εἰσιν σπαταλώδεις καὶ οὐκ ἐντείνονται)··καὶ παρὰ ἀπειρίαν δὲ τοῦ τίκτειν γίνεται [ὡς μὴ] συνεργεῖν τῇ ὠδῖνι··καὶ δι' ἐποχὴν δὲ διανοίας γίνεται, ἀμαυρᾶς γοῦν γινομένης τῆς ἀλγηδόνος (τοῦτο δ' ἄν τις εἴποι ἐπὶ τῶν ἀποπληκτικῶν γυναικῶν καὶ ληθαργικῶν)··καὶ διὰ ὑπόνοιαν δὲ τοῦ μὴ συνειληφέναι δυστοκία γίνεται.
66 Soranus 4.(1)17.(1)53: ἁμαρτάνει δὲ καὶ οὗτος μὴ πάντα τὰ αἴτια ἀναγράψας. Ἡρόφιλος δὲ ἐν τῷ Μαιωτικῷ λέγει 'δυστοκεῖσθαι γοῦν [παρὰ τὸ πλῆθος] † ὡς γὰρ Σίμωνος τοῦ Μάγνητος πολλάκις ὡράθη, ὅτι τρὶς ἀνὰ πέντε ἐκύησεν ἐργωδῶς.'
67 Soranus 4.(1)17.(2)54: ὁ δὲ Ἡροφίλειος Δημήτριος ἀντιδιαστέλλεται τοῖς ῥηθεῖσι λέγων τὰ αἴτια τῆς δυστοκίας τὰ μὲν παρ' αὐτὴν εἶναι τὴν τίκτουσαν, τὰ δὲ παρ' αὐτὸ εἶναι τὸ τικτόμενον, τὰ δὲ παρὰ τὸ δι' οὗ ἡ ἔκτεξις γίνεται.
68 Solinus 1.67.
69 Soranus 4.(1)17.(6)58: τῶν ῥηθέντων αἰτίων τῆς δυστοκίας ἃ μὲν ἐξ αὐτῶν ἐστι καταληπτέα, ἃ δὲ οὔ. λύπη μὲν γὰρ ἂν ὑπερτεταμένη, [ἢ] χαλᾷ καὶ ἀνίησιν, καὶ τὰ ἄλλα ψυχικὰ αἴτια ἐξ ἀνακρίσεως κατελήμφθη ὡς μὴ συνεργοῦντα τῇ εὐτοκίᾳ··κάρος δὲ καὶ λήθαργος πρόδηλά ἐστι, ἔτι δὲ τούτων σημεῖα ἐκ τοῦ περὶ ὀξέων μετάγεται τόπου.
70 Soranus 4(1)17(6)58: ἤδη δὲ καὶ τὸ μέγεθος τοῦ ἐμβρύου δυστοκίαν ποιοῦν σημειούμεθα ἐκ τοῦ ὄγκου τῆς κοιλίας··ἐὰν δὲ προπεσὸν μὴ κατὰ λόγον κουφίζῃ τὴν κοιλίαν, ὑποληπτέον πολλὰ εἶναι τὰ κυούμενα. ἤδη δὲ καὶ τὰ πλάγια καὶ τὰ προβάλλοντα τὰς χεῖρας, ἤτοι [τὰ παρὰ φύσιν] ἐσχηματισμένα, ταῖς καθέσεσι τῶν δακτύλων σημειούμεθα.
71 Plin. HN 7.4.37.
72 Soranus 1.8.33.
73 See Chapter 2 in this volume.
74 Soranus 4.(1)17.(3)55: τὸ γὰρ κατὰ φύσιν σχῆμα τοῖς γεννωμένοις τὸ ἐπὶ κεφαλήν ἐστι, παρατεταμένων τῶν χειρῶν τοῖς μηροῖς καὶ ἐπ' εὐθὺ φερομένου τοῦ ἐμβρύου· ... τῶν δὲ [λοιπῶν] σχηματισμῶν ἀμείνων ὁ ἐπὶ πόδας τέ ἐστι καὶ μάλιστα ὅταν ἐπ' εὐθείαν φέρηται, τῶν χειρῶν παρὰ τοὺς μηροὺς παρατεταμένων.
75 Solinus 1.65-7.
76 Soranus 4,(1)17.(3)55: τὰ δὲ δεδιπλωμένα φερόμενα χείριστος πάντων τῶν σχηματισμῶν ἐστιν, καὶ τούτων ὅσα ἐπὶ τὰ ἰσχία φέρεται. τριχῶς γὰρ καὶ τὰ δεδιπλωμένα σχηματίζεται··ἢ γὰρ πρὸς τῷ στόματι τῆς ὑστέρας τά τε σκέλη καὶ ἡ

κεφαλὴ ὑπάρχει ἢ τὸ ἐπιγάστριον ἢ τὰ ἰσχία. ἄμεινον δὲ τὴν κοιλίαν ἔχειν πρὸς τὸ στόμα τῆς ὑστέρας·· διελόντων γὰρ ἡμῶν τὸ ἐπιγάστριον καὶ κομισαμένων τὰ ἐντοσθίδια, συμπεσόντος τοῦ σώματος εὐχερὴς γίνεται ὁ μετασχηματισμός.

77 Soranus 4.(1)17.(8)60. For more on the midwife's actions in case of abnormal presentation, see Bonnet-Cadilhac 2004: 199–208.
78 Soranus 4(2)18.(8)60: πολλὰ γὰρ οὕτως δυστοκηθέντα βιώσαντα βλέπομεν.
79 Soranus 4.(1)17.(3)55.
80 Soranus 4.(2)18.(7)59.
81 Soranus 4.(3)19.(9)61: διόπερ τὸν μὲν ὑποκείμενον δεῖ προλέγειν κίνδυνον, πυρετῶν ἐπιγινομένων καὶ νευρικῆς συμπαθείας, ἔσθ' ὅπου δὲ καὶ φλεγμονῆς ὑπερβαλλούσης, καὶ γάγγραινα μάλιστα ὑποφαίνειν ὀλίγας ἐλπίδας ἔχειν.
82 Soranus 4.(3)19.(9)61: εἰ δὲ μὴ ἐπακούοι πρὸς τὴν διὰ τῶν χειρῶν ἐφολκὴν διὰ μέγεθος ἢ νέκρωσιν ἢ καθ' οἱονδηποτοῦν τρόπον σφήνωσιν, ἐπὶ τοὺς εὐτονωτέρους τρόπους δεῖ μετελθεῖν, τὸν τῆς ἐμβρυουλκίας καὶ τῆς ἐμβρυοτομίας· καὶ γάρ, εἰ τὸ κυηθὲν διαφθείρει, τὴν κυοφοροῦσαν τηρεῖν ἀναγκαῖον.
83 Soranus 4.(1)17.(6)58.
84 Tert. *De anima* 25. 4.
85 Blizqez 2015: 249–60 and 425–30, lists and describes the application of the several instruments of gynaecological surgery used in antiquity; see also Baker 1999: 141–51.
86 The Greeks call the *aeneum spiculum*, ἐμβρυοσφάκτης; there is no certainty as to what the instrument looked like, but it is sometimes identified with finds from the ancient Marcianopolis (Bulgaria), although L. J. Blizqez does not find that interpretation convincing, believing instead that Tertullian's *aeneum spiculum* is an ordinary scalpel or lancet. In his description of dismembering the foetus, and specifically piercing the head, Soranus uses ἐμβρυοτόμον, perhaps meaning a lancet-like knife; Blizqez 2015: 255–7.
87 Tert. *De anima* 25.5–6.
88 Soranus 4.(3)19.(9)61.
89 Soranus 4.(3)19.(10)62.
90 Soranus 4.(3)19.(10)62: εἶτα διδόναι τοὺς ἐμβρυουλκοὺς ἐμπείρῳ τινὶ κατέχειν καὶ παραινεῖν, ὅπως πειθηνίως δι' αὐτῶν ἐφέλκηται τὸ ἔμβρυον μήτε σπαράττων ἐν τοῖς ἐπισπασμοῖς μήτε πάλιν ἀνιείς (ἀνατρέχει γὰρ τὸ προκύψαν ἀνεθέν), ἀλλ', ὅταν δέῃ τὴν ἐφολκὴν ἐπισχεῖν.
91 Soranus 4.(3)19.(10)62: εὐθύνοντα τὸ ἑτεροκλινῶς φερόμενον, καὶ τοὺς τόπους ἐλαίῳ θερμῷ διαβρέχειν ἤ τινι τῶν εἰρημένων γλίσχρων ἀφεψημάτων.
92 Soranus 4.(3)19.(11)63.
93 Full description: Soranus 4.(3)19.(12)64.
94 CIL III 9632; English translation following Hug 2014: 278.

95 Soranus 4.(3)19.(13)65: τὰ δὲ προειρημένα βοηθήματα λύοντα τὸ πάθος καὶ τὴν ἐξ αὐτοῦ δυσέργειαν λύει.
96 Molleson, Cox 1988: 53–60; Gourevitch 2011: 159–61.
97 Mays, Robson-Brown, Vincent, Eyers, King, Roberts 2014: 111–15.
98 Speert 2004.
99 Dig. 11.8.2: negat lex regia mulierem, quae praegnas mortua sit, humari, antequam partus ei excidatur; qui contra fecerit, spem animantis cum gravida peremisse videtur.
100 Gourevitch 2001: 279.
101 Gourevitch 1987: 187–93.
102 Plin. HN 7.9.47; Solinus 1.68: A birth is more auspicious if the mother dies of it, as in the case of the first Scipio Africanus. His mother died, and because he was born by being cut from her womb, he was the first Roman to be called 'Caesar'.
103 Suder 1987: 621–8.
104 W. Suder notes that the placement of the highest women mortality on the age scale provides indirect information on the age of greatest fertility. Namely, in the provinces of Africa, Gaul and Spain, the lowest masculinization of the data, that is, highest female mortality, falls in the fifteen- to twenty-year-old age bracket. Thus this age group also presumably had the highest female fertility. Suder 1987: 628.
105 Gourevitch 1987: 187.
106 Plin. *Ep.* 4.21.1–2: Tristem et acerbum casum Helvidiarum sororum! Utraque a partu, utraque filiam enixa decessit. Adficior dolore, nec tamen supra modum doleo: ita mihi luctuosum videtur, quod puellas honestissimas in flore primo fecunditas abstulit. Angor infantium sorte, quae sunt parentibus statim et dum nascuntur orbatae, angor optimorum maritorum, angor etiam meo nomine.
107 Cic. *Att.* 12.30: quod Lentulum invisis valde gratum.
108 For a list of cases, see Hug 2014, esp. Table 2 pp. 273–80.
109 CIL XIV 2737: Rhanidi Sulpiciae l(ibertae) / delicio / nata brevi spatio partu subiecta nec ante / testatur busto tristia fata Rhanis / namque bis octonos nondum compleverat annos / et rapta est vitae rapta puerperio / parentis tumulus duo funera corpore in uno / exequias geminas nunc cinis unus habet // Sulpicia Trionis l(iberta) / Rhanis.
110 CIL III 3572: Hic sita sum matrona genus nomen/que Veturia Fortunati coniux de patre Vetu/rio nata ternovenos misera et nupta bis octo / per annos unicuba uniiuga quae post / sex partus uno superstite obit / T(itus) Iulius Fortunatus (centurio) leg(ionis) II ad(iutricis) p(iae) f(idelis) / coniugi incomparabili et insigni in se pietate.
111 AE 1991, 1076: Gemina D(ecimi) Pu/blici Subici ser(ua) an(norum) / XXV h(ic) s(itus) e(st) obit in / partu C(aius) Aerariu[s l(ibertus)] / posui[t ci]ppum pa/[rca fuer?]as mihi si qu[a] / inferi sapent ut m[e] / abduceres si me / amasti fac abdu/cas s(it) t(ibi) t(erra) l(euis).

112 AE 1976, 326; English translation foll. Hug 2014: 278.
113 CIL VIII 20288: D(is) M(anibus) s(acrum) / Rusticeia / Matrona / v(ixit) a(nnos) XXV / causa meae mortis partus fatu[mque malignum] / se⌈rd⌉ tu desine flere mihi kariss[ime coniux] / [et] fil(ii) nostri serva com[munis amorem] / [ad caeli] transivit spi[ritus astra] / [---] maritae [---].
114 CIL IX 3968: D(is) M(anibus) [s(acrum)] / Aediae [- - -] / haec tenet exanimam [tellus natalis in urbe] / quae nupsit Roma morbi [sed fraudibus atri] / post annos ueniens uisum La[ris arua paterni] / incidit infelixs(!) pregnax sa[luamque puellam] / enixa est misera acerbaq[ue decidit ipsa] / lugentesque suos miseros [cum prole reliquit] / et tulit Elysium uiginti e[t quattuor annis] / Eutyches et Hi[- - -.
115 CIL VI 5534.
116 CIL VIII 24734: Daphnis ego Hermetis coniunx sum libera facta / cum dominus vellet primu(m) Hermes liber ut esset / fato ego facta prior fato ego rapta prior / quae tuli quod genui gemitus uiro saepe reliqui / quae domino invito uitam dedi proxime nato / nunc quis alet natum quis uitam longa(m) ministrat / me Styga quod rapuit tam cito eni(m) a(d) superis / pia uixit annis XXV h(ic) s(ita) e(st).
117 AE 1995, 1793.
118 CIL III 272 = CIL III 6759: D(is) M(anibus) c(onstitutum?) / Aeturniae Zotic(a)e / Annius Flavianus / dec(urialis) lictor Fufid(i) / Pollionis leg(ati) Gal(atiae) / coniugi b(ene) m(erenti) vixit / ann(is) XV mens(ibus) V / dieb(us) XVIII quae / partu primo post / diem XVI relicto / filio decessit.
119 Carroll 2011: 99–120, esp. 112.
120 Carroll 2014: 159–78.
121 Carroll 2014: 159–78; the author believes that if both the mother's and the child's names are listed, it is likely that the child died later than eight to nine days after birth, that is, after the naming, whereas if the image is only accompanied by the mother's name, it is possible the child's death occurred during delivery or soon after, before the naming. See Chapter 2 this volume.
122 Ehmig 2013: 111–29; Aubert 2004: 187–98.
123 Turcan 2001: 18–21.
124 Horat. *Carmen Saec.* 13–20: Rite maturos aperire partus / lenis, Ilithyia, tuere matres, / sive tu Lucina probas vocari / seu Genitalis: / diva, producas subolem patrumque / prosperes decreta super iugandis / feminis prolisque novae feraci / lege marita.
125 Since childbirth would often take place by candlelight, it was assisted by the goddess Candelifera. Another goddess associated with life was Juno Lucina (Cic., *De natura deorum* 2.68: luna a lucendo nominata sit; eadem est enim Lucina, itaque ut apud Graecos Dianam eamque Luciferam sic apud nostros Iunonem Lucinam in pariendo invocant, quae eadem Diana Omnivaga dicitur non a venando sed quod in septem numeratur tamquam vagantibus). But if Candelifera's role could be

considered ancillary, Juno Lucina was seen by the Romans as the goddess who brought light to the newborn infant, that is, brought 'the gift of life' (Mart. Capella *De nuptiis Philologiae et Mercurii* 2.149: sive te Lucinam, quod lucem nascentibus tribuas, ac Lucetiam convenit nuncupare).

126 Tatarkiewicz 2015: 57–70.
127 Cid López 2007: 357–72.
128 Flambard 1987: 191–210 for the interpretation that Juno was worshipped at the site of present-day church of S. Lorenzo (St Lawrence) in Lucina.
129 Plin. NH 16.85.235: Romae vero lotos in Lucinae area, anno qui fuit sine magistratibus, CCCLXXIX urbis aede condita; incertum ipsa quanto vetustior; esse quidem vetustiorem non est dubium, cum ab eo luco Lucina nominetur. Another source confirming the existence of the temple is the inscription CIL VI 358: P(ublio) Servilio L(ucio) Antonio co(n)s(ulibus) / a(nte) d(iem) IIII K(alendas) Sext(iles) / locavit Q(uintus) Pedius q(uaestor) urb(anus) / murum Iunoni Lucinae / HS CCCLXXX (milibus) / eidemque probavit.
130 Ovid. *Fasti* 3.243–58.
131 Stat. *Silvae* 3.122–126.
132 Catullus, *Carm.* 34.14–18.
133 Terent. *Adelph.* 487–8.
134 Plaut. *Aul.* 692.
135 CIL II 676.
136 It was in the hope of gaining her favour for the imperial family that sacrifices were made and altars were erected to her, such as this altar from Rome: Iunoni Lucinae / pro salute domus Augustorum / Imp(eratoris) Caes(aris) M(arci) Aureli Antonini Aug(usti) Armeniaci Parthici maximi Medici et Faustinae Aug(ustae) eius et / Imp(eratoris) Caes(aris) L(uci) Aureli Veri Aug(usti) Armeniaci Parthici maximi Medici et Lucillae Augustae eius / liberorumque eorum / Fortunatus decurialium gerulorum dispensator aram cum base consecr(avit) // permissu / Maeci Rufi curat(oris) aedium // consecravit X K(alendas) Sept(embres) / [Q(uinto) Ser]vilio Pudente L(ucio) Fufidio Pollione co(n)s(ulibus) [CIL VI 360].
137 Julia Mamaea: RIC IV 341; RIC III 770; Lucilla: RIC III 771.
138 Ovid. *Fasti* 3.257–8: si qua tamen gravida est, resoluto crine precetur ut solvat partus molliter illa suos. Soranus 2.(2)21.(6)70: διὰ τοῦτο δὲ [καὶ] τὰς τρίχας λύειν διὰ δὲ τὴν προειρημένην αἰτίαν τάχα δὴ καὶ ἡ λύσις τῶν τριχῶν εὐτονίαν ἀποτελεῖ τῆς κεφαλῆς.
139 Engraved haematite 16 × 13.5 × 3 mm in size, dated to the third century CE; Michel 2001: 245, no. 387.
140 A red jasper amulet 17 × 15 × 2 mm in size, dated to the third century CE; Michel 2001: 246, no. 388.
141 Tomlin 2008: 219–24.

Chapter 6

1 Kampen 1994: 111–37.
2 For more on the gesture of *tollere liberos* and the debate on whether it meant actually picking up a child off the ground, or whether it should be understood as a set of gestures signifying that the child was accepted, see Köves-Zulauf 1990: 1–93; Dasen 2014: 231–3; see also Laes 2011: 64; Corbier 2001: 53–7; Shaw 2001: 31–77.
3 As Dasen thinks, according to this proposal the term pre-liminal would refer to all of pregnancy, but there were no religious rites in the liminal period for a child who died before the *dies lustricus*; see Dasen 2009; Brind'amour 1975: 17–58.
4 Dasen 2009: 202–7.
5 Soranus 2.(6)26.(10)79. Putting the child down on the ground is also mentioned by Pliny (HN 7.1): 'but man alone on the day of his birth she casts away naked on the naked ground, to burst at once into wailing and weeping, and none other among all the animals is more prone to tears, and that immediately at the very beginning of life.'
6 CIL II 1964; AE 2001 61: plures liberos haben/tem pauiores habenti praeferto priorem/que nuntiato ita ut bini liberi post no/men inpositum aut singuli puberes amis/ si vrive potentes amissae pro singulis / sospitibus numerentur.
7 Gell. 3.16.21: Memini ego Romae accurate hoc atque sollicite quaesitum, negotio non rei tunc parvae postulante, an octavo mense infans ex utero vivus editus et statim mortuus ius trium liberorum supplevisset, cum abortio quibusdam, non partus, videretur mensis octavi intempestivitas.
8 Zabłocki 1992: 204.
9 Dasen 2009: 202–7.
10 Dasen 2014: 238; Laes 2014: 364–83.
11 CIL VI 5534: Cornelia / Calliste mihi nomen erat / quod forma probavit annus / ut accedat ter mihi quintus / erat grata fui domino gemino / dilecta parenti septima [l]anguen/ti summaque visa dies causa / latet fati partum tamen esse / loquontur sed quaecumque / fuit tam cito non merui.
12 AE 1995, 1793: [Ha]nc struem perennis arae posuit his in sedibus / Iulius Festae Secundus coniugi karissimae / uixit annos sextriginta bisque uiginti dies / pondus uteri enisa decimum luce rapta est tertia / nata claro Rubriorum genere de primoribus / sancta mores pulchra uisu praecluens prudentia / exornata summo honore magno iudicio patrum / aurea uitta et corona Mauricae prouinciae / haec et diuum consecuta est summa pro meritis bona / quinque natos lacte mater ipsa quos aluit suo / sospites superstitesque liquit uotorum potens.
13 AE 1897, 43; CIL VIII 24734: Daphnis ego Hermetis coniunx sum libera facta / cum dominus vellet primu(m) Hermes liber ut esset / fato ego facta prior fato ego rapta prior / quae tuli quod genui gemitus uiro saepe reliqui / quae domino invito uitam

dedi proxime nato / nunc quis alet natum quis vitam longa(m) ministrat / me Styga quod rapuit tam cito eni(m) a(d) superis / pia uixit annis XXV h(ic) s(ita) e(st).

14 Cael. Aurel. 1.107.
15 Varro *De agric.* 2.9: nam in Illyrico hoc amplius, praegnatem saepe, cum venit pariendi tempus, non longe ab opere discedere ibique enixam puerum referre, quem non peperisse, sed invenisse putes.
16 Ael. *De animal.* 7.12: εἰ δὲ Λιγυστίνων αἱ γυναῖκες μέγα φρονοῦσιν, ὅτι κἀκεῖναι τὴν ὠδῖνα ἀπολύσασαι καὶ ἐξαναστᾶσαι τῶν ἔργων ἔχονται.
17 Works worth mentioning include those of Soranus of Ephesus, Galen, Oribasius, Aëtius of Amida and Paul of Aegina.
18 Dixon considers Soranus a well-known, influential person whose work can be regarded as up to the standards of his times, but we cannot be sure to what extent his advice was followed by an average Roman family: Dixon 1988: 108; Tatarkiewicz 2013: 49–62.
19 Dasen 2007: 49–62.
20 Valette-Cagnac 2003 http://terrain.revues.org/1534 (accessed on 20 September 2019). According to Plutarch, nothing was of more importance to Cato than helping his wife bathe and re-swaddle a child regardless of his civic duties, except perhaps some public matter (Plut. *Cato the Elder* 20).
21 Galanakis 1998: 2012–13. Although eighteen centuries apart, the two developed similar systems for evaluating newborn infants, with four out of five criteria the same. The one criterion Soranus did not take into consideration was the child's pulse rate, whereas Virginia Apgar's score ignores the condition of the mother while pregnant and the child's maturity.
22 Soranus 2.(6)26.(10)79.
23 Belmont 1973: 77–89; Dasen 2014: 234–6.
24 Oribasius, lib. Inc. 12 = Dar. (III) 117–18; Oribasius claimed, for instance, that crying was also considered ominous, even though it was the starting point of an infant's life. Therefore he advised his readers to reject all superstition and cut off the umbilical cord with a scalpel.
25 Catullus 64.307–19: Qui postquam niveis flexerunt sedibus artus / large multiplici constructae sunt dape mensae, / cum interea infirmo quatientes corpora motu / veridicos Parcae coeperunt edere cantus. / his corpus tremulum complectens undique vestis / candida purpurea talos incinxerat ora, / at roseae niveo residebant vertice vittae, / aeternumque manus carpebant rite laborem. / laeva colum molli lana retinebat amictum, / dextera tum leviter deducens fila supinis / formabat digitis, tum prono in pollice torquens / libratum tereti versabat turbine fusum, / atque ita decerpens aequabat semper opus dens, / laneaque aridulis haerebant morsa labellis, / quae prius in levi fuerant exstantia filo: / ante pedes autem candentis mollia lanae / vellera virgati custodibant calathisci.

26 Dasen 2011: 137; Breemer, Waszink 1947: 254–70; Dasen 2014: 235–6.
27 Soranus 2.(7)27.(11)80: τὰ γὰρ ἐπικαέντα περιωδυνίας καὶ φλεγμονὰς σφοδρὰς ὑπομένει. μὴ ἐξῃρημένου δὲ τοῦ χορίου κατὰ δύο τόπους ἀποβροχίζειν δεῖ τὸν οὐραχὸν καὶ τότε μεταξὺ διακόπτειν, ἵνα διὰ μὲν τοῦ ἑτέρου βρόχου τὴν τοῦ βρέφους αἱμορραγίαν προφυλαξώμεθα, διὰ δὲ θατέρου τὴν τῆς ἀποκεκυηκυίας·· ἔτι γὰρ αὐτῇ προσέχεται τὸ χόριον. The best-known example for a tragedy caused by this is the death of a child of empress Helena, or so reports Ammianus Marcellinus (16.10.19): 'For once before, in Gaul, when she had borne a baby boy, she lost it through this machination: a midwife had been bribed with a sum of money, and as soon as the child was born cut the umbilical cord more than was right, and so killed it.'
28 Soranus 2.(18)38.(41)110: καὶ πρῶτον μὲν μετὰ τρεῖς ἢ τέσσαρας ἡμέρας ἢ ὁποσασοῦν τοῦ ὀμφαλοῦ κατὰ μαρασμὸν ἀποπεσόντος τὸ ὑπολειφθὲν [καὶ] κατὰ τὴν βάσιν ἑλκύδριον ἀποθεραπεύειν; in Plutarch's opinion, it can take longer, as he believes that even one week before the umbilical cord is lost, the newborn child is more like a plant than an animal (*Mor.* 288C).
29 Soranus 2.(18)38.(41)110.
30 French 2005: 53–62.
31 Kampen 1981, catalogue III 21, 22, 23, 24, 25, 27.
32 Dasen 2014: 236–7.
33 Also discussed by Galen, *Hyg.* 1.33K: δεύτερον δέ, ὅπως ἄν τις, εἰ καὶ μὴ νεογενὲς εἴη τὸ παιδίον, ἀλλ' ἤδη παιδεύεσθαι δυνάμενον, ἐπιστατήσειεν αὐτοῦ· καὶ οὕτω καθ' ἑκάστην τῶν ἄλλων ἡλικιῶν. τὸ τοίνυν νεογενὲς παιδίον, τοῦτο δὴ τὸ ἄμεμπτον ἁπάσῃ τῇ παρασκευῇ, πρῶτον μὲν σπαργανούσθω, συμμέτροις ἁλσὶν περιπαττόμενον, ὅπως αὐτῷ στερρότερον καὶ πυκνότερον εἴη τὸ δέρμα τῶν ἔνδον μορίων. ἐν γὰρ τῷ κυΐσκεσθαι πάνθ' ὁμοίως ἦν μαλακὰ μήτε ψαύοντος αὐτοῦ τινος ἔξωθεν σκληροτέρου σώματος μήτ' ἀέρος ψυχροῦ προσπεσόντος, ὑφ' ὧν συναγόμενόν τε καὶ πιλούμενον γένοιτ' ἂν ἑαυτοῦ τε καὶ τῶν ἄλλων μορίων σκληρότερόν τε καὶ πυκνότερον. ἐπειδὰν δ' ἀποκυηθῇ, ἐξ ἀνάγκης ὁμιλεῖν μέλλει καὶ κρύει καὶ θάλπει καὶ πολλοῖς σκληροτέροις ἑαυτοῦ σώμασι. προσήκει διὰ ταῦτα τὸ σύμφυτον αὐτῷ σκέπασμα παρασκευασθῆναί πως ὑφ' ἡμῶν ἄριστον εἰς δυσπάθειαν. ἱκανὴ δὲ ἡ διὰ μόνων τῶν ἁλῶν παρασκευὴ τοῖς γε κατὰ φύσιν ἔχουσι βρέφεσιν. ὅσα γὰρ ἤτοι μυρίνης φύλλων ξηρῶν περιπαττομένων ἢ τινος ἑτέρου τοιούτου δεῖται, μοχθηρῶς δή που διάκειται. πρόκειται δ' ἡμῖν τό γε νῦν εἶναι περὶ τῶν ἄριστα κατεσκευασμένων τὸν λόγον ποιεῖσθαι. ταῦτ' οὖν, ὡς εἴρηται, σπαργανωθέντα γάλακτί τε χρήσθω τροφῇ καὶ λουτροῖς ὑδάτων χρηστῶν· ὑγρᾶς γὰρ χρῄζει τῆς συμπάσης διαίτης, ἅτε καὶ τὴν κρᾶσιν ὑγροτέραν ἔχοντα τῶν ἐν ταῖς ἄλλαις ἡλικίαις.
34 Soranus 2.(8)28.(13)82.
35 Soranus 2.(8)28.(13)82: κατὰ δὲ τοῦ ὀμφαλοῦ πτυγμάτιον ἐπιρρῖψαι ἐλαιοβραχὲς ἢ καὶ ἔριον, τὸ δὲ κύμινον ὡς δριμὺ παραιτεῖθσαι δεῖ.

36 Soranus 2.(16)36.(33)102: μετὰ δὲ ταῦτα διὰ τοῦ μεγάλου καὶ λιχανοῦ δακτύλου τὰ περὶ τὰ πυγαῖα ταῖς ἐμπιέσεσιν εὐπρεπείας ἕνεκα κοιλαινέτω, συνεστραμμένης δὲ τῆς χειρὸς ἐπαγωγῇ τὰ ὑπὲρ τὸν ἔσχατον τῆς ῥάχεως σπόνδυλον λεληθότως ἀπωθείσθω πρὸς τὸ μὴ γενέσθαι λόρδωσιν, οὕτω δὲ καὶ κατὰ νώτου καὶ μεταφρένου χάριν τοῦ δυσεξύβωτα καὶ [μὴ] ἀνώμαλα εἶναι. μετὰ δὲ ταῦτα τὸ κεφάλιον πρῶτον μὲν [κατὰ] περιαγωγὴν ἑκατέρᾳ χειρὶ τριβέτω στρογγύλως, δεύτερον δέ πως ὑποτυποῦτω ποτὲ μὲν ἐξ ἀντιθέτων τῶν χειρῶν ᾗ μὲν κατ' ἰνίου, ᾗ δὲ κατὰ μετώπου τασσομένῃ, ποτὲ δὲ ᾗ μὲν κατὰ κορυφῆς, ᾗ δὲ ὑπ' ἀνθερεῶνα. εὐρυθμιζέτω δὲ δεξιῶς τὸ κρανίον, ὥστε μὴ προμηκέστερον ἢ φοξὸν ἀποτελεσθῆναι. ποτὲ δὲ καὶ κινείτω προσεπαίρουσα τὸ κεφάλιον καὶ ἀποτεινέτω, γυμνασίας ἕνεκα τῶν τενόντων καὶ κινήσεως τῶν σπονδύλων, ἐπεὶ δι' αὐτοῦ ταῦτα τὰ μέρη κινεῖν ἀδυνατεῖ τὸ νήπιον.
37 Soranus 2.(16)36.(34)103: εἰ δὲ ἄρρεν τὸ νήπιον ὑπάρχον φαίνοιτο λειπόδερμον, τρυφερῶς ἐπισπάσθω τὴν ἀκροποσθίαν ἢ καὶ διὰ κροκύδος συνεχέτω πρὸς διακράτησιν· ἑλκομένη γὰρ ἐκ τοῦ πρὸς ὀλίγον καὶ συνεχῶς ἐπισπωμένη ῥᾳδίως ἐπιδίδωσι καὶ τὸ κατὰ φύσιν ἀπολαμβάνει μῆκος καλύπτουσα τὴν βάλανον καὶ συνεθιζομένη τὴν φυσικὴν εὐμορφίαν τηρεῖν. προσαναπλασσέτω δὲ καὶ τὸν ὄσχεον ἐκ τῶν συμμηριῶν, [καὶ] ἵνα μὴ θλίβηται, προϋποβάλλουσα ἔριον κατὰ τῶν μηρῶν οὕτως αὐτὸν ἀποτιθέτω. For the importance of the appearance of the foreskin, see Hodges 2001: 375–405.
38 Soranus 2.(16)36.(34)103: τούτων δὲ ἐπιμεληθεῖσα στρεφέτω τὸ βρέφος καὶ τὰ ἔμπροσθεν συναλειφέτω. καὶ διά τινων ἡμερῶν τοὺς ὀφθαλμοὺς ἐγχυματιζέτω, καὶ μὴ καθ' ἡμέραν, ὀφθαλμίαι γὰρ ἐντεῦθεν ἐνίοις ἐπακολουθοῦσιν ἑλκουμένων ποτὲ καὶ τῶν ὑμένων.
39 Soranus 2.(16)36.(34)103: τριβέτω δὲ τοῖς ἀντίχερσιν ἑκατέροις καὶ τοὺς ὀφθαλμοὺς [καὶ] περιπλασσέτω καὶ τὸν μυκτῆρα διεγείρουσα μὲν αὐτὸν ἐπὶ σιμῶν, θλίβουσα δὲ ἐπὶ γρυπῶν, προσαναστέλλουσα [μέν], ἐφ' ὧν τὸ γρυπόν, οὐ κατὰ μετεωρισμὸν ἐπὶ τοῦ ὑψώματος, κατὰ προπέτειαν δὲ τῶν περὶ τὸ σφαιρίον ἄκρων, ἐπισπωμένη δὲ ἀνεσταλμένα τὰ πτερυγώματα τῶν ῥινῶν.
40 Plut. *Mor.* 3D. See also Dasen 2007: 49–62.
41 Soranus 2.(9)29.(15)84.
42 Soranus 2.(9)29.(15)84; From the preserved images we can visualize what babies looked like when so swaddled, and see that different ways and styles of swaddling existed: Nissen 2006: 804–9; Deyts 2004: 227–37. One interesting type of source is made up of depictions of swaddled infants on coins bearing the image of Juno Lucina, although unfortunately they are very schematic, which is typical of numismatic sources. Coins with images of that goddess were minted to celebrate births in the imperial family, indicating that a request for help had been fulfilled. Because of her domain of influence, Juno Lucina is usually shown holding a newborn child, e.g. on RIC III, 771; RIC IV 341.

43 Argetsinger 1992: 175–93; Köves-Zulauf 1990; Cens. 2.1–3.
44 Rawson 2003: 108–13.
45 E.g. CIL IV 294: Iu(v)enilla nata diie Satu(rni) h(ora) secu(nda) v(espertina) IIII nonas Au(gustas); CIL IV 8149: Natus Cornelius Sabinus.
46 CIL IV 8149: Natus Cornelius Sabinus; CIL IV 294: Iu(v)enilla // nata / die Satu(rni) (h)ora secu(nda) v(espertina) / IIII Non(as) Au(gustas).
47 Stat. *Silv.* 4.8.35–42.
48 Iuv. *Sat.* 4.79.
49 Iuv. *Sat.* 9.85.
50 Gell. 12.1.1–2.
51 HA. *Marc.* 10.7–9; but a registry of birth existed long before Marcus Aurelius' times, being mentioned in two well-known decrees from Augustus' reign.
52 Legal aspects of the matter, sources and further reading in the studies of Fritz Schulz: Schulz 1943: 78–91; Schulz 1943a: 55–64; also Sanchez-Moreno Ellart 2004: 107–19; Parkin 2003: 175–82. Under Augustus, only the births of legitimate children were officially registered, but from the times of Marcus Aurelius on, all children were registered, whether born to married couples or not.
53 Apul. *Apol.* 89.
54 S. A. Takács incorrectly claims that the information is to be found in Dio (Takács 2008: 65). In fact, the source for offering a coin at Juno's temple after the birth of male progeny is Dionysius of Halicarnassus (AR 4.15:[5]).
55 Macrob. *Sat.*, 1.16.36: Est etiam Nundina Romanorum dea a nono die nascentium nuncupata, qui lustricus dicitur. Est autem dies lustricus quo infantes lustrantur et nomen accipiunt: sed is maribus nonus, octavus est feminis; Dasen 2014: 238–40.
56 Plutarch *Rom.* 102 (288C): διὰ τί τῶν παίδων τοῖς μὲν ἄρρεσιν ἐναταίοις, τοῖς δὲ θήλεσιν ὀγδοαίοις τὰ ὀνόματα τίθενται; ἢ τὸ μὲν προτέροις τοῖς θήλεσιν αἰτίαν ἔχει τὴν φύσιν; καὶ γὰρ αὔξεται τὸ θῆλυ καὶ ἀκμάζει καὶ τελειοῦται πρότερον τοῦ ἄρρενος. τῶν δ' ἡμερῶν τὰς μετὰ τὴν ἑβδόμην λαμβάνουσιν· ἡ γὰρ ἑβδόμη σφαλερὰ τοῖς νεογνοῖς πρός τε τἆλλα καὶ τὸν ὀμφαλόν· ἑβδομαῖος γὰρ ἀπολύεται τοῖς πλείστοις· ἕως δ' ἀπολυθῇ, φυτῷ μᾶλλον ἢ ζώῳ προσέοικε τὸ νήπιον.
57 Pers. *Sat.* 2.31–4.
58 Other authors merely mention naming celebrations but not the day they took place. Cf. Suet. *Nero* 6.2: Eiusdem futurae infelicitatis signum evidens die lustrico exstitit; nam C. Caesar, rogante sorore ut infanti quod vellet nomen daret, intuens Claudium paruum suum, a quo mox principe Nero adoptatus est, eius se dixit dare, neque ipse serio sed per iocum et aspernante Agrippina, quod tum Claudius inter ludibria aulae erat. Arnob. *adv. nat.* 3.4: Sed et illud rursus desideramus audire, a vobisne inposita habeant haec nomina quibus eos vocatis an ipsi haec sibi diebus imposuerint lustricis.
59 Tert. *De idol.* 16.1–2: Circa officia vero privatarum et communium sollemnitatum, ut togae purae, ut sponsalium, ut nuptialium, ut nominalium, nullum putem periculum

observari de flatu idololatriae, quae interuenit. Causae enim sunt considerandae, quibus praestatur officium.
60 CIL II 1964; AE 2001, 61: plures liberos haben/tem pauiores habenti praeferto priorem/que nuntiato ita ut bini liberi post no/men inpositum aut singuli puberes amis/ si vrive potentes amissae pro singulis / sospitibus numerentur.
61 van Gennep 2006: 37–50; Jaskulska 2013: 79–82; Laes 2014: 364–83.

Conclusion

1 CIL II 5965: Voto sum compos superest mihi plurima proles / coniugis ut volui sum [munus nacta supremum].
2 CIL VI 15346; *Remains of Old Latin, Volume IV: Archaic Inscriptions, transl.* E. H. Warmington, Cambridge 1940 (Loeb Classical Library).

Bibliography

Abel, E. L. (1999) 'Was the fetal alcohol syndrome recognized by the Greeks and Romans?', *Alcohol and Alcoholism* 34, 6: 868–72.

Alberici, L. A., Harlow, M. (2007) 'Age and Innocence: Female Transitions to Adulthood in Late Antiquity', *Hesperia Supplements* 41: 193–203.

Allély, A. (2003) 'Les enfants malformés et considéres comme prodigia à Rome et en Italie sous la République', *REA* 105: 127–56.

Allély, A. (2004) 'Les enfants malformés à Rome sous le Principate', *REA* 106: 73–101.

Alonso Alonso, A. (2011) 'Medicae y obstetrices en la epigrafía latina del imperio Romano. Apuntes en torno a un análisis comparativo', *Classica et Cristiana* 6: 267–96.

Ambrosini G. (1666) *Phytologiae hoc est de Plantis*, P. Prima, Tomus I, Bononiae.

Ambrosini, A., Stanghellini, G. (2012) 'Myths of motherhood. The role of culture in the development of postpartum depression', *Annali dell'Istituto superiore di sanità* 48, 3: 277–86.

Amundsen, D. W., Diers, C. J. (1969) 'The age of Menarche in Classical Greece and Rome', *Human Biology* 41, 1: 125–32.

Argetsinger, K. (1992) 'Birthday Rituals: Friends and Patrons in Roman Poetry and Cult', *Classical Antiquity* 11, 2: 175–93.

Arthur, N. A., Gowland, R. L. and R. C. Redfern (2016), 'Coming of age in Roman Britain: Osteological evidence for pubertal timing', *American Journal of Physical Anthropology*, 159, 4: 698–713.

Aubert, J. J. (2004) 'La procréation (divinement) assistée dans le monde gréco-romain' [in:] V. Dasen (ed.), *Naissance et petite enfance dans l'Antiquité. Actes du colloque de Fribourg, 28 novembre – 1er décembre 2001*: 259–76, Fribourg: Academic Press.

Augoustakis, A. (2010) *Motherhood and the Other: Fashioning Female Power in Flavian Epic. Oxford Studies in Classical Literature and Gender Theory*, Oxford: Oxford University Press.

Badinter, E. (1998) *Historia miłości macierzyńskiej*, transl. K. Choiński, Warszawa: Oficyna Wydawnicza Volumen.

Badinter, E. (2013) 'Konflikt: kobieta i matka', transl. J. Jedliński, Warszawa: Wydawnictwo Naukowe PWN.

Baggieri, G. (1998) 'Etruscan wombs', *The Lancet*: 352, 9130: 790.

Bagnall, R. S., Cribiore R. (2006) *Women's Letters from Ancient Egypt, 300 BC–AD 800*, Michigan: University of Michigan Press.

Baker, P. (1999) 'Soranus and the Pompeii Speculum: the Sociology of Gynaecology and the Roman Perceptions of the Female Body' [in:] P. Baker, C. Forcey, S. Jundi,

R. Witcher (eds) *Theoretical Roman Archaeology Conference* (TRAC 98), London: 141–51.

Barragán Nieto, J. P. (2009) 'El espacio de la mujer en la medicina Romana' [in:] F. de Oliveira, C. Teixeira, P. Barata Dias (eds) *Espaços e Paisagens. Antiguidade Clássica e Heranças Contemporâneas*, Vol. I, *Línguas e Literaturas. Grécia e Roma*: 83–9, Coimbra: Imprensa da Universidade de Coimbra.

Bauman, R. R. (1992) *Women and Politics in Ancient Rome*, London: Routledge.

Beard, M. (2017) *Women & Power: A Manifesto*, New York, London: Liveright.

Belmont, N. (1973) 'Levana, ou comment «élever» les enfants', *Annales. Économies, Sociétés, Civilisations* 28, 1: 77–89.

Bendz, G. (1943) 'Zu Caelius Aurelianus', *Eranos: acta philologica Suecana* 41: 65–76.

Bettini, M. (1999) *The Portrait of the Lover*, Berkeley: University of California Press.

Blizqez, L. J. (2015) *The Tools of Asclepius. Surgical Instruments in Greek and Roman Times*, Leiden: Brill.

Bodel, J. (1995) 'Minicia Marcella: Taken before Her Time', *The American Journal of Philology* 116, 3: 453–60.

Bonnet-Cadilhac, C. (1995) 'Les représentations du foetus in utero', *Medicina nei Secoli*, 7, 2: 339–50.

Bonnet-Cadilhac, C. (2004) 'Si l'enfant se trouve dans une présentation contre nature, que doit faire la sage-femme?' [in:] V. Dasen (ed.) *Naissance et petite enfance dans l'Antiquité. Actes du colloque de Fribourg, 28 novembre – 1er décembre 2001*: 199–208, Fribourg: Academic Press.

Bordenache Battaglia, G. (1983) *Corredi funerari di età imperiale e barbarica nel Museo Nazionale Romano*, Roma: Quasar.

Borg, B. (2013) *Crisis & Ambition. Tombs and Burial Customs in Third-Century CE Rome*, Oxford: Oxford University Press.

Bradley, M. (2011) 'Obesity, Corpulence and Emaciation in Roman Art', *Papers of the British School at Rome* 79: 1–41.

Breemer, S., Waszink, J. H. (1947) 'Fata Scribunda', *Mnemosyne* 13, 4: 254–70.

Brind'amour L. & P. (1975) 'Le dies lustricus, les oiseaux de l'aurore et l'amphidromie', *Latomus* 34: 17–58.

Brown P. (2008) *The Body and Society: Men, Women, and Sexual Renunciation in Early Christianity*, New York: Columbia University Press.

Bruun, Ch. (2010) 'Pliny, Pregnancies, and Prosopography: Vistilia and Her Seven Children', *Latomus* 69: 758–77.

Budin, S. L., MacIntosh Turfa, J. (eds) (2016) *Women in Antiquity: Real Women across the Ancient World*, London: Routledge.

Caldwell, J. C. (2004) 'Fertility control in the classical world: Was there an ancient fertility transition?', *Journal of Population Research* 21, 1: 1–17.

Caldwell, L. (2015) *Roman Girlhood and the Fashioning of Femininity*, Cambridge: Cambridge University Press.

Cantarella, E. (1987) *Pandora's Daughters: The Role and Status of Women in Greek and Roman Antiquity*, Baltimore: Johns Hopkins University Press.

Cantarella, E. (2002) 'Marriage and Sexuality in Republican Rome: A Roman Conjugal Love Story' [in:] M. Nussbaum, J. Sihvola (eds) *The Sleep of Reason. Erotic Experience and Sexual Ethics in Ancient Greece and Rome*: 269–82, Chicago: University of Chicago Press.

Carlon, J. M. (2009) *Pliny's Women: Constructing Virtue and Creating Identity in the Roman World*, Cambridge: Cambridge University Press.

Carroll, M. (2001) *Romans, Celts and Germans: The German Provinces of Rome*, Stroud: Tempus.

Carroll, M. (2011) 'Infant Death and Burial in Roman Italy', *Journal of Roman Archeology* 24: 99–120.

Carroll, M. (2014) 'Mother and Infant in Roman Funerary Commemoration' [in:] ed. M. Carroll and E.-J. Graham, *Infant Health and Death in Roman Italy and Beyond (Journal of Roman Archaeology, Suppl. 96)*: 159–78.

Chodorow, N. (1978) *The Reproduction of Mothering: Psychoanalysis and the Sociology of Gender*, Berkley: University of California Press.

Cid López, R. M. (2007) 'Imágenes y prácticas religiosas de la sumisión femenina en la antigua Roma. El culto de "Juno Lucina" y la fiesta de "Matronalia"', *Studia historica. Historia antigua* 25: 357–72.

Cilliers, L. (2004) 'Vindicianus' Gynaecia and Theories on Generation and Embryology from the Babylonians up to Graeco-Roman Times' [in:] Horstmanshoff, M., and Stol, M. (eds) *Magic and Rationality in Ancient Near Eastern and Graeco-Roman Medicine*: 343–67, Leiden: Brill.

Cilliers, L., Retief F. (2006) 'Medical practice in Graeco-Roman antiquity', *Curationis* 29, 2: 34–40.

Corbier, M. (2001) 'Child Exposure and Abandonment' [in:] S. Dixon (ed.) *Childhood, Class and Kin in the Roman World*: 53–7, London: Routledge.

Corvisier, J.-N. (1985) *Santé et société en Grèce ancienne*, Paris: Economica.

Coulon, G. (1994) *L'enfant en Gaule romaine*, Paris: Editions Errance.

Coulon, G. (2004) 'Images et imaginaire de la naissance dans l'Occident Romain' [in:] V. Dasen (ed.) *Naissance et petite enfance dans l'Antiquité, Actes du colloque de Fribourg, 28 novembre – 1er décembre 2001*: 209–225, Fribourg: Academic Press / Vandenhoeck & Ruprecht.

D'Ambra, E. (2014) 'Beauty for Roman Girls: Portraits and Dolls' [in:] S. Moraw, A. Kieburg (eds) *Mädchen im Altertum = Girls in antiquity*: 312–19, Münster: Waxmann.

Dasen, V. (1997), 'A propos de deux fragments de Deae nutrices à Avenches: Déesses-mères et jumeaux dans le monde italique et gallo-romain', *Bulletin de l'Association Pro Aventico* 39: 125–40.

Dasen, V. (1998) 'Les naissances multiples dans les textes médicaux antiques', *Gesnerus* 55: 183–204.

Dasen, V. (2005) *Jumeaux, jumelles dans l'Antiquité grecque et romaine*, Kilchberg: Akanthus Verlag für Archäologie.

Dasen, V. (2007) '"All Children are dwarfs". Medical Discourse and Iconography of Children's Bodies', *Oxford Journal of Archaeology* 27, 1: 49–62.

Dasen, V. (2009) 'Roman Birth Rites of Passage Revisited', *Journal of Roman Archeology* 22: 202–7.

Dasen, V. (2011) 'Le pouvoir des femmes: des Parques aux Matres', *Études de lettres*, 3–4: 115–46.

Dasen, V. (2013) 'Becoming Human: From the Embryo to the Newborn Child' [in:] J. Evans Grubbs and T. Parkin (eds) *The Oxford Handbook of Childhood and Education in the Classical World*: 17–39, Oxford: Oxford University Press.

Dasen, V. (2014) 'Iconographie et archéologie des rites de passage de la petite enfance dans le monde romain. Questions méthodologiques' [in:] A. Mouton, J. Patrier (eds) *Vivre, grandir et mourir dans l'antiquité: rites de passage individuels au Proche-Orient ancien et ses environs*: 231–3, Leiden: Nederlands Instituut voor het Nabije Oosten.

Dasen, V. (2015) *Le sourire d' Omphale. Maternité et petit enfance dans l'Antiquité*, Rennes: Presses universitaires de Rennes.

Dasen, V. (2016) 'Agir. Identité(s) des médecins antiques', *Histoire, médecine et santé* 16, 8: 9–15.

Dasen, V. (2016a) 'L'ars medica au féminin', *Eugesta, Revue sur le genre dans l'Antiquité* 6: 1–40.

Dasen, V. (ed.) (2004) *Naissance et petite enfance dans l'Antiquité*, Fribourg: Academic Press / Vandenhoeck. Ruprecht.

Dasen, V., Boudon-Millot, B., Marie, V. (eds) (2008) *Femmes en médecine. En l'honneur de D. Gourevitch*, Paris: De Boccard.

Deacy, S. (2013) 'Uxoricide in Pregnancy: Ancient Greek Domestic Violence in Evolutionary Perspective', *Evolutionary Psychology*, 11, 5: 994–1010.

Denooz, J. (2010) 'Uxor chez Pline le Jeune', *L'antiquité classique* 79: 163–72.

Devine, A. M. (1985) 'The Low Birth-rate in Ancient Rome: A Possible Contributing Factor', *Rheinisches Museum für Philologie* 128, 3–4: 313–17.

Deyts, S. (2004) 'La femme et l'enfant au maillot en Gaule: iconographie et épigraphie' [in:] V. Dasen (ed.) *Naissance et petite enfance dans l'Antiquité. Actes du colloque de Fribourg, 28 novembre – 1er décembre 2001*: 227–37, Fribourg: Academic Press / Vandenhoeck & Ruprecht.

Dierichs, A. (2002) *Von der Götter Geburt und der Frauen Niederkunft*, Mainz: Philipp von Zabern.

Dixon, S. (1988) *The Roman Mother*, London: Croom Helm.

Dixon, S. (1992) *The Roman Family*, Baltimore: Johns Hopkins University Press.

Dixon, S. (2001) *Reading Roman Women*, London: Bloomsbury Publishing.

Dixon, S. (2003) 'Sex and the Married Woman in Ancient Rome' [in:] D. L. Balch and C. Osiek (eds) *Early Christian Families in Context: An Interdisciplinary Dialogue*: 111–29, Cambridge:William B. Eerdmans Publishing Company.

Dolansky, F. (2012) 'Playing with Gender: Girls, Dolls, and Adult Ideals in the Roman World', *Classical Antiquity* 31, 2: 256–92.
Drabkin, I. E. (1944) 'On medical education in Greece and Rome', *Bulletin of the History of Medicine* 15: 333–51.
Drabkin, I. E. (1957) 'Medical Education in Ancient Greece and Rome', *Journal of Medical Education* 32, 4: 286–96.
Ducaté-Paarmann, S. (2005) 'Rites de fécondité: le recours au divin' [in:] D. Gourevitch, A. Moirin and N. Rouquet (eds) *Maternité et petite enfence en Gaule romaine*: 33–5, Bourges Éditions du CEDARC.
Durand, M., Finon C. (2000) 'Catalogue des ex-voto anatomiques du temple gallo-romain de la forêt d'Halatte (Oise)', *Revue archéologique de Picardie. Numéro spécial* 18: 9–91.
Durry, M. (1955) 'Le mariage des filles impubères à Rome', *Comptes rendus des séances de l'Académie des Inscriptions et Belles-Lettres* 99, 1: 84–91.
Duval, P. M. (1989) 'Médecins et médecine de Gaule' [in:] *Travaux sur la Gaule (1946–1986)*: 1163–73, Rome: École française de Rome.
Dyjakowska, M. (2014) 'Orbitas omni fugienda nisu – rozważania Publiusza Papiniusza Stacjusza o rodzinie rzymskiej', *Studia Prawnicze KUL* 1, 57: 7–22.
Ehmig, U. (2013), 'Risikobewältigung bei Schwangerschaft und Geburt in der römischen Antike: lateinische dokumentarische und archäologische Zeugnisse', *Arctos* 47: 111–29.
Engels, D. (1980) 'The Problem of Female Infanticide in the Greco-Roman World', *Classical Philology* 75, 2: 112–20.
Evans Grubbs, J. (1995) *Law and Family in Late Antiquity: The Emperor Constantine's Marriage Legislation*, Oxford: Oxford University Press.
Eyben, E. (1972) 'Antiquity's View of Puberty', *Latomus* 31, 3: 677–97.
Eyben, E. (1980) 'Family Planning in Graeco-Roman Antiquity', *Ancient Society* 11–12: 5–82.
Flambard, J. M. (1987) 'Deux toponymes du Champ de Mars: ad Ciconias, ad Nixas' [in:] *L'Urbs: espace urbain et histoire (Ier siècle av. J.-C. – IIIe siècle ap. J.-C.). Actes du colloque international de Rome (8–12 mai 1985)*: 191–210, Rome: École Française de Rome.
Flemming, R. (2000) *Medicine and the Making of Roman Women: Gender, Nature, and Authority from Celsus to Galen*, Oxford: Oxford University Press.
Flemming, R. (2007) 'Women, Writing and Medicine in the Classical World', *The Classical Quarterly* 57, 1: 257–79.
Flemming, R. (2013) 'Gendering Medical Provision in the Cities of the Roman West' [in:] E. Hemelrijk and G. Woolf (eds) *Women and the Roman City in the Latin West*: 271–95, Leiden Brill.
Foxhall, L. (2013) *Studying Gender in Classical Antiquity*, Cambridge: Cambridge University Press.
Fratantuono, L. (2015) *A Reading of Lucretius' 'De rerum natura'*, London: Lexington Books.

French, V. (1986) 'Midwives and Maternity Care in the Graeco-Roman World', *Helios, New Series* 13, 2: 69–84.

French, V. (2005) 'Midwives and Maternity Care in the Roman World' [in:] E. van Teijlingen, G. Lowis, P. McCaffery and M. Porter (eds) *Midwifery and the Medicalization Of Childbirth: Comparative Perspectives*: 53–62, New York: Nova.

Frier, B. W. (1994) 'Natural Fertility and Family Limitation in Roman Marriage', *Classical Philology* 89, 4: 318–33.

Frier, B. W. (2015) 'Roman law and the marriage of underage girls', *Journal of Roman Studies* 28: 652–65.

Galanakis, E. (1998) 'Apgar score and Soranus of Ephesus', *The Lancet* 352, issue 9145: 2012–13.

Garsney, P. (1999) *Food and Society in Classical Antiquity*, Cambridge: Cambridge University Press.

Gillmeister, A. (2013) 'Foucault i matrony. Kobiety w religii rzymskiej: między potestas a potentia', *Klio. Czasopismo poświęcone dziejom Polski i powszechnym* 24, 1: 3–16.

Gillmeister, A. (2015) '"Cum tacita virgine". Westalki – kobiecość – religia w republikańskim Rzymie' [in:] B. Czwojdrak and A. A. Kluczek (eds) *Kobiety i władza w czasach dawnych:* 22–32, Katowice: Wydawnictwo Uniwersytetu Śląskiego.

Golden, M. (1998) 'Did the ancients care when their children died?', *Greece and Rome* 35: 152–63.

Gourevitch, D. (1984) *Le mal d'être femme. La femme et la médicine dans la Rome antique*, Paris: Les Belles Lettres.

Gourevitch, D. (1987) 'La mort de la femme en couches et dans les suites de couches' [in:] F. Hinard (ed.) *La mort, les morts et l'au-delà dans le monde romain*: 187–93, Caen: Université de Caen.

Gourevitch, D. (1990) 'Se marier por avoir des enfants: le point de vue du médecin' [in:] J. Andreau and H. Bruhns (eds) *Parenté et stratégies familiales dans l'Antiquité Romaine:* 139–51, Paris: École française de Rome.

Gourevitch, D. (1994) 'Moi, Vipsania, j'attends un enfant', *Acta Belgica Historiae Medicinae* 7, 4: 200–6.

Gourevitch, D. (1995) 'L'alimentation animale de la femme enceinte, de la nourrice et du bébé sevré' [in:] R. Chevallier (ed.) *Caesarodunum, Actes du colloque de Nantes 1991, Homme et animal dans l'Antiquité romaine*: 283–93, Tours: Centre de Recherches A. Piganiol.

Gourevitch, D. (2001) 'Problèmes d'obstétrique à Rome: césarienne, version, embryotomie et drogue de la dernière chance' [in:] J. N. Corvisier, Ch. Didier, M. Valdher (ed.) *Thérapies, médecine et démographie antiques:* 277–92, Amiens: Artois Presses Université.

Gourevitch, D. (2003) 'La mère qui mange et le foetus qui réagit: une allusion méconnue à la sensorialité foetale', *Revue de philologie, de littérature et d'histoire anciennes* 76, 2: 219–23.

Gourevitch, D. (2004) 'Soranos, adieu Soranos', *Cahiers de la villa Kérylos* 15: 135–61.

Gourevitch, D. (2009) 'La matrone romaine poussée à la procréation' [in:] F. Briquel-Chatonnet, S. Farès and B. Michel (eds) *Femmes cultures et sociétés dans les civilisations méditerranéennes et proche-orientales de l'Antiquité*, (Topoi. Supplement 10): 115–25, Lyon: Maison de l'Orient et de la Méditerranée.

Gourevitch, D. (2011) *Pour une archéologie de la médicine romaine,* Paris: De Boccard.

Gourevitch, D., Ricciardetto, A. (2018) 'Moi, Téreus, enceinte et battue', *La revue du praticien* 68: 690–4.

Green, M. (2008) *Making Women's Medicine Masculine: The Rise of Male Authority in Pre-Modern Gynaecology*, Oxford: Oxford University Press.

Green, M. H., Hanson, A. E. (1994) 'Soranus of Ephesus: Methodicorum princeps', [in:] W. Haase (ed.) *ANRW 37, 2, Philosophie, Wissenschaften, Technik. Wissenschaften*: 968–1076, Berlin: de Gruyter.

Gromkowska-Melosik, A. (2013) *Kobieta epoki wiktoriańskiej. Tożsamość, ciało, medykalizacja*, Kraków: Oficyna Wydawnicza Impuls.

Hackworth Petersen, L., Salzman-Mitchell, P. (2010) *Mothering and Motherhood in Ancient Greece and Rome*, Austin: University of Texas Press.

Haentjens, A. M. E. (2000) 'Reflections on Female Infanticide in the Greco-Roman World', *L'antiquité classique* 69: 261–4.

Hallet, J. (1984) *Fathers and Daughters in Roman Society*, Princeton: Princeton University Press.

Hänninen, M. L. (2005) 'From Womb to Family. Rituals and Social Conventions to Roman Birth' [in:] K. Mustakallio, J. Hanska, H. L. Sainio and V. Vuolanto (eds) *Hoping for Continuity: Childhood, Education and Death in Antiquity and the Middle Ages*: 49–60, Roma: Institutum Romanum Finlandiae.

Hanson, A. E. (1987) 'The Eight Months' Child and the Etiquette of Birth: obsit omen!', *Bulletin of the History of Medicine*, 61, 4: 589–602.

Harlow, M. (2012) 'Death and the Maiden: Reprising the Burials of Roman Girls and Young Women' [in:] M. Carroll and J. P. Wild (eds) *Dressing the Dead in Classical Antiquity*: 148–57, Stroud: Amberley.

Harlow, M., Laurence, R. (2002) *Growing Up and Growing Old in Ancient Rome: a life course approach*, London: Routledge.

Harris, W. V. (1994) 'Child Exposure in the Roman Empire', *Journal of Roman Studies* 84: 1–22.

Hawkins, J. N. (2015) 'Parrhesia and Pudenda: Speaking Genitals and Satiric Speech' [in:] C. W. Marshall and T. Hawkins (eds) *Athenian Comedy in the Roman Empire*: 43–68, London: Bloomsbury.

Hemelrijk, E. A. (1999) '*Matrona Docta*': *Educated Women in the Roman Elite from Cornelia to Julia Domna*, London: Routledge.

Hemelrijk, E. A. (2020) *Women and Society in the Roman World: A Sourcebook of Inscriptions from the Roman West*, Cambridge: Cambridge University Press.

Hemelrijk, E., Woolf, G. (eds) (2013) *Women and the Roman City in the Latin West*, Leiden: Brill.

Hersch, K. K. (2010) *The Roman Wedding: Ritual and Meaning in Antiquity*, Cambridge: Cambridge University Press.

Hibbard, B. (2001) *The Obstetrician's Armamentarium: Historical Obstetric Instruments and Their Inventors*, San Anselmo: Norman Publishing.

Hindermann, J. (2013) '"Mulier", "femina", "uxor", "coniunx": die begriffliche Kategorisierung von Frauen in den Briefen von Cicero und Plinius dem Jüngeren', *Eugesta* 3: 143–61.

Hodges, F. M. (2001) 'The Ideal Prepuce in Ancient Greece and Rome: Male Genital Aesthetics and Their Relation to Lipodermos, Circumcision, Foreskin Restoration, and the Kynodesme', *Bulletin of the History of Medicine* 75, 3: 375–405.

Hoepken, C. (2007) 'Frühromische Gräber in Köln' [in:] G. Uelsberg (ed.) *Krieg und Frieden. Kelten, Römer und Germanen*: 298–9, Bonn: Primus.

Hopkins, M. K. (1965) 'Contraception in the Roman Empire', *Comparative Studies in Society and History*, 8, 1: 124–51.

Hopkins, M. K. (1965a) 'The Age of Roman Girls at Marriage', *Population Studies* 18, 3: 309–27.

Hopwood, N. Flemming, R. and Kassell, L. (eds) (2019) *Reproduction: from Antiquity to the present day*, Cambridge: Cambridge University Press.

Hufnagel, G. L. (2012) *A History of Women's Menstruation From Ancient Greece to the Twenty-first Century: Psychological, Social, Medical, Religious, and Educational Issues*, Lewiston: Edwin Mellen Press.

Hug A. (2014) *Fecunditas, Sterilitas, and the Politics of Reproduction at Rome*, Toronto. (unpubl.diss.)

Irving, J. (2012) 'Restituta: The Training of the Female Physician', *Melbourne Historical Journal* 40, 2: 45–56.

James, L., Dillon, S. (eds) (2012) *A Companion to Women in the Ancient World*, Oxford: Wiley-Blackwell.

Jaskulska, S. (2013) '"Rytuał przejścia" jako kategoria analityczna. Przyczynek do dyskusji nad badaniem rytualnego oblicza rzeczywistości', *Studia Edukacyjne* 26: 79–82.

Jońca, M., Szarek, P. (2010) 'Rodzina i prawo w rzymskich papirusach', *Zeszyty Prawnicze UKSW* 10, 1: 311–14.

Jurewicz, A. (1997) 'Postumus' w "Noctes Atticae" Aulusa Gelliusa, *Prawo Kanoniczne*, 40, 1–2: 255–62.

Jurewicz, A. (2006) 'Domniemanie ojcostwa – "ratio decidendi" ustawodawcy', *Zeszyty Prawnicze*, 6, 1: 95–119.

Kampen, N. (1981) *Image and Status: Roman Working Women in Ostia*, Berlin: Mann.

Kampen, N. (1994) 'Material Girl: Feminist Confrontations with Roman Art', *Arethusa* 27, 1: 111–37.

Kapparis, K. A. (2002) *Abortion in the ancient world*, London: Duckworth Academic.

Kelley A. (2013) *Glorified Daughters. The Glorification of Daughters on Roman Epitaphs*, Kent State University.

King, H. (1986) 'Agnodike and the Profession of Medicine', *Proceedings of the Cambridge Philosophical Society* 32: 53–77.
King, H. (1995) 'Medical texts as a source for women's history' [in:] A. Powell (ed.) *The Greek World*. Routledge Worlds: 199–218. London: Routledge.
Klęczar, A. (2013) *Katullus, Poezje wszystkie*, Kraków: Homini.
Kokoszko, M. (ed.) (2014) *Dietetyka i sztuka kulinarna antyku i wczesnego Bizancjum (II–VII w.)*, Łódź: Wydawnictwo Uniwersytetu Łódzkiego.
Kokoszko, M., Jagusiak K., Rzeźnicka Z. (2014) *Dietetyka i sztuka kulinarna antyku i wczesnego Bizancjum (II–VII w.). Zboża i produkty zbożowe w źródłach medycznych antyku i wczesnego Bizancjum*, Łódź: Wydawnictwo Uniwersytetu Łódzkiego.
Kollesch, J. (1979) 'Ärztliche Ausbildung in der Antike', *Klio* 61, 2: 507–13.
Kołosowski, T. (2013) 'Etyczno-antropologiczne aspekty aborcji w świetle wybranych dzieł antycznej literatury Grecji i Rzymu', *Seminare. Poszukiwania naukowe* 33: 251–62.
Kompa, A. (2015) 'Kobieta rzymska, kobieta bizantyńska — co studia klasyczne mogą zaoferować dzisiejszym gender studies?' [in:] B. Czwojdrak and A. A. Kluczek (eds) *Kobiety i władza w czasach dawnych*: 49–69, Katowice: Wydawnictwo Uniwersytetu Śląskiego.
Korpela, J. (1987) *Das Medizinalpersonal im Antiken Rom*, Helsinki: Finnish Academy of Sciences.
Köves-Zulauf, T. (1990) *Römische Geburtsriten*, München: Beck.
Krenkel, W. A. (1987) 'Familienplanung und Familienpolitik in der Antike', *Würzburger Jahrbücher für die Altertumswissenschaft* 4: 197–203.
Künzl, E., Engelmann H. (1997) 'Römische Ärztinnen und Chirurginnen. Beiträge zu einem antiken Frauenberufsbild', *Antike Welt* 28, 5: 375–9.
Kursa, S. P. (2012) 'Repudium i jego skutki prawne w świetle kodyfikacji Justyniana', *Czasopismo Prawno-Historyczne* 64, 2: 60–80.
Kuryłowicz, M. (2011) 'Rozwój historyczny rzymskiej adopcji', *Studia Iuridica Lublinensia* 16: 35–53.
Lacan, J. (2007) *La relazione d'oggetto e le strutture freudiane. Seminario, Libro IV*, Torino: Biblioteca Einaudi.
Laes, Ch. (2010) 'The Educated Midwife in the Roman Empire: an Example of Differential Equations', [in:] M. Horstmanshoff (ed.) *Hippocrates and Medical education: Selected Papers Read at the 12th International Hippocrates Colloquium Universiteit Leiden, 24–26 August 2005*: 261–8, Leiden: Brill.
Laes, Ch. (2011) *Children in the Roman Empire: Outsiders Within*, Cambridge: Cambridge University Press.
Laes, Ch. (2012) 'Latin Inscriptions and the Life Course. Regio III (Bruttium and Lucania) as a Test Case' *Arctos* 46: 93–111.
Laes, Ch. (2014) 'Infants between Biological and Social Birth in Antiquity: a Phenomenon of the Longue Durée', *Historia* 63, 3: 364–83.
Laes, Ch. (2016) *Impotence*, in: R. S. Bagnall, K. Brodersen, C. B. Champion, A. Erskine, S. R. Huebner (eds), *The Encyclopedia of Ancient History*, Oxford: Wiley-Blackwell.

Lambert, G. R. (1982) 'Childless By Choice: Graeco-Roman Arguments and Their Uses', *Prudentia* 14: 123–38.

Leiwo, M., Halla-Aho, H. (2002) 'A Marriage Contract: Aspects of Latin-Greek Language Contact (P. Mich. VII 434 and P. Ryl. IV 612 = ChLA IV 249)', *Mnemosyne* 55, 5: 560–80.

Lelis, A., Percy, W., Verstraete, B. (2003) *The Age of Marriage in Ancient Rome*, Lewiston: Edwin Mellen Press.

Lewandowska, D. (2021) *Ciąża mnoga i wieloraczki w starożytności*, Warszawa: Wydawnictwo UW.

López Eire, A., Cortés Gabaudan, F. (eds) (2006) *Estudios y traduccion Dioscorides. Sobre los remedios medicinales. Manuscrito de Salamanca*, Salamanca: Ediciones de la Universidad de Salamanca.

Mancini, G. (1930) 'Scoperta della tomba della Vergine Vestale Tiburtina Cossina', *Notizie degli Scavi*: 353–69.

Marcone, A. (ed.) (2018) *Lavoro, lavoratori e dinamiche sociali in Roma antica*, Roma: Castelvecchi.

Mastrocinque, A. (2014) *Bona Dea and the Cults of Roman Women*, Stuttgart: Franz Steiner Verlag.

Mays, S., Robson-Brown, K., Vincent, S., Eyers J., King H., Roberts A. (2014) 'An Infant Femur Bearing Cut Marks from Roman Hambleden, England', *International Journal of Osteoarchaeology* 24, 1: 111–15.

McGinn, T. (2015) 'Child Brides at Rome'. *Iura: Rivista internazionale di diritto romano e antico* 63: 107–55.

Michel, S. (2001) *Die Magischen Gemmen im Britischen Museum*, London: British Museum Press.

Milnor, K. (2005) *Gender, Domesticity, and the Age of Augustus: Inventing Private Life*, Oxford: Oxford University Press.

Molleson, T., Cox, M. (1988) 'A Neonate with Cut Bones from Poundbury Camp, 4th century AD', *Bulletin de la Société royale Belge d'Anthropologie et de Préhistoire* 99: 53–60.

Moog, F. P. (2004), 'Herophilos von Kalchedon' [in:] W. E. Gerabek (ed.) *Enzyklopädie Medizingeschichte*: 575–9, Berlin: De Gruyter.

Moraw, S., Kieburg A. (eds) (2014) *Girls in Antiquity*, Münster: Waxmann.

Morelli, A. L. (2009) *Madri di uomini e di dèi. La rappresentazione della maternità attraverso la documentazione numismatica di epoca romana*, Bologna: Ante Quem.

Morgan, K. (1991) 'Ovid, "Amores 2.13.18": A Solution', *The Classical World* 85, 2: 95–100.

Morice, P., Josset, P., Chapron, Ch., Dubuisson, J. B. (1995) 'History of infertility', *Human Reproduction* 1: 497–504.

Morillo Cerdán, A. (1999) *Lucernas romanas en la región septentrional de la península ibérica: contribución al conocimiento de la implantación romana en Hispania*, vol. 2, Montagnac: Editions M. Mergoil.

Musca, D. A. (1988) 'La donna nel mondo pagano e nel mondo cristiano: le punte minime dell'età matrimoniale attraverso il materiale epigrafico (Urbs Roma)' [in:] *Atti Accad. Romanistica Costantiniana: VII Convegno*: 176–81, Napoli: Edizioni Scientifiche Italiane.

Musiał, D. (2013) 'Kobieta i mężczyzna w świecie antycznym: uwagi o starych sporach i nowych oczekiwaniach', *Klio. Czasopismo poświęcone dziejom Polski i powszechnym* 26, 3: 5–22.

Newby, Z. (2018) 'The Grottarossa Doll and her Mistress: Hope and Consolation in a Roman Tomb' [in:] Newby, Z. and R. Toulson (eds) *The Materiality of Mourning, Cross-disciplinary Perspectives*: 77–102, London: Routledge.

Nickel, D. (1979) 'Berufsvorstellungen über weibliche Medizinalpersonen in der Antike', *Klio* 61, 2: 515–18.

Niczyporuk, P. (2014) 'Zawarcie małżeństwa "liberorum procreandorum causa" w prawie rzymskim', *Zeszyty Prawnicze* 14, 3: 193–220.

Nifosi, A. (2019) *Becoming a Woman and Mother in Greco-Roman Egypt: Women's Bodies, Society and Domestic Space*, Abingdon: Routledge

Nissen, C. (2006) 'Les offrandes liées à la fécondité et à la maternité dans la Gaule romaine', *La revue du practicien* 56: 804–9.

Nussbaum, M. C. (1998) *Cultivating humanity: a classical defense of reform in liberal education*, Cambridge: Harvard University Press.

Oberhelman, S. M. (2014) 'Anatomical Votive Reliefs as Evidence for Specialization at Healing Sanctuaries in the Ancient Mediterranean World', *Athens Journal of Health* 1: 47–62.

Olszewski, L. (2002) 'Upadłe i boskie: ubóstwienie cesarzowych i księżniczek z dynastii julijsko-klaudyjskiej (30 rok przed Chr. – 68 rok po Chr.)' (an unpublished dissertation available at the library of the Adam Mickiewicz University), Poznań.

Oria Segura, M. (2016) 'Figurilla feminina embarazada com simbolo astral en la antigua Caura¿Sulpica privada a Dea Caelestis', *Lucentum* 35: 99–115.

Papadimitriou, A. (2016) 'The Evolution of the Age at Menarche from Prehistorical to Modern Times', *Journal of Pediatric and Adolescent Gynecology* 29, 6: 527–30.

Parker, H. N. (1997) 'Women Doctors in Greece, Rome and the Byzantine Empire' [in:] L. R. Furst (ed.) *Women Healers and Physicians: Climbing a Long Hill*: 131–50, Kentucky: University Press of Kentucky.

Parkin, T. (2003) *Old Age in the Roman World: A Cultural and Social History*, Maryland: Johns Hopkins University Press.

Pawlak, M. (2015) *Herodes Attyk. Sofista, dobroczyńca, tyran,* Toruń: Wydawnictwo Naukowe UMK.

Perkins, P. (2012) 'The bucchero childbirth stamp on a late Orientalizing period shard from Poggio Colla'. *Etruscan Studies*, 15 (2): 146–201.

Pinault, J. R. (1992) 'The Medical Case for Virginity in the Early Second Century C.E.: Soranus of Ephesus, Gynecology 1.32', *Helios* 19, 1: 123–39.

Pomeroy, S. B. (1975) *Goddesses, Whores, Wives, and Slaves: women in classical antiquity*, London: The Bodley Head Ltd.

Pomeroy, S. B. (1978) 'Plato and the Female Physician (Republic 454d)', *The American Journal of Philology* 99, 4: 496–500.

Pomeroy, S. B. (1991) *Women's History and Ancient History*, Chapel Hill: University of North Carolina Press.

Pomeroy, S. B. (2002) *Spartan women*, Oxford: Oxford University Press.

Pomeroy, S. B. (2007) *The Murder of Regilla*, Cambridge: Harvard University Press.

Prenner, A. (2012) *Mustione 'traduttore' di Sorano di Efeso. L'ostetrica, la donna, la gestazione*, Napoli: Liguori.

Rabinowitz, N. S., Richlin, A. (1993) *Feminist Theory and the Classics*, New York: Routledge.

Rawson, B. (2003) *Children and childhood in Roman Italy*, Oxford: Oxford University Press.

Reiss, R. E., Ask, A. D. (1988) 'The Eighth-month Fetus: Classical Sources for a Modern Superstition', *Obstetrics and Gynaecology* 71, 2: 270–3.

Retief, F. P. (2005) 'The Healing Hand: The Role of Women in Ancient Medicine', *Acta Theologica Supplementum* 7: 166–91.

Riddle, J. M. (1992) *Contraception and Abortion from the Ancient World to the Renaissance*, Cambridge: Harvard University Press.

Rowlandson, J. (1998) *Women and Society in Greek and Roman Egypt. A Sourcebook*, Cambridge: Cambridge University Press.

Rudolf, E. I. (2016) 'Zdrowie reprodukcyjne kobiet – rozważania terminologiczne' [in:] A. Szlagowska (ed.) *Problemy zdrowia reprodukcyjnego kobiet. Wstęp do badań*, Wrocław: Wydawnictwo Uniwersytetu Medycznego im. Piastów Śląskich.

Richlin, A. (1997) 'Pliny's Brassiere' [in:] J. Hallett, M. Skinner (eds) *Roman Sexualities*: 197–220, Princeton: Princeton University Press.

Richlin, A. (2014) *Arguments with Silence: Writing the History of Roman Women*, Ann Arbor: University of Michigan Press.

Sanchez-Moreno Ellart, C. (2004) 'Notes on some new issues concerning the birth certificates of Roman citizens', *Journal of Juristic Papyrology* 34: 107–19.

Sanders, H. A. (1938) 'A Latin Marriage Contract', *Transactions and Proceedings of the American Philological Association* 69: 104–16.

Scheidel, W. (2001) 'Progress and Problems in Roman Demography' [in:] W. Scheidel (ed.) *Debating Roman Demography*: 1–81, Leiden: Brill.

Schulz, F. (1943) 'Roman Register of Birth and Birth Certificates', *Journal of Roman Studies* 32: 78–91.

Schulz, F. (1943a) 'Roman Register of Birth and Birth Certificates II', *Journal of Roman Studies* 33: 55–64.

Schumacher, L. (2001) *Sklaverei in der Antike. Alltag und Schicksal der Unfreien*, München: C. H. Beck.

Scott, E. (2000) 'Unpicking a Myth: the infanticide of female and disabled infants in antiquity' [in:] G. Davies, A. Gardner and K. Lockyear (eds) *Theoretical Roman Archaeology Conference (TRAC 2000)*: 143–51, London: Oxbow Books.

Shail, A., Howie, G. (eds) (2005) *Menstruation. A Cultural History*, Houndmills 2005: Palgrave Macmillan.

Sharrock, A., Keith, A. (eds) (2020) *Maternal Conceptions in Classical Literature and Philosophy*, Toronto: University of Toronto Press.

Shaw, B. (2002) 'With whom I lived: measuring Roman marriage', *Ancient Society* 32: 195–242.

Shelton, J. A. (2013) *The Women of Pliny's Letters*, London: Routledge.

Sherwin-White, A. N. (1966) *The Letters of Pliny. A Historical and Social Commentary*, Oxford: Clarendon Press.

Shotter, D. C. A. (1966) 'Tiberius' Part in the Trial of Aemilia Lepida', *Historia: Zeitschrift Für Alte Geschichte* 15, 3: 312–17.

Sissa, G. (2013) 'The Hymen is a Problem, Still. Virginity, Imperforation, and Contraception, from Greece to Rome', *Eugesta* 3: 67–123.

Speert, H. (2004) *Obstetrics and Gynecology: a History and Iconography*, New York: CRC Press.

Staples, A. (1998) *From Good Goddess to Vestal Virgins: Sex and Category in Roman Religion*, London: Routledge.

Stawowska-Jundziłł, B. (2011) 'Zaślubione śmierci. Pochówki młodych kobiet z okresu Cesarstwa Rzymskiego zmarłych przed ślubem' [in:] B. Stawowska-Jundziłł (ed.) *Kultura, edukacja, rodzina, gender studies*: 49–83, Bydgoszcz: Wydawnictwo Uniwersytetu Kazimierza Wielkiego.

Stern, D. N., Bruschweiler-Stern, N., Freeland A. (1999) *Birth of a mother: how the motherhood experience changes you forever*, New York: Basic Books.

Strong, A. K. (2016) *Prostitutes and Matrons in the Roman World*, Cambridge: Cambridge University Press.

Suder, W. (1987) 'Umieralność okołoporodowa kobiet w Cesarstwie Rzymskim', *Przegląd Historyczny* 78, 4: 621–8.

Suder, W. (1993) 'Molucrum, fausse grossesse de la jeune fille (Afranius, Virgo, 338–340)', *Revue de philologie* 67: 89–94.

Suder, W. (1994) *Kloto, Lachesis, Atropos. Studia społeczno-demograficzne i medyczne z historii starożytnego Rzymu*, Wrocław: Wydawnictwo Uniwersytetu Wrocławskiego.

Suder, W. (1998) 'A partu, utriaque filiam enixa decessit. Mortalité maternelle dans l'empire Romain' [in:] ed. G. Sabatth *Études de médicine romaine*, Saint-Etienne 1998: 161–6.

Suder, W. (2004) 'Propaganda i legislacja matrymonialna Augusta' [in:] L. Morawiecki and P. Berdowski (eds) *Ideologia i propaganda w starożytności*: 357–9, Rzeszów: Biblioteka FRAZY.

Suder, W. (2005) 'Propaganda e legislazione matrimonial di Augusto', *Antiquitas* 28, 67–87.

Suder, W. (2007) 'Być kobietą w starożytnym Rzymie. Prawo i medycyna w ustawach małżeńskich cesarza Oktawiana' [in:] B. Płonka-Syroka, J. Radziszewska and A. Szlagowska (eds) *Oczekiwania kobiet i wobec kobiet. Stereotypy i wzorce kobiecości w kulturze europejskiej i amerykańskiej*: 3–11, Warszawa: DiG.

Suder, W., Stankiewicz, L. (1994) 'Molucrum – ciąża molarna młodej dziewczyny. Afraniusz, *Virgo*, 338–340', *Medycyna Nowożytna* 1, 1: 163–75.

Szram, M. (2001) *Duchowy sens liczb w alegorycznej egzegezie aleksandryjskiej (II–V w.)*, Lublin: RW KUL.

Tadajczyk, K. T (2014) *Status społeczno-prawny i odpowiedzialność lekarza w prawie rzymskim*, Łódź.

Takács, S. A. (2008) *Vestal Virgins, Sibyls, and Matrons: Women in Roman Religion*, Austin: University of Texas Press.

Tan, D. A., Haththotuwa, R., Fraser, I. S. (2017) 'Cultural aspects and mythologies surrounding menstruation and abnormal uterine bleeding', *Best Practice & Research Clinical Obstetrics & Gynaecology* 40: 121–33.

Tansey, P. (2013) 'Marcia Catonis and the flumen clarum', *The Classical Quarterly*, 63, 1: 423–6.

Tarwacka, A. (2009) 'Rozwód Oktawii i Nerona, czyli nowa Lukrecja', *Zeszyty Prawnicze 2009*, 9, 1: 171–5.

Tarwacka, A. (2011) '*Censoria potestas* Oktawiana Augusta', *Zeszyty Prawnicze UKSW* 11, 1: 359–75.

Tarwacka, A. (2013) 'As Far as the Bedroom… The Censor's Mark in Family Matters in Republican Rome', Zeszyty Prawnicze 13, 2: 187–201.

Tarwacka, A. (2014) 'O tym, że nie było skarg o zwrot posagu w mieście Rzymie przed rozwodem Carviliusa; i w związku z tym, co właściwie znaczy "paelex" i jakie jest pochodzenie tego słowa Aulus Gellius, "Noce Attyckie" 4, 3. Tekst – tłumaczenie – komentarz', *Zeszyty Prawnicze* 14, 2: 235–40.

Tatarkiewicz, A. (2013) 'Childbirth under the Care of a Midwife in Rome. The Ideal of Soranus and the Reality of Inscriptions. An Outline of the Problem' [in:] K. Kłodziński, Sz. Olszaniec, P. Wojciechowski, M. Pawlak, K. Królczyk and A. Tatarkiewicz (eds) *Society and religions. Studies in Greek and Roman History*, vol. 4: *The Roman Empire in the Light of Epigraphical and Normative Sources*: 127–51, Toruń: Wydawnictwo Naukowe UMK.

Tatarkiewicz, A. (2013a) 'Higiena i pielęgnacja noworodka w starożytnym Rzymie. Rady Soranosa z Efezu' [in:] W. Korpalska and W. Ślusarczyk (eds) *Czystość i brud. Higiena w starożytności*: 49–62, Toruń: Wydawnictwo Naukowe UMK.

Tatarkiewicz, A. (2015) 'Ciąża, poród i połóg pod opieką rzymskich bogów' [in:] K. Kochańczyk-Bonińska, L. Misiarczyk (eds), *W kręgu religii śródziemnomorskich* (vol. 19 of *Studia Antiquitatis Christianae*): 57–70, Warszawa: Wydawnictwo UKSW.

Tatarkiewicz, A. (2015a) 'Przedstawienia porodu w Rzymie w świetle źródeł medycznych i ikonograficznych', *Medycyna Nowożytna* 21: 175–90.

Tatarkiewicz, A. (2017) 'Żeby urodzić... rady lekarzy i wsparcie bogów w przygotowaniach do ciąży w czasach rzymskich' [in:] B. Płonka-Syroka and M. Dąsal (eds) *Medycyna i religia:* 23–33, Warszawa: DiG.

Tatarkiewicz, A. (2018) *'Mater in statu nascendi'. Społeczne i medyczne aspekty zdrowia reprodukcyjnego kobiet w starożytnym Rzymie*, Poznań: Instytut Historii UAM.

Tatarkiewicz, A. (2021) 'Les espoirs perdus... de jeunes filles mortes avant leur mariage' [w:] K. Balbuza, M. Duch, Z. Kaczmarek, K. Królczyk, A. Tatarkiewicz (eds) *Antiquitas Aeterna Classical Studies Dedicated to Leszek Mrozewicz on His 70th Birthday*: 407–12, Wiesbaden: Harrassowitz Verlag.

Tatarkiewicz, A. (2021a) 'Souffrances des accouchées. Les moyens antiques d'avancer l'accouchementet de calmer ses douleurs', *Ágora. Estudos Clássicos em Debate*, 23 (1): 49–64.

Thylander, H. (1952) *Inscriptions du port d'Ostie*, Lund: C. W. K. Gleerup.

Todman, D. (2008) 'Tombstone Memorial for a Female Physician (Medica), First Century AD', *Journal of Medical Biography* 16, 2: 108.

Tombeur, P. (2005) 'Maternitas dans la tradition latine', *Clio. Histoire, femmes et sociétés* 21: 139–49.

Tomlin, R. S. O. (2008) 'Special Delivery: A Graeco-Roman Gold Amulet for Healthy Childbirth', *ZPE* 167: 219–24.

Touwaide, A. (2002) *Metrodora, Brill's New Pauly* 8: 132.

Treggiari, S. (1991) *Roman Marriage. 'Iusti Coniuges' from the Time of Cicero to the Time of Ulpian*, Oxford: Oxford University Press.

Tsoucalas, G. Kousoulis, A. A., Androutsos, G. (2012) 'Innovative Surgical Techniques of Aspasia, the Early Greek Gynecologist', *Surgical Innovation* 19, 3: 337–8.

Tsoucalas, G., Sgantzos, M. (2016) 'Aspasia and Cleopatra Metrodora, Two Majestic Female Physician-Surgeons in the Early Byzantine Era', *Journal of Universal Surgery* 4, 3, 55: 1–5.

Turcan, R. (2001) *The Gods of Ancient Rome: Religion in Everyday Life from Archaic to Imperial Times*, New York: Routledge.

Turfa, J. M. (1986) 'Anatomical votive terracottas from Etruscan and Italic sanctuaries' [in:] J. Swaddling (ed.) *Italian Iron Age Artefacts in the British Museum: Papers of the Sixth British Museum Classical Colloquium*: 205–13, London: British Museum.

Turgut, M. (2011) 'Ancient medical schools in Knidos and Kos', *Child's Nervous System* 27, 2: 197–200.

Valette-Cagnac, E. (2008), 'Etre enfant à Rome', *Terrain* 40, URL: http://terrain.revues.org/1534.

van Gennep, A. (2006) *Obrzędy przejścia. Systematyczne studium ceremonii*, Warszawa: PIW.

Vons, J. (2000) *L'image de la femme dans l'œuvre de Pline l'Ancien*, Bruxelles: Latomus.

Wainwright, E. M. (2006) *Women Healing / Healing Women: The Genderization of Healing in Early Christianity*, London: Routledge.

Watson, P. (1983) '*Puella* and *virgo*', *Glotta* 61: 119–43.

Watts, W. J. (1973) 'Ovid, the Law and Roman Society on Abortion', *Acta Classica* 16: 89–101.

Winsbury, R. (2013) *Pliny the Younger. A Life in Roman Letters,* London: Bloomsbury.

Wołodkiewicz, W., Zabłocka, M. (1996) *Prawo rzymskie. Instytucje,* Warszawa: C.H. Beck.

Wood, S. (2000) *Imperial Women: A Study in Public Images, 40 BC–AD 68,* Leiden: Brill.

Zabłocki, J. (1992) 'In decem mensibus gigni hominem', *Prawo Kanoniczne* 35, 3–4: 197–210.

Index

abortion 56, 8, 21–6, 29–31, 53, 98, 99, 135, 160, 173 n.43, 173 n.51, 175 n.94, 199 n.22
Afranius 97, 98, 202 n.65
Ammianus Marcellinus 11, 79, 222 n.27
Apgar score 75, 148
Apuleius 11, 80, 156, 168
Artemidorus 11, 96
Augustus 16–22, 38, 59, 95, 96, 156, 170 n.14, 171 n.24, 186 n.134, 224 n.51–2
Aulus Gellius 2, 7, 11, 15, 95, 104, 144, 155, 170 n.16, 171 n.33

birth 2–13, 16, 18, 24–5, 29, 45, 48, 51–3, 60, 62, 63, 65, 73–5, 81, 82, 88–90, 95–7, 102–3, 105, 111, 112–25, 133, 135, 137, 140, 142–3, 146, 149, 155, 157, 196 n.90, 197 n.110, 201 n.42, 203 n.59, 211 n.12–15, 217 n.102, 220 n.5, 223 n.42, 224 n.51
birthing chair 75, 112, 140, 141, 211 n.15

Caelius Aurelianus 10, 84, 146
caesarean section 134–5
Cassius Dio 11, 38, 103
Censorinus 11, 88, 104–5, 200 n.39
childbirth 1, 6, 9, 22, 23, 38, 46, 52, 78, 79, 102, 109, 114, 120, 135–44, 159–63, 165 n.3, 169 n.79, 177 n.12, 190 n.3, 218 n.125
childhood 1, 2, 4, 5, 37, 46, 49, 51, 160
childless 22, 53, 55, 66, 174 n.71
children 22–3, 25, 31, 38, 45, 47, 53–7, 59, 60, 61, 65, 67, 69, 75, 88, 89, 93, 95–7, 101, 103–7, 122, 125–6, 136, 144, 156, 160, 170 n.15, 172 n.37, 175 n. 94, 177 n.12, 189 n. 184, 196 n.90, 198 n.9, 202 n. 59, 205 n.114, 208 n.132

Cicero 11, 16, 25, 37, 69, 103, 135, 145, 202 n.59
conceive 10, 26, 28, 44, 46, 53, 56, 59, 65, 67
conception 8, 26–9, 41, 56, 57, 59, 62, 65, 66, 69, 85, 89, 93, 104, 160
contraception 8, 21, 26, 31, 38, 160, 175 n.94
contraceptives 9, 26, 29
cursus laborum 2, 159
Cyranides 27, 64, 116, 120

death 9, 25, 30, 31, 39, 47–51, 65, 79, 95, 98–101, 106, 115, 122, 128, 135–8, 204 n.98, 208 n.132, 218
delivery 10, 78, 90, 94, 103, 107, 111, 114, 117–18, 120, 122, 124, 126, 128, 135, 137, 139, 140, 146, 149, 202, 210–11, 218 n.121
dies lustricus 5, 10, 51, 143, 144, 157–9, 163
Dionysius of Halicarnassus 11, 15, 21, 95, 157, 159
divorce 2, 8, 17, 23, 53–5, 62, 75, 160, 188 n.169
doctor 9, 25, 41, 71, 72, 77, 80–2, 92, 94, 97, 99, 103, 114, 121, 123, 127, 129, 134, 146, 162, 197 n. 110, 197 n.115
doll 46–7, 51–2, 181 n.69

father 2, 4, 16, 25, 49, 57, 61, 63, 88, 103, 118, 143, 148, 156, 167 n.40, 176 n.10, 188 n.169, 208 n.132
fertile 8, 21, 29, 39, 53, 55, 58, 65, 96, 174 n.71
fertility 8, 9, 12, 18, 20, 29, 31, 38, 44, 45, 53–5, 59–60, 62, 65–6, 69, 95, 98, 137, 160, 177 n.12
foetus 30, 40, 46, 66, 86, 89, 91, 93, 99, 100, 104–5, 111, 120, 123–8, 130, 169 n.79, 202 n. 57, 216 n.86

Galen 147, 205
Gargilius 30, 40, 116
genitals 6, 29, 30, 81, 94, 99, 116, 130, 146, 185 n.124
girl 1, 2, 5, 24, 37–9, 45, 47, 49, 51–2, 82, 87–9, 96, 106, 135–7, 157, 161, 177 n.17, 198 n.9

Hippocrates 29, 40, 59, 89, 100, 105, 116, 121, 178, 197 n.115, 205 n.114
Horace 11, 17
Hyginus 82–3

impotence 62–5, 187 n. 162, 188 n.165
infertile *see* infertility
infertility 6, 8, 28, 31, 41, 53–5, 58–65, 69, 100, 160, 188 n.169
intercourse 10, 26–8, 41, 56, 59, 60–1, 64, 94, 160, 167 n.26, 185 n.117
ius trium liberorum 18, 20, 53, 105, 144, 160

Juvenal 11, 20, 22, 28, 31, 63, 155

labour 5, 8, 9, 22, 26, 46, 59, 66, 73, 75, 80, 89, 93, 111–23, 127, 133, 147, 163, 167, 201 n.42 (*see also* childbirth)
Lucretius 11, 16, 28, 58, 60

marriage 15–20, 37–9, 45–9, 54–5, 62–5, 102–3, 143, 160, 176, 181 n.65, 182 n.81
Martial 11, 18, 63
medicae 2, 9, 71–2, 75, 77, 80–1, 162
menstrual 41–5, 58, 69, 78, 103, 160, 167
menstruation 41, 45, 56, 66, 85, 161, 178 n.24, 178 n.33, 179 n.43
midwives 9, 11, 42, 44, 46, 71, 73–82, 119, 150, 162, 194 n.46, 196 n.90, 198 n.117
miscarriage 25–6, 29, 31, 44, 65, 90, 99–101, 105, 120, 144, 188 n.166, 202 n.63
motherhood 4, 8, 11, 51, 95, 135, 138, 158, 160–1, 163, 165, 169 n.79, 181 n.69

newborn 10, 13, 51, 75, 88, 93, 111, 114, 116–17, 122, 143–4, 148, 153, 157, 221 n.21
nurse 46, 71, 93, 132, 140, 150, 161
nursing *see* nurse

obstetrices 71, 73, 76, 78, 80–3, 162 (*see also* midwives)
offspring 8, 11, 15, 16, 18, 21–2, 24, 47, 53–4, 69, 90, 98, 107, 160, 189 n.184
Ovid 11, 12, 24, 31, 66, 138

paediatrics 73, 148
  Dioscorides 30, 32, 99
physician 1, 8–10, 16, 42, 46, 56, 65, 71–3, 77, 80–3, 93, 104, 111, 116, 121, 123, 159, 161, 190 n.3, 202 n.57
Pliny the Elder 11, 65, 78, 92, 96
Pliny the Younger 11, 18, 31, 46, 47, 65, 90, 135
Plutarch 3, 7, 65, 95, 98, 101, 157, 221 n.20
postpartum 5, 78, 115, 135, 137, 145–6, 163
pregnancy 5–8, 10, 12–3,16, 22, 26, 28–9, 31, 38, 40, 44, 46, 59, 65, 80, 85–109, 118–19, 123, 124–38, 144, 158, 160, 162, 189 n.184, 204 n.98, 205 n.114
puerperium 5, 135, 145–7

Quintilian 22, 24

reproductive 5–6, 8, 10, 12, 17, 22, 24, 38, 45, 71, 135, 152, 159, 161

Solinus 11, 42–3, 60–1, 85, 89, 123–5
Soranus 8, 9–11, 26–7, 29, 30–1, 40–1, 45–6, 55, 58, 60, 73, 75, 78, 81, 90–3, 98, 111, 114–16, 121, 123, 125, 127, 133, 135, 147, 149, 151, 154, 162
Suetonius 15, 31, 59, 133
swaddling 75, 145, 148, 151–3, 223 n.42

Tacitus 21, 31, 38, 95, 119
Tertullian 66, 127–8, 158, 169 n.79, 188 n.173
triplets 95–7, 201 n.54, 202 n.57
twins 26, 95, 97, 124, 189 n.184

umbilical cord 79, 86, 116, 149, 222 n.27
uterus 86, 89, 91, 94, 97, 111–12, 116, 125–8, 130–2, 147

vagina 26, 27, 30, 59, 113, 116, 185 n.117
virgin *see* virginity

virginity 8, 37–8, 46, 51, 82, 97, 176 n.10, 181 n.60

womb 24, 26, 66, 69, 81, 86, 89, 111, 115, 120, 127–8, 133–4, 139, 165, 201 n.39, 202 n.63, 203 n.66, 205 n.114, 217 n.102

www.ingramcontent.com/pod-product-compliance
Lightning Source LLC
Chambersburg PA
CBHW062139300426
44115CB00012BA/1983